Principles of Proteomics

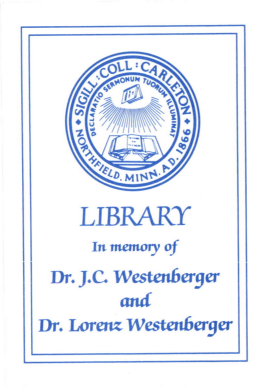

Principles of Proteomics

R. M. Twyman

Department of Biological Sciences,
University of York, York, UK

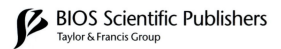
BIOS Scientific Publishers
Taylor & Francis Group

© **Garland Science/BIOS Scientific Publishers, 2004**

First published 2004

A CIP catalogue record for this book is available from the British Library.

ISBN 1 85996 273 4

Garland Science/BIOS Scientific Publishers
4 Park Square, Milton Park, Abingdon, Oxon OX14 4RN, UK and
270 Madison Avenue, New York, NY 10016, USA
World Wide Web home page: www.garlandscience.com

Garland Science/BIOS Scientific Publishers is a member of the Taylor & Francis Group

Distributed in the USA by
Fulfilment Center
Taylor & Francis
10650 Toebben Drive
Independence, KY 41051, USA
Toll Free Tel.: +1 800 634 7064; E-mail: taylorandfrancis@thomsonlearning.com

Distributed in Canada by
Taylor & Francis
74 Rolark Drive
Scarborough, Ontario M1R 4G2, Canada
Toll Free Tel.: +1 877 226 2237; E-mail: tal_fran@istar.ca

Distributed in the rest of the world by
Thomson Publishing Services
Cheriton House
North Way
Andover, Hampshire SP10 5BE, UK
Tel.: +44 (0)1264 332424; E-mail: salesorder.tandf@thomsonpublishingservices.co.uk

Library of Congress Cataloging-in-Publication Data

Twyman, Richard M.
    Principles of proteomics / Richard M. Twyman.
        p. cm. — (Advanced texts)
    ISBN 1-85996-273-4
    1. Proteomics.   I. Title.   II. Series.

    QP551.T94 2004
    572'.6—dc22

                                    2004011210

Production Editor: Catherine Jones
Typeset by Phoenix Photosetting, Chatham, Kent, UK
Printed and bound by Cromwell Press, Trowbridge, UK

Cover image courtesy of Paul Travers

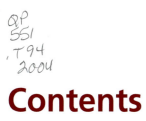

Contents

Color plates can be found between pages 18 and 19, 82 and 83, 114 and 115, 146 and 147, 210 and 212

Abbreviations

2DGE	two-dimensional gel electrophoresis
3D-PSSM	three dimensional position specific scoring matrix
AC	affinity chromatography
ADP	adenosine diphosphate
AFM	atomic force microscopy
ATP	adenosine triphosphate
BCA	bicinchoninic acid
BCG	Bacille Clamette-Guérin
BLAST	basic local alignment search tool
CATH	class, architecture, topology and homologous superfamily
CBP	calmodulin-binding protein
CCD	charge-coupled device
CD	circular dichroism
cDNA	complementary DNA
CDS	circular dichroism spectroscopy
CE	capillary electrophoresis
CF	chromatofocusing
CGE	capillary gel electrophoresis
CHAPS	3-[(3-Cholamidopropyl)dimethylammonio]-1-propanesulfonate
CHS	chalcone synthase
CID	collision-induced dissociation
COSY	correlation spectroscopy
cRNA	complementary RNA
DALPC	direct analysis of large protein complexes
DDBJ	DNA database of Japan
DHFR	dihydrofolate reductase
DIGE	difference gel electrophoresis
DNA	deoxyribonucleic acid
dsRNA	double-stranded RNA
DTT	dithiothreitol
EDC	N, N′ dimethylaminopropylethylcarbodiimide
EGF	epidermal growth factor
EGFR	epidermal growth factor receptor
EGTA	ethylene glycol-bis-(2-aminoethyl)-N, N, N′, N′ tetraacetic acid
eIF	eukaryotic initiation factor
ELISA	enzyme-linked immunosorbent assay
EM	electron microscopy
ER	endoplasmic reticulum
ESI	electrospray ionization
EST	expressed sequence tag
FMN	falvin mononucleotide
fnII	fibronectin type II domain
FRET	fluorescence resonance energy transfer
FT-ICR	Fourier transform ion-cyclotron resonance

GM	genetically modified
GPI	glycosylphosphatidylinositol
GST	glutathione-S-transferase
HMM	hidden Markov model
HPLC	high-performance liquid chromatography
HTI	high-throughput imaging
ICAT	isotope-coded affinity tag
IEC (IEX)	ion exchange chromatography
IEF	isoelectric focusing
IMAC	immobilized metal-affinity chromatography
IPG	immobilized pH gradient
LC	liquid chromatography
LCM	laser capture microdissection
MAD	multiple wavelength anomalous dispersion
MALDI	matrix-assisted laser desorption/ionization
MCAT	mass-coded abundance tag
MIP	molecular imprinted polymer
MIR	multiple isomorphous replacement
μLC-MS	microcapillary liquid chromatography-mass spectrometry analysis
MPSS	massively parallel signature sequencing
mRNA	messenger RNA
MS	mass spectrometry
MS/MS	tandem mass spectrometry
MudPIT	multidimensional protein identification technology
Multi D-LC	multidimensional liquid chromatography
NAD	nicotinamide adenine dinucleotide
NEPHGE	nonequilibrium pH gradient electrophoresis
NIGMS	National Institute of General Medical Sciences
NMR	nuclear magnetic resonance
NOE	nuclear Overhauser effect
NOESY	NOE spectroscopy
NTA	nitrilotriacetate
OPA	o-phthaldialdehyde
ORF	open reading frame
PAGE	polyacrylamide gel electrophoresis
PAL	phenylalanine ammonia lyase
PAS	periodic acid/Schiff
PCA	protein complementation assay
PCR	polymerase chain reaction
PDB	Protein Databank
PDMS	polydimethysiloxane
PGC	porous graphitic carbon
PISA	protein *in situ* array
PLP	pyridoxal phosphate
PMF	peptide mass fingerprinting
PNGase	peptide-N-glycosidase
PPi	pyrophosphate
PQL	protein quantity locus
PS	position shift
PSD	post-source decay
PSI-BLAST	position-specific iterated BLAST
PTM	post-translational modification

PVDF	polyvinylidenedifluoride
QTL	quantitative trait locus
RCA	rolling circle amplification
RISC	RNA-induced silencing complex
RMSD	root mean square deviation
RNA	ribonucleic acid
RNAi	RNA interference
RRS	Ras recruitment system
RT-PCR	reverse transcriptase polymerase chain reaction
SAGE	serial analysis of gene expression
scFv	single chain fragment variable
SCOP	Structural Classification of Proteins
SDS	sodium dodecylsulfate
SEC	size exclusion chromatography
SELDI	surface-enhanced laser desorption/ionization
SEND	surface-enhanced neat desorption
SGA	synthetic genetic array
SH2	Src homology 2
SH3	Src homology 3
SILAC	stable isotope labeling with amino acids in cell culture
siRNA	small interfering RNA
SIRAS	single isomorphous replacement with anomalous scattering
SNP	single nucleotide polymorphism
SOS	son of sevenless
SPR	surface plasmon resonance
SRCD	synchrotron radiation circular dichroism
SRS	SOS recruitment system
TAP	tandem affinity purification
TEV	tobacco etch virus
TIM	triose phosphate isomerase
TLC	thin layer chromatography
TNF	tumor necrosis factor
TOCSY	total correlation spectroscopy
TOF	time of flight
TPA	tissue plasminogen activator
TQ	triple quadrupole
tRNA	transfer RNA
UPA	universal protein array
USPS	ubiquitin-based split protein sensor
UV	ultraviolet
XRC	x-ray crystallography

Preface

Proteomics, a word in use for less than a decade, now describes a rapidly growing and maturing scientific discipline, and a burgeoning industry. Proteomics is the global analysis of proteins. It seeks to achieve what other large-scale enterprises in the life sciences cannot: a complete description of living cells in terms of all their functional components, brought about by the direct analysis of those components rather than the genes that encode them. The field of proteomics has grown rapidly in a short time, yet promises to provide more information about living systems than even the genomics revolution that started ten years before. The reason for this is the richness of proteomics data. Genes have sequences, but proteins have sequences, structures, biochemical and physiological functions, and their activities are influenced by chemical modification, localization within or without the cell, and perhaps most importantly of all, their interactions with other molecules. If genes are the instruction carriers, proteins are the molecules that execute those instructions. Genes are the instruments of change over evolutionary timescales, but proteins are the molecules that define which changes are accepted and which are discarded. It is from proteins that we shall learn how living cells and organisms are built and maintained, and how they fail when things go wrong.

As is the case for any emerging scientific field, proteomics makes a lot of sense to those performing large-scale protein analysis on a day-to-day basis, and much less sense to those looking in from the outside. Proteomics abounds with jargon and acronyms. New technologies and variations appear on what can seem to be a daily basis. It can be difficult to keep up, and even specialists in one area of proteomics sometimes have difficulties applying their knowledge in other specialized areas. It is my hope that this book will be useful to those who need a broad overview of proteomics and what it has to offer. It is not meant to provide expertise in any particular area: there are plenty of books on electrophoresis, mass spectrometry, bioinformatics etc. for the reader needing detailed treatment of particular technologies. However, this book pulls together disparate information concerning the different proteomics technologies and their applications, and presents them in what I hope is a simple and user-friendly manner. After a brief introductory chapter, the various proteomics technologies are discussed in more detail: two-dimensional gel electrophoresis, multidimensional liquid chromatography, mass spectrometry, sequence analysis, structural analysis, methods for studying protein interactions, modifications, localization and function. Protein chips, an emerging and promising recent addition to the proteomics armory, are described in the penultimate chapter. The final chapter presents a few examples of how proteomics is being applied, particularly in the medical and pharmaceutical fields. Again, this is not intended to be comprehensive coverage, but is provided so the reader has an overview of the scope of proteomics and its potential. At the end of each chapter is a short bibliography, containing some classic papers and useful reviews for those wanting to delve deeper into the subject. I have assumed that the reader has a working knowledge of molecular biology and biochemistry.

This book would not have been possible without the help and support of many people, not least the team at Garland/BIOS for their patience, persistence and optimism in the face of tight deadlines. I'd like to thank the many friends and colleagues who offered opinions on the individual chapters and pointed out potential errors or omissions, and in particular, I would like to thank all at the Fraunhofer Institute of Molecular Biology and

Applied Ecology, the Technical University in Aachen and the Department of Biological Sciences, University of York.

As ever, this book is dedicated with love to my parents, Peter and Irene, and my children, Emily and Lucy.

Richard M. Twyman

From genomics to proteomics

1.1   Introduction

Proteomics is a rapidly growing area of molecular biology that is concerned with the systematic, large-scale analysis of proteins. It is based on the concept of the proteome as a complete set of proteins produced by a given cell or organism under a defined set of conditions. Proteins are involved in almost every biological function, so a comprehensive analysis of the proteins in the cell provides a unique global perspective on how these molecules interact and cooperate to create and maintain a working biological system. The cell responds to internal and external changes by regulating the level and activity of its proteins, so changes in the proteome, either qualitative or quantitative, provide a snapshot of the cell in action. The proteome is a complex and dynamic entity that can be defined in terms of the sequence, structure, abundance, localization, modification, interaction and biochemical function of its components, providing a rich and varied source of data. The analysis of these various properties of the proteome requires an equally diverse range of technologies.

This introductory chapter considers the importance of proteomics in the context of systems biology, discusses some of the major goals of proteomic analysis and introduces the major technology platforms. We begin by tracing the origins of proteomics in the genomics revolution of the 1990s and following its evolution from a concept to a mainstream technology with a current market value of over $1.5 billion.

1.2   The birth of large-scale biology

The overall goal of molecular biology research is to determine the functions of genes and their products, allowing them to be linked into pathways and networks, and ultimately providing a detailed understanding of how biological systems work. For most of the last 50 years, research in molecular biology has focused on the isolation and characterization of individual genes and proteins because there was neither the information nor the technology available for larger scale investigations. The only way to study biological systems was to break them down into their components, look at these individually, and attempt to reassemble each system from the bottom up. This approach is known as reductionism, and it dominated the molecular life sciences until the early 1990s.

The face of biological research began to change in the 1990s as technological breakthroughs made it possible to carry out large-scale DNA sequencing. Until this point, the sequences of individual genes and proteins had accumulated slowly and steadily as researchers cataloged their new discoveries. This can be seen from the steady growth in the

GenBank sequence database from 1980–1990 (*Figure 1.1*). The 1990s saw the advent of factory-style automated DNA sequencing, resulting in a massive explosion of sequence data (*Figure 1.1*). In the early 1990s, much of the new sequence data was represented by expressed sequence tags (ESTs), short fragments of DNA obtained by the random sequencing of cDNA libraries. In 1995, the first complete cellular genome sequence was published, that of the bacterium *Haemophilus influenzae*. In the next few years, over 100 further genome sequences were completed, including our own human genome which was essentially finished in 2003.

The large-scale sequencing projects ushered in the genomics era, which effectively removed the information bottleneck and brought about the realization that biological systems, while large and very complex, were ultimately finite. The idea began to emerge that it might be possible to study biological systems in a holistic manner simply by cataloging and enumerating the components if sufficient amounts of data could be collected and analyzed. Unfortunately, while the technology for genome sequencing had advanced rapidly, the technology for studying the functions of the newly discovered genes lagged far behind. The sequence databases became clogged with anonymous sequences and gene fragments, and the problem was exacerbated by the

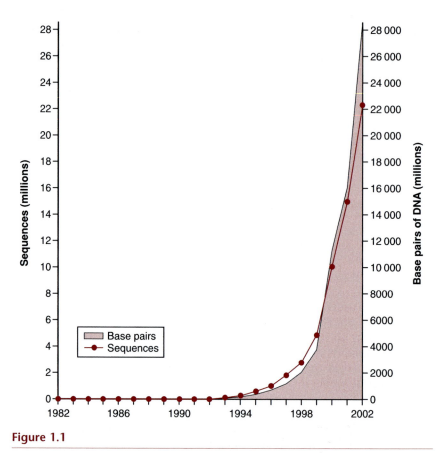

Figure 1.1

Growth of the GenBank database in its first 20 years. Courtesy of GenBank.

unexpectedly large number of new genes found even in well-characterized organisms. As an example, consider the bakers' yeast *Saccharomyces cerevisiae*, which was thought to be one of the best-characterized model organisms prior to the completion of the genome-sequencing project in 1996. Over 2000 genes had been characterized in traditional experiments and it was thought that genome sequencing would identify at most a few hundred more. Scientists got a shock when they found the yeast genome contained over 6000 genes, nearly a third of which were unrelated to any previously identified sequence. Such genes were described as orphans because they could not be assigned to any classical gene family (*Figure 1.2*).

The availability of masses of anonymous sequence data for hundreds of different organisms has precipitated a number of fundamental changes in the way research is conducted in the molecular life sciences. Traditionally gene function had been studied by moving from phenotype to gene, an approach sometimes called forward genetics. An observed mutant phenotype (or purified protein) was used as the starting point to map and identify the corresponding gene, and this led to the functional analysis of that gene and its product. The opposite approach, sometimes termed reverse genetics, is to take an uncharacterized gene sequence and modify it to see the effect on phenotype. As more uncharacterized sequences have accumulated in databases, the focus of research has shifted from forward to reverse genetics. Similarly, most research prior to 1995 was hypothesis-driven, in that the researcher put forward a hypothesis to explain a given observation, and then designed experiments to prove or disprove it. The genomics revolution instigated a progressive change towards discovery-driven research, in which the components of the system under investigation are collected irrespective of any hypothesis about how they might work. The final paradigm shift concerns the sheer volume of data generated in today's experiments. Whereas in the past researchers have focused on individual gene products and generated rather small amounts of data,

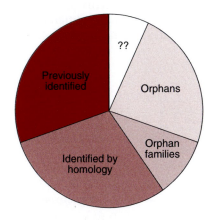

Figure 1.2

Distribution of yeast genes by annotation status in the aftermath of the *Saccharomyces cerevisiae* genome project. (?? shows questionable open reading frames.)

now the trend is towards the analysis of many genes and their products and the generation of enormous datasets that must be mined for salient information using computers. Advances in genomics have thus forced parallel advances in bioinformatics, the computer-aided handling, analysis, extraction, storage and presentation of biological data.

1.3   The genome, transcriptome and proteome

As systems biology has supplanted the reductionist approach, so it has been necessary to re-evaluate the central dogma of molecular biology, which states that a gene is transcribed into RNA and then translated into protein (*Figure 1.3a*). The new paradigm is that the genome (all the genes in the organism) gives rise to the transcriptome (the complete set of mRNA in any given cell) which is then translated to produce the proteome (the complete collection of proteins in any given cell) (*Figure 1.3b*).

The genome is a static information resource with a defined gene content that, with few exceptions, remains the same regardless of cell type or environmental conditions. In contrast, both the transcriptome and proteome are dynamic entities, whose content can fluctuate dramatically under different conditions due to the regulation of transcription, RNA processing, protein synthesis and protein modification. The transcriptome and proteome are much more complex than the genome because a single gene can produce many different mRNAs and proteins. Different transcripts can be generated by alternative splicing, alternative promoter or polyadenylation site usage, and special processing strategies like RNA editing. Different proteins can be generated by alternative use of start and stop codons and the proteins synthesized from these mRNAs can be modified in various different ways during or after translation. Some types of modification, such as glycosylation, are generally permanent. Others, such as phosphorylation, are transient and are often used in a regulatory manner. The same protein can be modified in many different ways giving rise to innumerable variants. For example, about 70% of human proteins are thought to be glycosylated and the glycan chains can have many different structures. Often there are several glycosylation sites on the same protein, and different glycan

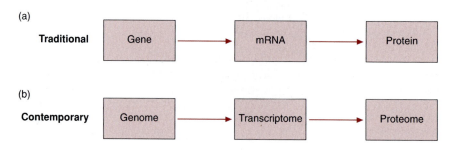

(a)

Traditional   Gene   →   mRNA   →   Protein

(b)

Contemporary   Genome   →   Transcriptome   →   Proteome

Figure 1.3

The new paradigm in molecular biology – the focus on single genes and their products has been replaced by global analysis.

chains can be added to each site. The largest recorded number of glycosylation sites on a single polypeptide is over 20, giving the potential for millions of potential glycoforms. Over 400 different types of post-translational modification have been documented adding significantly to the diversity of the proteome. For example, while it is estimated that the human genome contains about 30 000 genes, it is likely that the proteome catalog comprises more than a million proteins when post-translational modification is taken into account. Indeed, only by increasing diversity at the transcriptome and proteome levels can the increased biological complexity of humans be explained compared to nematodes (18 000 genes), fruit flies (12 000 genes) and yeast (6000 genes).

1.4   Functional genomics at the DNA and RNA levels

The complete genome sequences that are now available for a large number of important organisms provide potential access to every single gene and therefore pave the way for functional analysis at the systems level, an approach often termed functional genomics. However, even complete gene catalogs provide at best a list of components, and no more explain how a biological system works than a list of parts explains the workings of a machine. Before we can begin to understand how these components build a bacterial cell, a mouse, an apple tree or a human being, we must understand not only what they do as individual entities, but also how they interact and cooperate with each other. Because the genome is a static information resource, functional relationships among genes must be studied at the levels of the transcriptome and proteome. The need for such analysis has encouraged the development of novel technologies that allow large numbers of mRNA and protein molecules to be studied simultaneously.

1.4.1   Transcriptomics

Because the genomics revolution saw technological advances in large-scale cloning and sequencing methods, it made good sense to put these technologies to work in the functional analysis of genes. The first functional genomics methods were therefore based on DNA sequencing, and were used to study mRNA expression profiles on a global scale (transcriptomics). The expression profile of a gene can reveal a lot about its role in the cell and can also help to identify functional links to other genes. For example, the expression of many genes is restricted to specific cells or developing structures, often showing that the genes have particular functions in those places. Other genes are expressed in response to external stimuli. For example, they might be switched on or switched off in cells exposed to endogenous signals such as growth factors or environmental molecules such as DNA-damaging chemicals. Genes with similar expression profiles are likely to be involved in similar processes, and in this way showing that an orphan gene has a similar expression profile to a characterized gene may allow a function to be predicted on the basis of 'guilt by association'. Furthermore, mutating one gene may affect the expression profiles of others, helping to link those genes into functional pathways and networks. The two major technologies for large-scale expression analysis that emerged from genomics were large-scale cDNA sequence sampling, based on standard DNA-sequencing methods, and the use of DNA arrays for expression analysis by hybridization.

Sequence sampling is probably the most direct way to study the transcriptome. In the most basic approach, clones are randomly picked from cDNA libraries and 200–300 bp of sequence is obtained, allowing the clones to be identified by comparison with sequence databases. The number of times each clone appears in the sample is then determined. The abundance of each clone represents the abundance of the corresponding transcript in the transcriptome of the original biological material. If enough clones are sequenced, statistical analysis provides a rough guide to the relative mRNA levels and comparisons can be made across two or more samples if suitable cDNA libraries are available. This approach has been used to identify differentially expressed genes but is laborious and expensive because large-scale sequencing is required. A potential short cut is to take very short sequence samples, known as sequence signatures, and read many of them at the same time. Several techniques have been developed for high-throughput signature recognition but the one that has had the most impact thus far is serial analysis of gene expression (SAGE) (*Figure 1.4*). The principles of several sequence sampling techniques are outlined briefly in *Box 1.1*.

Although sequence sampling is a powerful technique for expression analysis, the method of choice in transcriptomics is the use of DNA microarrays. These are miniature devices onto which many different DNA sequences are immobilized in the form of a grid. There are two major types, one made by the mechanical spotting of DNA molecules onto a coated glass slide and one produced by *in situ* oligonucleotide synthesis (the latter is also known as a high-density oligonucleotide chip). Although manufactured in completely different ways, the principles of mRNA analysis are much the same for each device. Expression analysis is based on multiplex hybridization using a complex population of labeled DNA or RNA molecules (*Plate 1*). For both devices, a population of mRNA molecules from a particular source is reverse transcribed *en masse* to form a representative complex cDNA population. In the case of spotted microarrays, a fluorophore-conjugated nucleotide is included in the reaction mix so that the cDNA population is universally labeled. In the case of oligonucleotide chips, the unlabeled cDNA is converted into

Figure 1.4 – opposite

Serial analysis of gene expression (SAGE). The basis of the method is to reduce each cDNA molecule to a representative short sequence tag (nine to fifteen nucleotides long). Individual tags are then joined together (concatenated) into a single long DNA clone as shown at the bottom of the diagram. Sequencing of the clone provides information on the different sequence tags which can identify the presence of corresponding mRNA sequences. The mRNA is converted to cDNA using an oligo (dT) primer with an attached biotin group (Ⓑ) and the biotinylated cDNA is cleaved with a frequently cutting restriction nuclease (the anchoring enzyme, shown as a downward triangle). The resulting 3′ end fragments which contain a biotin group are then selectively recovered by binding to streptavidin-coated beads (pink circles), separated into two pools and then individually ligated to one of two double-stranded oligonucleotide linkers,

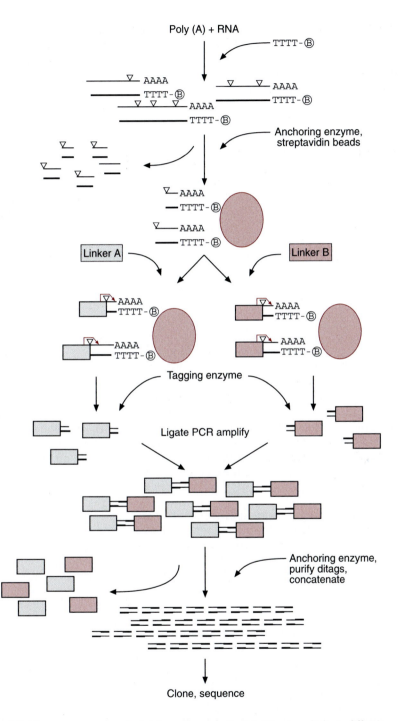

A and B (shown as gray and pink boxes respectively). The two linkers differ in sequence except that they have a 3' CTAG overhang and immediately adjacent to it, a common recognition site for the type IIs restriction nuclease which will serve as the tagging enzyme (shown as an extended red arrow). Cleavage with the tagging enzyme generates a short sequence tag from each mRNA and fragments from the separate pools can be brought together to form 'ditags' then concatenated as shown.

BOX 1.1

Sequence sampling techniques for the global analysis of gene expression

Random sampling of cDNA libraries
Randomly picked clones are sequenced and searched against databases to identify the corresponding genes. The frequency with which each sequence is represented provides a rough guide to the relative abundances of different mRNAs in the original sample. This is a very labor-intensive approach, particularly where several cDNA libraries need to be compared.

Analysis of EST databases
ESTs are signatures generated by the single-pass sequencing of random cDNA clones. If EST data are available for a given library, the abundance of different transcripts can be estimated by determining the representation of each sequence in the database. This is a rapid approach, advantageous because it can be carried out entirely *in silico*, but it relies on the availability of EST data for relevant samples.

Differential display PCR
This procedure was devised for the rapid identification of cDNA sequences that are differentially expressed across two or more samples. The method has insufficient resolution to cope with the entire transcriptome in one experiment, so populations of labeled cDNA fragments are generated by RT-PCR using one oligo-dT primer and one arbitrary primer, producing pools of cDNA fragments representing subfractions of the transcriptome. The equivalent amplification products from two biological samples (i.e. products amplified using the same primer combination) are then run side by side on a sequencing gel, and differentially expressed cDNAs are revealed by quantitative differences in band intensities. This technique homes in on differentially expressed genes but false positives are common and other methods must be used to confirm the predicted expression profiles.

Serial analysis of gene expression (SAGE)
In this technique, very short sequence signatures (sequence tags) are collected from many cDNAs. The tags are ligated together to form long concatemers and these concatemers are sequenced. The representation of each transcript is determined by the number of times a particular tag is counted. Although technically demanding, SAGE is much more efficient than standard cDNA sampling because 50–100 tags can be counted for each sequencing reaction. The method is shown in detail in *Figure 1.4*.

Massively parallel signature sequencing (MPSS)
Like SAGE, the MPSS technique involves the collection of short sequence tags from many cDNAs. However, unlike SAGE (where the tags are cloned in series) MPSS relies on the parallel analysis of thousands of cDNAs attached to microbeads in a flow cell. The principle of the method is that a restriction enzyme is used to expose a four-base overhang on each cDNA. There are 16 possible four-base sequences, which are detected by hybridization to a set of 16 different adapter oligonucleotides. Each adapter hybridizes to a different decoder oligonucleotide defined by a specific fluorescent tag. Another four-base overhang is then exposed, and the process is repeated. By imaging the microbeads after each round of cleavage and hybridization, thousands of cDNA sequences can be read in four-nucleotide chunks. As with SAGE, the number of times each sequence is recorded can be used to determine relative gene expression levels. The method is outlined in *Figure 1.5*.

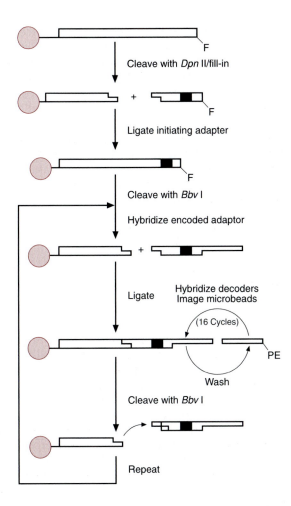

Figure 1.5

Massively parallel signature sequencing (MPSS). A cDNA sequence attached to a bead is cleaved with the enzyme *Dpn* II, and an adapter with a matching *Dpn* II sticky end is ligated to it. The adapter contains a fluorescent label (F) and the recognition site for the type IIs restriction enzyme *Bbv* I. This cleaves a specific number of base pairs downstream from its recognition site, and leaves a four-base overhang in the original cDNA sequence. The sequence of the four-base overhang is determined by hybridization to a mixture of 16 encoded adapters, which have reciprocal overhangs comprising all 16 possible combinations of four bases. Each encoded adapter also has a short single-stranded region which is recognized by 16 decoder oligonucleotides carrying different fluorescent labels (PE). After 16 rounds of hybridization and imaging, the first four-base sequence of millions of cDNAs attached to different beads can be determined. The encoded adapter also contains a *Bbv* I restriction site, so the process can be repeated on a further four-base segment of the cDNA. ©Nature Publishing Group, Nature Biotechnology, Vol 18: 630-634, 'Gene expression analysis by massively parallel signature sequencing (MPSS) on microbead arrays' by Brenner S. *et al.*

a labeled cRNA (complementary RNA) population by the incorporation of biotin, which is later detected with fluorophore-conjugated avidin. The complex population of labeled nucleic acids is then applied to the array and allowed to hybridize. Each individual feature or spot on the array contains 10^6–10^9 copies of the same DNA sequence, and is therefore unlikely to be completely saturated in the hybridization reaction. Under these conditions, the intensity of the hybridizing signal at each address on the array is proportional to the relative abundance of that particular cDNA or cRNA in the mixture, which in turn reflects the abundance of the corresponding mRNA in the original source population. Therefore, the relative levels of thousands of different transcripts can be monitored in one experiment. Comparisons between samples may be achieved by hybridizing labeled cDNA or cRNA prepared from each of the samples to identical microarrays, but in the case of spotted microarrays it is preferable to use different fluorophores to label alternative samples and hybridize both labeled populations to the same array. By scanning the array at different wavelengths, the relative levels of mRNAs can be compared across multiple samples (*Plate 1*).

1.4.2   Large-scale mutagenesis

One of the clearest ways to establish the function of a gene is to mutate it and observe the effect on phenotype. Mutations have been at the forefront of biological research since the beginning of the 20th century but only in the 1990s did it become practical to generate comprehensive mutant libraries, i.e. collections of organisms with systematically produced mutations affecting every gene in the genome. Like transcriptomics, such developments relied on prior advances in large-scale clone preparation and sequencing.

Mutagenesis strategies can be divided into two approaches. The first is genome-wide mutagenesis by homologous recombination, which involves the deliberate and systematic inactivation of each gene in the genome through replacement with a DNA cassette containing a nonfunctional sequence (*Figure 1.6*). This form of gene replacement, often called 'gene knockout', produces null mutations that result in complete loss-of-function phenotypes, although due to genetic redundancy it is often the case that no phenotype is observed. This approach can be used on a genome-wide scale only where the organism in question has a fully sequenced genome and is amenable to homologous recombination. Thus far, systematic homologous recombination has been restricted to the relatively small genomes of yeast and bacteria

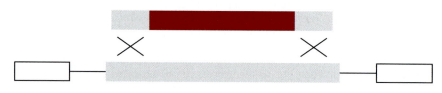

Figure 1.6

Large-scale mutagenesis by gene knockout in yeast has been achieved by systematically replacing each endogenous gene (gray bar) with a nonfunctional sequence or marker (red bar) inserted within a homology cassette. Recombination occurs at the homologous flanking regions (X) leading to the replacement of the functional endogenous gene with its nonfunctional counterpart.

because individual mutagenesis cassettes are required for every gene. While homologous recombination can be achieved in the fruit fly *Drosophila melanogaster*, in the mouse and in a moss called *Physcomitrella patens*, genome-wide gene knockout projects for these organisms have yet to be carried out.

The second approach is genome-wide random mutagenesis by irradiation, the application of mutagenic chemicals or by the random insertion of DNA sequences. While this is not as comprehensive as systematic homologous recombination, it is applicable in a wider range of organisms, it does not require a completed genome sequence and it is much easier to perform. Insertional mutant libraries have been produced in several species, including bacteria, yeast, *D. melanogaster*, the mouse and many plants, and these can produce both null mutations with complete loss-of-function phenotypes as well as partial loss-of-function mutations caused by splicing errors and other phenomena. In contrast, irradiation and chemical mutagenesis produce more subtle point mutations that can allow gene function to be studied in more detail. A key advantage of using insertional DNA elements rather than radiation or chemicals is that the interrupted gene is tagged with a DNA sequence that can be isolated by hybridization or PCR, allowing the mutated gene to be mapped and identified. Furthermore, the insertional construct can be designed to collect information about the gene in addition to its mutant phenotype (*Box 1.2*). Transcriptional and translational fusions can be used to monitor the expression of the interrupted gene and localize the protein, while the inclusion of a strong, outward-facing promoter can activate genes adjacent to the insertion site generating strong, gain-of-function phenotypes caused by overexpression or ectopic expression. An example of a highly modified insertional construct used in yeast is shown in *Figure 1.7*.

1.4.3   RNA interference

RNA interference (RNAi) is a highly conserved cellular defense mechanism, which appears to have evolved to protect cells from viruses. The effect is triggered by double-stranded RNA (dsRNA), which many viruses use as a replicative intermediate, and results in the rapid degradation of the inducing dsRNA molecule and any single-stranded RNA in the cell with the same sequence. In the context of functional genomics, RNAi is useful because the introduction of a dsRNA molecule homologous to an endogenous gene results in the rapid destruction of any corresponding mRNA and hence the potent silencing of that gene at the post-transcriptional level.

The mechanism of RNA interference is complex, but involves the degradation of the dsRNA molecule into short duplexes, about 21–25 bp in length, by a dsRNA-specific endonuclease called Dicer (*Figure 1.8*). The short duplexes are known as small interfering RNAs (siRNAs). These molecules bind to the corresponding mRNA and assemble a sequence-specific RNA endonuclease known as the RNA-induced silencing complex (RISC), which is extremely active and reduces the mRNA of most genes to undetectable levels. RNA interference can be used in both cells and embryos because it is a systemic phenomenon – the siRNAs appear to be able to move between cells so that dsRNA introduced into

BOX 1.2

Advanced insertional elements for functional genomics

Gene traps

The gene trap is an insertion element that contains a reporter gene downstream of a splice acceptor site. A reporter gene encodes a product that can be detected and visualized using a simple assay. For example, the *lacZ* gene encodes the enzyme β-galactosidase, which converts the colorless substrate X-gal into a dark blue product. If the gene trap integrates within the transcription unit of an endogenous gene, the splice acceptor site causes the reporter gene to be recognized as an exon allowing it to be incorporated into a transcriptional fusion product. Because this fusion transcript is expressed under the control of the interrupted gene's promoter, the expression pattern revealed by the reporter gene is often identical to that of the interrupted endogenous gene. Early gene trap vectors depended on in-frame insertion, but the incorporation of internal ribosome entry sites, which allow independent translation of the reporter gene, circumvents this limitation.

Enhancer traps

The enhancer trap is an insertion construct in which the reporter gene lies downstream of a minimal promoter. Under normal circumstances, the promoter is too weak to activate the reporter gene, which is therefore not expressed. However, if the construct integrates in the vicinity of an endogenous enhancer, the marker is activated and reports the expression profile driven by the enhancer.

Activation traps

The activation trap is an insertion construct containing a strong, outward-facing promoter. If the element integrates adjacent to an endogenous gene, that gene will be activated by the promoter. Unlike other insertion vectors, which cause loss-of-function by interrupting genes, an activation tag causes gain of function through overexpression or ectopic expression.

Protein localization traps

These are insertion constructs that identify particular classes of protein based on their localization in the cell. For example, a construct has been described in which the reporter gene is expressed as a fusion to the transmembrane domain of the CD4 type I protein. If this inserts into a gene encoding a secreted product, the resulting fusion protein contains a signal peptide and is inserted into the membrane of the endoplasmic reticulum in the correct orientation to maintain β-galactosidase activity. However, if the construct inserts into a different type of gene, the fusion product is inserted into the ER membrane in the opposite orientation and β-galactosidase activity is lost.

one part of the embryo can cause silencing throughout. As well as introducing dsRNA directly into cells or embryos it is possible to express dual transgenes for the sense and antisense RNAs, to express an inverted repeat construct that generates hairpin RNAs that act as substrates for Dicer, or to introduce siRNA directly. The ease with which RNAi can be initiated has allowed large-scale RNAi programs to be carried out, most notably in the nematode worm *Caenorhabditis elegans* where the phenomenon was discovered. These experiments involved the synthesis of thousands of dsRNA molecules and their systematic administration to

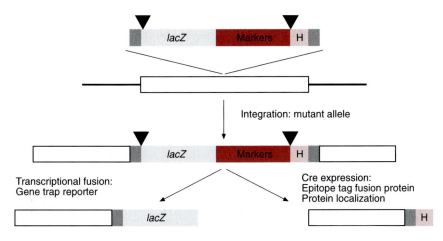

Figure 1.7

Multifunctional *E. coli* Tn*3* cassette used for random mutagenesis in yeast. The cassette comprises Tn*3* components (dark gray), *lacZ* (light gray), selectable markers (red) and an epitope tag such as His₆ (pink, H). The *lacZ* gene and markers are flanked by *loxP* sites (black triangles). Integration generates a mutant allele which may or may not reveal a mutant phenotype. The presence of the *lacZ* gene at the 5′ end of the construct allows transcriptional fusions to be generated, so the insert can be used as a reporter construct to reveal the normal expression profile of the interrupted gene. If Cre recombinase is provided, the *lacZ* gene and markers are deleted leaving the endogenous gene joined to the epitope tag, allowing protein localization to be studied.

worms either by microinjection, soaking or feeding. Most recently, a screen was carried out in which nearly 17 000 bacterial strains were generated and fed to worms, each strain expressing a different dsRNA, representing 86% of the genes in the *C. elegans* genome (see Further Reading). The expression of siRNA is also being used for the functional analysis of human genes in cultured cells.

1.5 The need for proteomics

Transcriptome analysis, genome-wide mutagenesis and RNA interference have risen quickly to dominate functional genomics technologies because they are all based on high-throughput clone generation and sequencing, two of the technology platforms that saw rapid development in the genome-sequencing era. But what do they really tell us about the working of biological systems? Nucleic acids, while undoubtedly important molecules in the cell, are only information-carriers. Therefore, the analysis of genes (by mutation) or of mRNA (by RNA interference or transcriptomics) can only tell us about protein function indirectly. Proteins are the actual functional molecules of the cell (*Box 1.3*). They are responsible for almost all the biochemical activity of the cell and achieve this by interacting with each other and with a diverse spectrum of other molecules. In this sense, they are functionally the most relevant components of biological systems and a true understanding of such systems can only come from the direct study of proteins.

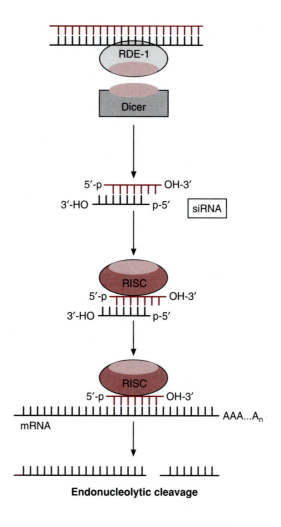

Figure 1.8

The mechanism of RNA interference. Double-stranded RNA (dsRNA) is recognized by the protein RDE-1, which recruits a nuclease known as Dicer. This cleaves the dsRNA into short fragments, 21–23 bp in length with two-base overhangs. The fragments are known as short interfering RNAs (siRNAs). The siRNA is incorporated into the RNA-induced silencing complex (RISC). The siRNA serves as guide for RISC and, upon perfect base pairing, the target mRNA is cleaved in the middle of the duplex formed with the siRNA. Reprinted from Current Opinion in Plant Biology, Vol. 5, Vionnet, 'RNA silencing: small RNAs as ubiquitous regulators of gene expression', pp 444–451, ©2002, with permission from Elsevier.

The importance of proteomics in systems biology can be summarized as follows:

- *The function of a protein depends on its structure and interactions, neither of which can be predicted accurately based on sequence information alone.* Only by looking at the structure and interactions of the protein directly can definitive functional information be obtained.
- *Mutations and RNA interference are coarse tools for large-scale functional analysis.* If the structure and function of a protein are already

understood in fairly good detail, very precise mutations can be introduced to investigate its function further. However, for the large-scale
analysis of gene function, the typical strategy is to completely inacti-
vate each gene (resulting in the absence of the protein) or to
overexpress it (resulting in overabundance or ectopic activity). In
each case, the resulting phenotype may not be informative. For
example, the loss of many proteins is lethal, and while this tells us
the protein is essential it does not tell us what the protein actually
does. Random mutagenesis can produce informative mutations
serendipitously, but there is no systematic way to achieve this. Some
proteins have multiple functions in different times and/or places, or
have multiple domains with different functions, and these cannot be
separated by blanket mutagenesis approaches.

- *The abundance of a given transcript may not reflect the abundance of the*
  corresponding protein. Transcriptome analysis tells us the relative abundance of different transcripts in the cell, and from this we infer the
  abundance of the corresponding protein. However, the two may not
  be related because of post-transcriptional gene regulation. Not all the
  mRNAs in the cell are translated, so the transcriptome may include
  gene products that are not found in the proteome. Similarly, rates of
  protein synthesis and protein turnover differ among transcripts,
  therefore the abundance of a transcript does not necessarily correspond to the abundance of the encoded protein. The transcriptome
  may not accurately represent the proteome either qualitatively or
  quantitatively.

- *Protein diversity is generated post-transcriptionally.* Many genes, particularly in eukaryotic systems, give rise to multiple transcripts by
  alternative splicing. These transcripts often produce proteins with
  different functions. Mutations, acting at the gene level, may
  therefore abolish the functions of several proteins at once. Splice
  variants are represented by different transcripts so it should be
  possible to distinguish them by RNA interference and transcriptome
  analysis, but some transcripts give rise to multiple proteins whose
  individual functions cannot be studied other than at the protein
  level.

- *Protein activity often depends on post-translational modifications, which*
  are not predictable from the level of the corresponding transcript. Many
  proteins are present in the cell as inert molecules, which need to be
  activated by processes such as proteolytic cleavage or phosphorylation. In cases where variations in the abundance of a specific
  post-translational variant are significant, this means that only
  proteomics provides the information required to establish the function of a particular protein.

- *The function of a protein often depends on its localization.* While there
  are some examples of mRNA localization in the cell, particularly in
  early development, most trafficking of gene products occurs at the
  protein level. The activity of a protein often depends on its location,
  and many proteins are shuttled between compartments (e.g. the
  cytosol and the nucleus) as a form of regulation. The abundance of a
  given protein in the cell as a whole may therefore tell only part of
  the story. In some cases, it is the distribution of a protein rather than
  its absolute abundance that is important.

- *Some biological samples do not contain nucleic acids.* One practical reason for studying the proteome rather than the genome or transcriptome is that many important samples do not contain nucleic acids. Most body fluids, including serum, cerebrospinal fluid and urine, fall into this category, but the protein levels in such fluids are often important determinants of disease progression (e.g. proteins shed into the urine can be used to follow the progress of bladder cancer). Although nucleic acids are present in fixed biological specimens, they are often degraded or cross-linked beyond use, and protein analysis provides the only feasible means to study such material. It has also recently been shown that proteins may be better preserved than nucleic acids in ancient biological specimens, such as Neanderthal bones.
- *Proteins are the most therapeutically relevant molecules in the body.* Although there has been recent success in the development of drugs (particularly antivirals) that target nucleic acids, most therapeutic targets are proteins and this is likely to remain so for the foreseeable future. Proteins also represent useful biomarkers and may be therapeutic in their own right.

BOX 1.3

The central importance of proteins

The term *protein* was introduced into the language in 1938 by the Swedish chemist Jöns Jacob Berzelius to describe a particular class of macromolecules, abundant in living organisms, and made up of linear chains of amino acids. The term is derived from the Greek word *proteios* meaning 'of the first order' and was chosen to convey the central importance of proteins in the human body. As our knowledge of this class of macromolecules has grown, this definition seems all the more appropriate. We have discovered that proteins are vital components of almost every biological system in every living organism. There are thousands of different proteins in even the simplest of cells and they form the basis of every conceivable biological function.

Most of the biochemical reactions in living cells are catalyzed by proteins called enzymes, which bind their substrates with great specificity and increase the reaction rates millions or billions of times. Several thousand enzymes have been cataloged. Some catalyze very simple reactions, such as phosphorylation or dephosphorylation, while others orchestrate incredibly complex and intricate processes such as DNA replication and transcription. Proteins can also transport or store other molecules. Examples include ion channels (which allow ions to pass across otherwise impermeable membranes), ferritin (which stores iron in a bioavailable form), hemoglobin (which transports oxygen) and the component proteins of larger structures such as nuclear pores and plasmodesmata.

Other proteins have a structural or mechanical role. All eukaryotic cells possess a cytoskeleton comprising three types of protein filament – microtubules made of tubulin, microfilaments made of actin, and intermediate filaments made of specialized proteins such as keratin. Unlike enzymes and storage proteins, which tend to be globular in structure and soluble in aqueous solvents, the cytoskeletal proteins are fibrous and can link into bundles and networks. Such proteins not only provide mechanical support to the cell, but they can also control intracellular transport, cell shape and cell motility. For example, microtubule networks help to separate chromosomes during mitosis and to transport vesicles and other organelles from site to site within the cell. They also form the core structures of cilia and flagella. Actin filaments form contractile units in association with proteins of the myosin family. This actin–myosin interaction provides muscle cells with their immense contractile power. In other cells, actin filaments have a more general role in facilitating cell movement and changing cell shape, e.g. by forming a contractile ring during cell division. In multicellular organisms, further structural proteins are deposited in the extracellular matrix, which consists of protein fibers embedded in a complex gel of carbohydrates. Such proteins, which include collagen, elastin and laminin, contribute to the mechanical properties of tissues. Cell adhesion proteins, such as cadherins and integrins, help to stick cells together and to their substrates.

Another important role for proteins is communication and regulation. Most cells bristle with receptors for various molecules allowing them to respond to changes in the environment. These receptors are specialized proteins that either span the membrane, with domains poking out each side, or are tethered to it. In some cases, the ligands that bind to these receptors are also proteins: many hormones are proteins (e.g. growth hormone, insulin) as are most developmental regulators, growth factors and cytokines. In this way, a protein secreted by one cell can bind to a receptor on the outside of another and influence its behavior. Inside the cell, further proteins are involved in signal transduction, the process by which a signal arriving at the surface of the cell mediates a specific effect inside. Often, the ultimate effect is to change the pattern of gene expression in the responding cell by influencing the activity of regulatory molecules called transcription factors, which are also proteins. Other proteins are required for mRNA processing, translation, protein sorting in the cell and secretion. More specialized examples of proteins involved in communication include the light-sensitive protein rhodopsin, which is required for light perception in the retina, and the voltage-gated ion channels required for the transmission of nerve impulses along axons.

A final category of proteins encompasses those involved in 'species interactions', i.e. attack, defense and cooperation. All pathogenic microorganisms produce proteins that interact with the proteins of their host to enable infection and reproduction. For example, viruses have proteins that allow them to bind to the cell surface and facilitate entry, and some may have further proteins that interact with the machinery that controls cell division and protein synthesis, hijacking these processes for their own needs. Bacterial toxins, such as the cholera, tetanus and diphtheria toxins, are proteins. And the molecules we use to protect ourselves against invaders – e.g. antibodies, complement, etc. – are also proteins.

1.6 The scope of proteomics

Proteins are diverse molecules that can be studied in various different contexts, including sequence, structure, interactions, expression, localization and modification. Proteomics is divided into several major but overlapping branches, which embrace these different contexts and help to synthesize the information into a comprehensive understanding of biological systems.

1.6.1 Sequence and structural proteomics

Although proteomics as we understand it today would not have been possible without advances in DNA sequencing, it is worth remembering that the first protein sequence (insulin, 51 amino acids, completed in 1956) was determined 10 years before the first RNA sequence (a yeast tRNA, 77 bases, completed in 1966) and 13 years before the first DNA sequence (the *E. coli lac* operator in 1969). Until DNA sequencing became routine in the late 1970s and early 1980s, it was usually the protein sequence that was determined first, allowing the design of probes or primers that could be used to isolate the corresponding cDNA or genomic sequence. Protein sequencing by Edman degradation (see Chapter 3) often provided a crucial link between the activity of a protein and the genetic basis of a particular phenotype, and it was not until the mid 1980s that it first became commonplace to predict protein sequences from genes rather than to use protein sequences for gene isolation.

The increasing numbers of stored protein and nucleic acid sequences, and the recognition that functionally related proteins often had similar sequences, catalyzed the development of statistical techniques for sequence comparison which underlie many of the core bioinformatic methods used in proteomics today (Chapter 5). Nucleic acid sequences are stored in three primary sequence databases – GenBank, the EMBL nucleotide sequence database and the DNA database of Japan (DDBJ) – which exchange data every day. These databases also contain protein sequences that have been translated from DNA sequences. A dedicated protein sequence database, SWISS-PROT, was founded in 1986 and contains highly curated data concerning over 70 000 proteins. A related database, TrEMBL, contains automatic translations of the nucleotide sequences in the EMBL database and is not manually curated.

Since similar sequences give rise to similar structures, it is clear that protein sequence, structure and function are often intimately linked. The study of three-dimensional protein structure is underpinned by technologies such as X-ray crystallography and nuclear magnetic resonance spectroscopy, and has given rise to another branch of bioinformatics concerned with the storage, presentation, comparison and prediction of structures (Chapter 6). The Protein Data Bank was the first protein structure database (www.rscb.org) and now contains more than 10 000 structures. Technological developments in structural proteomics have centered on increasing the throughput of structural determination and the initiation of systematic projects for proteome-wide structural analysis.

1.6.2　Expression proteomics

Expression proteomics is devoted to the analysis of protein abundance and involves the separation of complex protein mixtures, the identification of individual components and their systematic quantitative analysis (*Figure 1.9*). Methods for the separation of protein mixtures based on two-dimensional gel electrophoresis (2DGE) were first developed in the 1970s and even at this time it was envisaged that databases could be created to catalog the proteins in different cells and look for differences representing alternative states, such as health and disease. Many of the statistical analysis methods which are usually associated with microarray analysis, such as clustering algorithms and multivariate statistics, were developed originally in the context of 2DGE protein analysis.

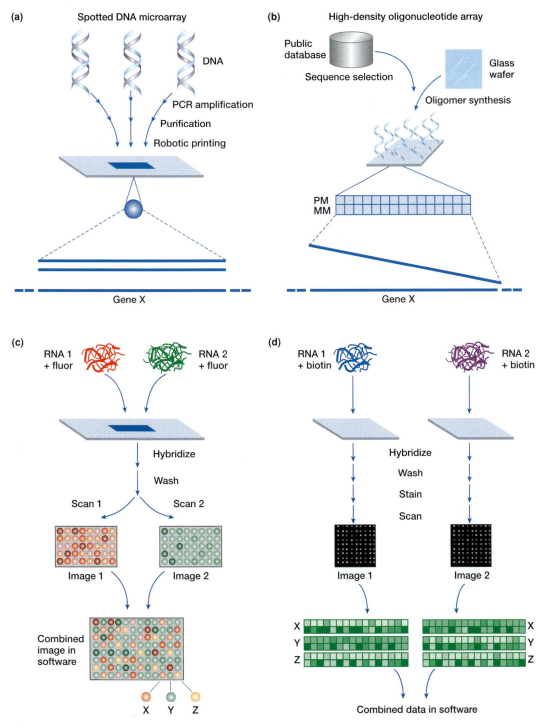

Plate 1

Expression analysis with DNA microarrays. (a) Spotted microarrays are produced by the robotic printing of amplified cDNA molecules onto glass slides. Each spot or feature corresponds to a contiguous gene fragment of several hundred base pairs or more. (b) High-density oligonucleotide chips are manufactured using a process of light-directed combinatorial chemical synthesis to produce thousands of different sequences in a highly ordered array on a small glass chip. Genes are represented by 15–20 different oligonucleotide pairs (PM, perfectly matched and MM, mismatched)

continued overleaf

continued from previous page

on the array. (c) On spotted arrays, comparative expression assays are usually carried out by differentially labeling two mRNA or cDNA samples with different fluorophores. These are hybridized to features on the glass slide and then scanned to detect both fluorophores independently. Colored dots labeled x, y and z at the bottom of the image correspond to transcripts present at increased levels in sample 1 (x), increased levels in sample 2 (y), and similar levels in samples 1 and 2 (z). (d) On Affymetrix GeneChips, biotinylated cRNA is hybridized to the array and stained with a fluorophore conjugated to avidin. The signal is detected by laser scanning. Sets of paired oligonucleotides for hypothetical genes present at increased levels in sample 1 (x), increased levels in sample 2 (y) and similar levels in samples 1 and 2 (z) are shown. Reprinted from Current Opinion in Microbiology, Vol. 3, Harrington et al. 'Monitoring gene expression using DNA microarrays', pp 285–291, ©2000, with permission from Elsevier.

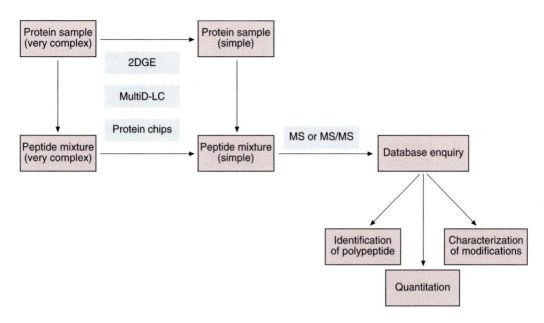

Figure 1.9

Expression proteomics is concerned with protein identification and qualitative analysis. This figure shows the aims of expression proteomics and major technology platforms used. See Chapters 2–4 and 8–9 for further information. 2DGE, two-dimensional gel electrophoresis; HPLC, high-performance liquid chromatography; MS, mass spectrometry; MS/MS, tandem mass spectrometry; MultiD-LC, multidimensional liquid chromatography.

Unfortunately, there were severe technical limitations, such as the difficulty in achieving reproducible separations and identifying separated proteins. The major breakthrough in expression proteomics was made in the early 1990s when mass spectrometry techniques were adapted for protein identification, and algorithms were designed for database searching using mass spectrometry data (Chapter 3). Today, thousands of proteins can be separated, quantified and rapidly identified. This can be used to catalog the proteins produced in a given cell type, identify proteins that are differentially expressed among different samples and characterize post-translational modifications. The key technologies in expression proteomics are 2D-gel electrophoresis and multidimensional liquid chromatography for protein separation (Chapter 2), mass spectrometry for protein identification (Chapter 3) and image analysis or mass spectrometry for protein quantitation (Chapter 4). The application of these techniques in the analysis of post-translational modifications is considered in Chapter 8. An emerging trend in expression proteomics, and a rapidly growing business sector within the proteomics market, is the use of protein chips for analysis and quantitation (Chapter 9).

1.6.3 Interaction proteomics

This branch of proteomics considers the genetic and physical interactions among proteins as well as interactions between proteins and nucleic acids or small molecules. The analysis of protein interactions can provide information not only about the function of individual proteins but also about how proteins function in pathways, networks, and complexes. It is a field that relies on many different technology platforms to provide diverse information, and is closely linked with functional proteomics and the large-scale analysis of protein localization (*Figure 1.10*). Conceptually the most ambitious aspect of interaction proteomics is the creation of proteome linkage maps based on binary interactions between individual proteins and higher-order interactions determined by the systematic analysis of protein complexes. Key technologies in this area include the yeast two-hybrid system (a genetic assay for binary interactions) and mass spectrometry for the analysis of protein complexes (Chapter 7). Interactions between proteins and nucleic acids underlie many important processes including gene regulation, while protein interactions with small molecules are also of interest, e.g. enzymes interacting with their substrates and receptors with their ligands. These types of interactions are often investigated using biochemical assays and structural analysis methods such as X-ray crystallography. The characterization of protein interactions with small molecules can play an important role in the drug development process.

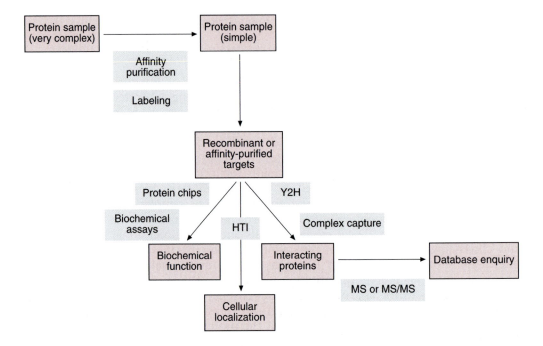

Figure 1.10

Functional proteomics is concerned with the investigation of protein interactions and biochemical, cellular and system functions. This figure shows the aims of functional proteomics and major technology platforms used. See Chapters 7 and 9 for further information. HTI, high-throughput imaging; Y2H, yeast two hybrid system; MS, mass spectrometry, MS/MS, tandem mass spectrometry.

1.6.4 Functional proteomics

The most straightforward way to establish the function of a protein is to test that function directly. Functional proteomics is a relatively new development in which protein functions are tested directly but on a large scale. An example is the systematic testing of expressed proteins for different enzymatic activities, as described in a landmark publication by Martzen and colleagues (see Further Reading). The development of functional protein chips, which allow high-throughput functional assays to be carried out in a simple fashion, is discussed in Chapter 9.

1.7 The challenges of proteomics

Proteomics encompasses a range of technological approaches for the large-scale characterization of proteins and it is clear that no one form of technology is suitable for every application. The different technologies have different strengths and weaknesses and a significant challenge is their integration and automation, a factor that underpinned the success of the large-scale DNA-sequencing projects. Important hurdles must be overcome at every stage of analysis, from sample preparation through to database management (*Figure 1.11*). One of the major drawbacks of proteomics is the lack of an amplification method, equivalent to the PCR, for the preparation of scarce proteins. This means that sensitivity is a key issue and that proteins with the lowest abundance are always going to be difficult to detect. Sensitivity is especially important considering the dynamic range of protein abundances in typical biological samples, which has been estimated at 10^5 for tissues and up to 10^9 for body fluids such as serum. Some of the key technologies also suffer from high rates of false-positive and false-negative results, e.g. the yeast two-hybrid system for the detection of binary protein interactions (Chapter 7). It should be emphasized that proteomics is a young science, many of the technologies used in proteomics are still prototypical and that better

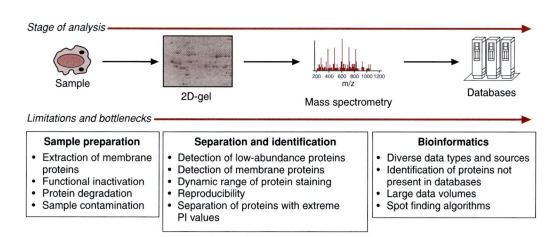

Figure 1.11

Challenges facing proteomics with current technology.

materials, instrument design and methodology are expected to improve sensitivity, resolution and repeatability in the future. Such advances will be required if proteomics is to be used to provide a comprehensive analysis of complex biological systems.

Further reading

Anderson, N.G. and Anderson, N.L. (1998) Proteome and proteomics: New technologies, new concepts, new words. *Electrophoresis* **19**: 1853–1861.

Blackstock, W. and Weir, M. (1999) Proteomics: quantitative and physical mapping of cellular proteins. *Trends Biotechnol* **17**: 121–127.

Coelho, P.S.R., Kumar, A. and Snyder, M. (2000) Genome-wide mutant collections: toolboxes for functional genomics. *Curr Opin Microbiol* **3**: 309–315.

Gygi, S.P., Rochon, Y., Franza, B.R. and Aebersold, R. (1999) Correlation between protein and mRNA abundance in yeast. *Mol Cell Biol* **19**: 1720–1730.

Kamath, R.S., Fraser, A.G., Dong, Y., *et al.* (2003) Systematic functional analysis of the *Caenorhabditis elegans* genome using RNAi. *Nature* **421**: 231–237.

Lee, K.H. (2001) Proteomics: a technology-driven and technology-limited discovery science. *Trends Biotechnol* **19**: 217–222.

Martzen, M.R., McCraith, S.M., Spinelli, S.L., *et al.* (1999) A biochemical genomics approach for identifying genes by the activity of their products. *Science* **286**: 1153–1155.

Pandey, A. and Mann, M. (2000) Proteomics to study genes and genomes. *Nature* **405**: 837–846.

Patterson, S.D. and Aebersold, R.H. (2003) Proteomics: the first decade and beyond. *Nature Genet* **33** (Suppl): 311–323.

Reif, D.M., White, B.C. and Moore, J.H. (2004) Integrated analysis of genetic, genomic and proteomic data. *Expert Rev. Proteomics* **1**: 67–75.

Tyers, M. and Mann, M. (2003) From genomics to proteomics. *Nature* **422**: 193–197.

Various authors (2002) The Chipping Forecast II. *Nature Genet* **32** (Suppl): 465–551.

Velculescu, V.E., Zhang, L., Vogelstein, B. and Kinzler, K.W. (1995) Serial analysis of gene expression. *Science* **270**: 484–487.

Strategies for protein separation

2

2.1 Introduction

The analysis of proteins, whether on a small or large scale, requires methods for the separation of protein mixtures into their individual components. Protein separation methods can be placed on a sliding scale from fully selective to fully nonselective. Selective methods aim to isolate individual proteins from a mixture usually by exploiting very specific properties such as their binding specificity or biochemical function. Such methods are particularly useful for studying protein interactions or functions, and are discussed in more detail in Chapter 7. They also form the basis of protein chip technology, which is considered in Chapter 9. In this chapter, however, we focus on nonselective separation methods, which aim to take a complex protein mixture and fractionate it in such a manner that all the individual proteins, or at least a substantial subfraction, are available for further analysis. Such methods lie at the heart of proteomics and exploit very general properties of proteins, such as their mass or net charge.

In proteomics, protein separation technology is pushed to its limits. The ultimate goal is to resolve all the individual proteins in the cell. As stated in Chapter 1, in a eukaryotic cell, this may represent 50 000–100 000 or more different types of protein when post-translational modifications are taken into consideration. These proteins are chemically very diverse and thus it is difficult to devise a separation method that will represent all proteins equally. At the current time, even the most sophisticated separation methods result in the under-representation of certain protein classes and are therefore at least partially selective.

Whether protein separation is selective, partially selective or nonselective, it is important to remember that the underlying principle is always the exploitation of physical and chemical differences between proteins which cause them to behave differently in particular environments. These physical and chemical differences are determined by the number, type and order of amino acids in the protein, and by any post-translational modifications that have taken place.

2.2 Protein separation in proteomics – general principles

Many techniques can be used to separate complex protein mixtures in what at least approaches a nonselective fashion, but not all of these techniques are suitable for proteomics. One major requirement is high resolution. The separation technique should produce fractions that comprise very simple mixtures of proteins, and ideally each fraction should contain an individual protein. This essentially rules out one-dimensional techniques, i.e. those that exploit a single chemical or physical property as the basis for separation, since this simply does not provide enough resolving power. All the techniques discussed in this chapter are multi-dimensional, i.e. two or more different fractionation principles are employed one after another. The other major requirement in proteomics is high throughput. The separation technique should resolve all the proteins in one experiment and should ideally be easy to automate. The most suitable methods for automation are those that rely on differential rates of migration to produce fractions that can be displayed or collected, a process generally described as separative transport. A final requirement is that the fractionation procedure should be compatible with downstream analysis by mass spectrometry, as this is the major technology platform for high-throughput protein identification (Chapter 3). The two groups of techniques that have come to dominate proteomics are two-dimensional gel electrophoresis (2DGE) and multidimensional liquid chromatography, the latter often combined with further liquid-based separations techniques such as capillary electrophoresis or chromatofocusing.

2.3 Principles of two-dimensional gel electrophoresis

2.3.1 General principles of protein separation by electrophoresis

Any charged molecule in solution will migrate in an applied electric field, a phenomenon known as electrophoresis. The rate of migration depends on the strength of the electric field and the charge density of the molecule, i.e. the ratio of charge to mass. Since dissolved proteins carry a net charge, a protein mixture in solution can in theory be fractionated by electrophoresis because different proteins, with different charge densities, migrate towards the appropriate electrodes at different rates. In practice, however, effective separation is never achieved because all the proteins are initially distributed throughout the solution.

The answer to this problem is to load the protein mixture in one place within the electrophoresis buffer, allowing proteins with different charge densities to migrate as discrete zones. However, there are many practical reasons why standard electrophoresis is not carried out in free solution. One is that any disturbance to the solution will disrupt the electrophoresis zones. Even if extreme precautions are taken to avoid shocks and vibrations from outside, electrophoresis generates heat and the convection currents within the buffer will disperse the zones quite effectively. Another reason is that the narrow protein zones generated by electrophoresis are broadened by diffusion, which acts quickly to homogenize the protein mixture once the electric field is removed (*Figure 2.1*). These effects are minimized if electrophoresis is carried out in very narrow vessels (capillary electrophoresis, *Box 2.1*) and/or within a stabilizing matrix such as paper or gel, since the latter also allows the separated proteins to be fixed in place once the procedure is complete. Polyacrylamide gels are favored because they facilitate separation by sieving the proteins on the basis of their size. Gels with different pore sizes can be produced easily and reproducibly by varying the concentration of acrylamide in the polymerization mixture, allowing the preferential separation of proteins with a particular range of molecular masses (p. 29). Polyacrylamide gel electrophoresis (PAGE) is therefore

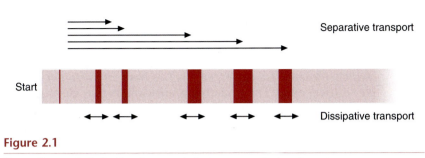

Figure 2.1

Separative and dissipative transport during zone electrophoresis.

one of the most widely used protein separation techniques in molecular biology.

As discussed above, all high-resolution protein fractionation methods employ multidimensional separation processes that exploit different properties of proteins for separation in each dimension. Although PAGE separates proteins according to both charge and mass, exploiting both these principles in the same dimension still results in a low-resolution separation. It would be better to apply these principles one after the other in orthogonal dimensions. It has therefore been necessary to devise modifications of gel electrophoresis that achieve separation on the basis of charge alone and on the basis of mass alone. These modified techniques are applied consecutively in two-dimensional gel electrophoresis, which is therefore also known as ISO-DALT (isoelectric focusing, and Dalton, the unit of protein mass).

BOX 2.1

Capillary electrophoresis in proteomics

Capillary electrophoresis (CE) is carried out in glass tubes that are typically about 50 μm in diameter and up to 1 m in length. The tubes may or may not be filled with gel, but the presence of gel facilitates sieving of the proteins or peptides and enhances size-dependent separation (capillary gel electrophoresis, CGE). The thin tubes are efficient at dissipating heat, allowing the use of very strong electric fields. The separations are thus rapid, efficient and can be monitored in real time rather than at the experiment's end point. The narrow diameter of the capillary tubes requires very small sample volumes. Therefore, the major application of capillary electrophoresis in proteomics has been the separation of peptides in relatively simple mixtures, such as the tryptic digests of purified proteins or spots excised from 2D-gels.

More recently, the limited loading capacity of CE tubes has been circumvented by drying and concentrating larger samples, or by coupling CE to a solid-phase extraction system. If such steps are taken, CE can also be applied to the separation of more complex mixtures of proteins or peptides, and can be used downstream of other liquid-phase separation methods (such as size exclusion chromatography and reversed phase HPLC, p. 39) in multidimensional separations.

2.3.2 Separation according to charge but not mass – isoelectric focusing

The first dimension separation in 2DGE is usually isoelectric focusing (IEF), in which proteins are separated on the basis of their net charge irrespective of their mass. The underlying principle is that electrophoresis is carried out in a pH gradient, allowing each protein to migrate to its isoelectric point, i.e. the point at which its pI value is equivalent to the surrounding pH and its net charge is zero (*Figure 2.2*). In standard electrophoresis, there is no pH gradient because the electrophoresis buffer has a uniform pH. Therefore, the charge density of each protein remains the same during electrophoresis and, in time, each protein reaches either the anode or the cathode. In the case of IEF, the charge density of each protein decreases as it moves along the pH gradient towards its isoelectric point. When the isoelectric point is reached, the protein's charge density is zero and it comes to a halt. Diffusion still acts against this tendency to focus at a single position in the gel, but a protein diffusing away from its isoelectric point becomes charged and therefore moves back towards its focus. Proteins with different pI values, as determined by the number and type of acidic and basic amino acid residues they contain, therefore focus at different positions in the pH gradient. Although there may be an initial sieving effect which separates the proteins on the basis of their size, running the gel for a suitably long period of time ensures that all proteins reach their isoelectric points and size-independent separation is achieved.

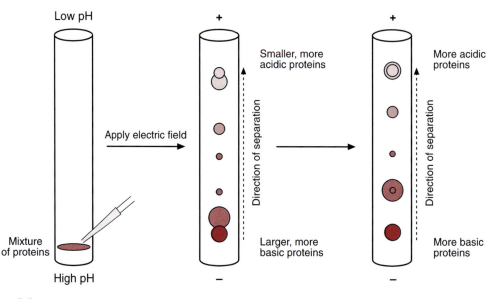

Figure 2.2

The principle of isoelectric focusing. A mixture of proteins is loaded at the basic end of a gel that has a pH gradient. An electric field is applied and the proteins separate according to their charge, focusing at positions where the pI value is equivalent to the surrounding pH. Larger proteins will move more slowly through the gel, but with sufficient time will catch up with small proteins of equal charge. The circles represent proteins, with shading to indicate protein pI values and diameters representing molecular mass.

The pH gradient in an IEF gel can be established in two ways. The first is to use synthetic carrier ampholytes, which are collections of small amphoteric molecules with pI values corresponding to a given pH range (*Figure 2.3a*). Initially, there is no pH gradient in the gel because all the ampholytes are evenly distributed; the pH of the electrophoresis buffer is the average of that of the ampholyte molecules. When the electric field is applied, however, the ampholytes themselves are subject to electrophoresis. The most acidic ampholyte moves towards the anode, the most basic ampholyte moves towards the cathode and all the other ampholytes establish intermediate zones according to their pI values. Once this stacking process is completed, the system has reached an equilibrium characterized by a continuous pH gradient. Proteins, which migrate much more slowly than the ampholyte molecules, then begin to move towards their isoelectric points in the gel. The proteins can be added to the gel before the electric field is applied or after a period of prefocusing.

There are several problems with the use of ampholytes, and these lead to poor reproducibility in 2DGE experiments. One of the most serious limitations is cathodic drift, where the ampholytes themselves migrate to

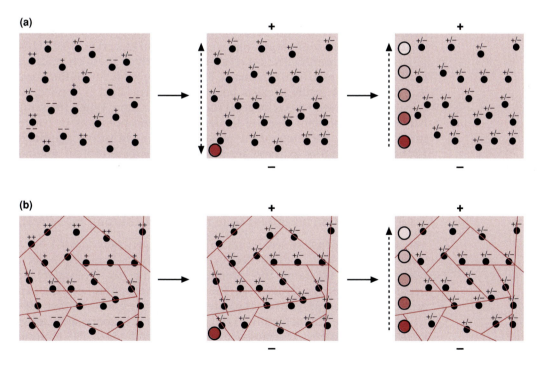

Figure 2.3

Different ways of forming a pH gradient for isoelectric focusing. (a) With ampholytes, the buffering molecules are free to diffuse and initially are distributed evenly so there is no pH gradient. When an electric field is applied, the ampholytes establish a pH gradient and become charge neutral. This leads to separation of proteins according to pI values. (b) In the case of an immobilized pH gradient, the buffering molecules are attached to the polyacrylamide gel matrix. No movement of the buffering molecules occurs when the electric field is applied but proteins are separated. Dotted arrows show direction of separation. Shading indicates protein pI values.

the cathode due to a phenomenon called electro-osmotic flow (bulk solvent movement towards the cathode). This results in pH gradient instability as basic ampholytes are progressively lost from the system. In practical terms, it is difficult to maintain a pH gradient that extends far beyond pH 7–8, resulting in the loss of many basic proteins.

One way in which the problem of cathodic drift has been addressed is a procedure known as nonequilibrium pH gradient electrophoresis (NEPHGE). In this method, the protein sample is applied to the acidic end of the gel (rather than the basic end, which is generally the case for standard isoelectric focusing) so that all the proteins are positively charged at the beginning of the gel run. If run to completion, the basic ampholytes and the basic proteins would still run off the end of the gel but the essential principle of NEPHGE is that the gel is not run for long enough to allow the system to reach equilibrium. Rather, the proteins are separated in a rapidly forming pH gradient that never becomes stable. For this reason, the conditions of separation are extremely difficult to reproduce.

Both these problems – cathodic drift and poor reproducibility – have been addressed by the development of immobilized pH gradient (IPG) gels, in which the buffering groups are attached to the polyacrylamide matrix of the gel (*Figure 2.3b*). This is now the standard approach in proteomics, where reproducibility is a key issue. The IPG is established using Immobilines, a collection of nonamphoteric molecules that contain a weak acid- or base-buffering group at one end, and an acrylic double bond to facilitate the immobilization reaction at the other. These chemicals are available from Amersham Pharmacia Biotech. The gel is run in the normal way but the pH gradient exists before the electric field is applied, and remains stable even when the gel is run for a long time. When the sample is loaded, the proteins migrate to their isoelectric points as in conventional isoelectric focusing. Many researchers also add carrier ampholytes to the IPG gel buffer as these are thought to increase protein solubility and prevent nonproductive interactions between proteins and the Immobiline reagents.

2.3.3   Separation according to mass but not charge – SDS-PAGE

The second dimension separation in 2DGE is generally carried out by standard SDS-PAGE (sodium dodecylsulfate polyacrylamide gel electrophoresis) and separates the proteins according to molecular mass irrespective of charge (*Figure 2.4*). The basis of the technique is the exposure of denatured proteins to the detergent sodium dodecylsulfate (SDS), which binds stoichiometrically to the polypeptide backbone and carries a large negative charge. The presence of tens or hundreds of SDS molecules on each polypeptide dwarfs any intrinsic charge carried by the proteins themselves, and stoichiometric binding means that larger proteins bind more SDS than smaller proteins. This has two important consequences that ensure separation on the basis of mass alone. First, all protein–SDS complexes have essentially the same charge density, and second, the relative differences in mass between proteins are maintained in the protein–SDS complexes.

The gel enhances the size-dependent separation by sieving the proteins as they migrate. The sieving effect depends on the pore size of the

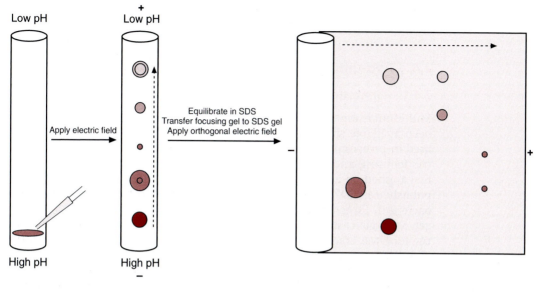

Figure 2.4

Two-dimensional electrophoresis using a tube gel for isoelectric focusing and a slab gel for SDS-PAGE. The proteins are separated in the first dimension on the basis of charge and in the second dimension on the basis of molecular mass. The circles represent proteins, with shading to indicate protein pl values and diameters representing molecular mass. The dotted line shows the direction of separation.

gel, which is in turn dependent on the gel concentration (total concentration of monomer as a percentage of the gel volume before it is cast, defined as %T). In the case of polyacrylamide gels, the monomer is made up of the gelling agent acrylamide and the cross-linking agent *bis*-acrylamide. The pore size also depends to a certain extent on the proportion of the monomer, by mass, that is represented by *bis*-acrylamide (defined as %C). Generally, as %T increases, the pore size decreases because more of the gelling agent is present per unit volume of the gel. In standard gels (where %T ≤ 15%), the minimum pore size is achieved when %C is approximately 5%. Below this value, there are fewer crosslinks and the minimum pore size is larger. Above this value, the acrylamide molecules become overlinked and form dense bundles interspersed with large cavities, and the minimum pore size again becomes larger. Therefore, by holding the amount of *bis*-acrylamide at 5%, the pore size of the gel can be effectively controlled by varying the total concentration of the monomer. The optimum value for %C, i.e. the value required to achieve minimum pore size, increases above 5% when %T > 15%. Gels can be cast with %T values ranging from 1% to over 30%. Gels with concentrations lower than about 3% are required for the sieving of very large proteins ($M_r \geq 10^6$) but are very fragile, and are generally stabilized by the inclusion of agarose (which does not sieve the proteins but provides a firm support matrix). Gels with concentrations over 30% can sieve very small proteins ($M_r = 10^3$). The mass of the proteins in the sample can be estimated by including, in one of the lanes of the gel, a series of protein markers whose masses are known.

2.4 Two-dimensional gel electrophoresis in proteomics

2.4.1 Limitations of 2DGE in proteomics

Multidimensional electrophoretic protein separation techniques have been available since the 1950s but the origin of the 2DGE method now used in proteomics is more recent. Protocols involving sequential isoelectric focusing and SDS-PAGE were developed in the mid 1970s and were first applied on a proteomic scale by Patrick O'Farrell in a landmark paper published in 1975 (see Further Reading). In this study, proteins from the bacterium *Escherichia coli* were separated by isoelectric focusing in a tube gel, i.e. a gel cast in a thin plastic tube. When the IEF run was complete, the tube was cracked open and the proteins exposed to SDS by immersion of the gel in an SDS solution. The tube gel was then attached to a SDS-PAGE slab gel, i.e. a flat gel cast between two plates, and the focused proteins were separated in the orthogonal dimension on the basis of size. After nonselective staining, the result was a two-dimensional protein profile in which approximately 1000 individual fractions were distributed over the gel as a series of spots, which represents approximately 20% of the *E. coli* proteome.

The basic procedure for 2DGE has changed little since this time, although the rather cumbersome tube gels have been largely replaced by IPG strip gels, which are easier to handle and give more reproducible separations. However, proteomics takes the power of 2DGE to its limits and a number of operational problems have been identified. These fall into four major areas: resolution, sensitivity, representation and automation. The limitations are discussed in more detail below together with strategies that have been used to overcome them. Variations on the standard theme of 2DGE are discussed briefly in *Box 2.2*.

2.4.2 Improving the resolution of 2DGE

Today's standard 2DGE systems, which are based on first-dimension isoelectric focusing using IPG strips followed by second-dimension SDS-PAGE, are capable of resolving approximately 2500 protein spots on a routine basis (*Figure 2.5*). However, the proteome of a complex eukaryotic cell may be more than an order of magnitude greater than this. Even in the case of a simple eukaryotic system such as yeast, where alternative splicing and post-translational protein modifications are the exception rather than the rule, individual protein spots on standard 2D-gels may comprise several different co-migrating proteins which can make downstream analysis very complex.

The resolution of 2DGE depends on the separation length in both dimensions, and can thus be increased if very large format gels are used. For example, IEF tube gels and IPG strips > 30 cm in length have been used to achieve maximal separation in the first dimension, in combination with very large SDS gels that also provide a separation distance of > 30 cm. Although such gels can be difficult to handle, they do allow the separation of up to 10 000 protein spots. Another way to increase the resolution of

BOX 2.2

Variations on the standard approach to 2DGE

Reverse 2DGE
In the vast majority of 2DGE procedures, isoelectric focusing is used in the first dimension followed by SDS-PAGE in the second dimension. Occasional experiments have been described in which the order of the separations is reversed, but this is not popular because SDS interferes with the isoelectric focusing step, and it is very difficult to remove SDS from proteins completely once they have been exposed.

IEF-MS
In this approach, the SDS-PAGE separation step is replaced with MALDI-TOF mass spectrometry. Mass spectrometry is used primarily for protein identification, as discussed in detail in Chapter 3. In this variant application, however, the technique is used simply to list the masses of the different proteins found in each region of the IEF gel, therefore providing a virtual 2D separation. The procedure involves soaking the IEF gel in a matrix compound suitable for MALDI analysis (Chapter 3) and scanning the dried gel at close intervals to ionize the proteins and determine their masses. While rapid and easy to automate, large proteins tend not to be detected because they are difficult to ionize. Also, there appears to be no easy way to integrate this form of protein separation with conventional downstream MS analysis for protein identification.

SDS-PAGE-MS/MS
This variation of the classical proteomics strategy omits the isoelectric focusing step. It is used primarily for the analysis of very simple protein mixtures, such as affinity-purified complexes, and is therefore employed in the study of protein interactions (discussed further in Chapter 7). When the protein mixture is simple, it can be presumed that each SDS-PAGE band contains only one protein. In a second application, however, SDS-PAGE-MS/MS is applied to complex protein mixtures and each band on the gel contains many different proteins. The goal in this case is simply to build a list of proteins in a particular sample; it is not possible to derive any quantitative data from such experiments.

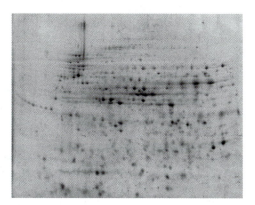

Figure 2.5

Separation of 240 μg of *E. coli* protein by 2DGE, pH range 4-7 and mass range 10 to 120 kD. The gel was stained with ruthenium II tris (bathophenantroline disulfonate) and scanned with a Fuji FLA-3000 laser scanner, with blue SHG-laser. Image supplied by Dr Micheal Lieber, raytest GmbH (see http://www.raytest.com).

2DGE is to use multiple IEF gels, each with a narrow pH range (*Figure 2.6*). These are known as zoom gels. Following second-dimension SDS-PAGE and image analysis, the images of the separate zoom gels can be stitched together by computer to produce a composite of the entire proteome. In one demonstration, the use of six zoom gels allowed the separation of 3000 proteins from *E. coli*, representing approximately 70% of the proteome. The combination of long separation distances and narrow pH ranges can be used to maximize the resolution of such gels. Alternatively, to increase the resolution of proteins within a particular pH range, gels with nonlinear pH gradients can be produced. This is achieved simply by increasing the spacing between the appropriate Immobiline reagents, and is often used to 'flatten' the pH gradient between pH 4 and 7, which accounts for the majority of proteins in the proteome (*Figure 2.7*). Finally, resolution can be increased by various forms of prefractionation prior to electrophoresis, to simplify the protein mixture that is being analyzed. This can be achieved, for example, by one or more rounds of chromatography (p. 35), by sucrose density centrifugation or by the affinity-based enrichment or depletion of particular proteins. Prefractionation is critical for the successful use of narrow range pH gels because proteins representing pI values outside the pH range of the zoom gel tend to precipitate in very concentrated zones at the electrodes and distort the focusing of the remaining proteins due to osmotic effects.

2.4.3 Improving the sensitivity of 2DGE

The proteins in a cell differ in abundance over four to six orders of magnitude, with most of the total protein content represented by a relatively small

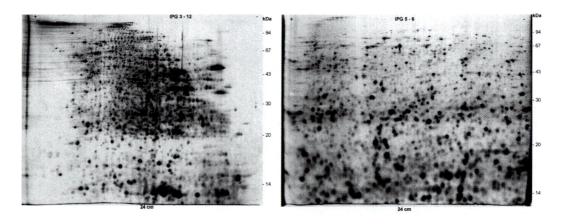

Figure 2.6

Both images represent mouse liver proteins separated by two-dimensional gel electrophoresis and silver stained to reveal individual protein spots. The left image is a wide pH range gel (pH 3–12) while the right image is a narrow pH range gel, which zooms proteins in the pH 5–6 range. Note that in the wider range gel, most proteins are clustered in the middle, reflecting the fact that most proteins have pI values in the 4–7 range. ©Swiss Institute of Bioinformatics, Geneva, Switzerland.

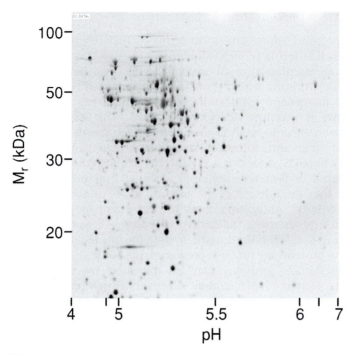

Figure 2.7

Higher-resolution separation can be achieved by flattening the pH gradient between pH 4 and pH 7, which accounts for the majority of proteins. ©Swiss Institute of Bioinformatics, Geneva, Switzerland.

number of abundant or superabundant proteins. In yeast, for example, it is estimated that 50% of the proteome comprises the output of just 100 genes and that the most abundant proteins are present at levels exceeding 1 000 000 copies per cell. The remaining proteins range from those that are moderately abundant (perhaps 100 000 copies in the cell) to those that are vanishingly rare (fewer than 1000 copies per cell). This latter class includes some of the functionally most relevant gene products, including transcription factors and other regulatory proteins. In body fluids, the range of protein concentration values may be even higher (nine orders of magnitude has been estimated).

The sensitivity problems of 2DGE fall into two categories. The first is the difficulty in detecting the rarest proteins at all, which reflects the sensitivity of protein staining, detection and quantitation methods (Chapter 4). The second problem is the tendency of the spots produced by abundant proteins to mask or obscure those produced by scarce proteins. Therefore, some sensitivity problems can be addressed by increasing the resolution of 2D-gels (see above) since this facilitates better separation of proteins with similar electrophoretic properties. The use of narrow-range IPG gels in combination with prefractionation or affinity-depletion of very abundant proteins goes a long way to resolving the problems caused by masking, particularly because this allows larger amounts of the sample to be loaded.

2.4.4 The representation of proteins on 2D-gels

Because proteins are so diverse in terms of their chemical and physical properties, it is virtually impossible to devise a method that leads to the unbiased representation of all proteins on a 2D-gel. The most important factor in determining which proteins are represented is the solubilization step, and for general applications the procedure has not changed very much since it was first developed in 1975. The standard lysis buffer includes a chaotropic agent to disrupt hydrogen bonds (urea, or a combination of urea and thiourea), a nonionic detergent such as NP-40 (definitely not SDS, since this is highly charged!), a reducing agent (usually dithiothreitol or β-mercaptoethanol, although these are charged molecules and they migrate out of the gel during IEF; noncharged alternatives such as tributyl phosphine may be more suitable) and, if desired, ampholytes representing the desired pH range. These conditions are not suitable for the solubilization of membrane proteins and this is why membrane proteins are under-represented on standard 2D-gels. The recovery of membrane proteins can be increased by choosing stronger detergents, such as CHAPS, and by selectively enriching the initial sample for membrane proteins, e.g. by preparing membrane fractions.

Other classes of proteins that are traditionally very difficult to separate by standard 2DGE include histones, other chromatin proteins and ribosomal proteins. Special separation methods have been devised in these cases. For example, a 2DGE approach that has been widely used for the separation of histones involves a first separation carried out on an acid–urea gel (which separates the proteins on the basis of size) and the second-dimension separation carried out on an acid–urea–Triton gel. Triton is a detergent that binds differentially to histones depending on their degree of hydrophobicity, thus the more hydrophobic histones have a greatly reduced mobility. A specific problem with nuclear proteins is their tendency to aggregate under normal electrophoresis conditions and modified buffers are thus used to avoid this.

2.4.5 The automation of 2DGE

The data produced by 2DGE experiments are visual in nature, so downstream analysis involves capturing the images from stained 2D-gels and then isolating particular spots for further processing and mass spectrometry. This process is difficult to automate and therefore constitutes the most significant bottleneck in proteomic research. Until quite recently, manual analysis and spot picking from gels was very common. However, there are now various software packages available that produce high-quality digitized gel images and incorporate methods to evaluate quantitative differences between spots on different gels (Chapter 4). These can be integrated with spot excision robots that use plastic or steel picking tips to transfer gel slices to microtiter plates for automated digestion, clean-up, concentration and transfer to the mass spectrometer. Several commercially available systems can fully automate the analysis and processing of 2D-gels, and can handle 200–300 protein spots per hour. Sections of a silver-stained gel before and after processing with a spot excision robot are shown, as an example, in *Figure 2.8*.

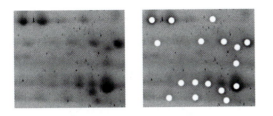

Figure 2.8

Section of a silver-stained 2D gel before and after processing with spot excision robot using a 2-mm plastic picking tip.

2.5 Principles of liquid chromatography in proteomics

2.5.1 General principles of protein and peptide separation by chromatography

Any separation technique that distributes the components of a mixture between two phases, a fixed stationary phase and a free-moving mobile phase, is known as chromatography. There are many chromatography formats, including paper chromatography, thin-layer chromatography, liquid chromatography and gas chromatography, but all depend on the same underlying principle. A mixture of molecules is dissolved in a solvent and fed into the chromatography process. As the mobile phase moves over the stationary phase, the components of the mixture can interact with the molecules of both the solvent and the stationary matrix. Different components in the mixture move at different rates because of their differing affinities for each phase. Molecules with the lowest affinity for the stationary phase will move the most quickly because they tend to remain in the solvent, while molecules with the highest affinity move the most slowly because they tend to stay associated with the stationary phase and are left behind. This results in the mixture being partitioned into a series of fractions, which can be eluted and collected individually.

In proteomics, liquid chromatography (LC) is used more often than other chromatography formats because of its versatility and compatibility with mass spectrometry (Chapter 3). Unlike gel electrophoresis, liquid chromatography is suitable for the separation of both proteins and peptides, and can therefore be applied either upstream of 2DGE to prefractionate the sample, downstream of 2DGE to separate the peptide mixtures from single excised spots, or instead of 2DGE as the major protein separation technology (*Figure 2.9*). Alternative LC methods can exploit different separation principles, such as size, charge, hydrophobicity and affinity for particular ligands. As is the case for electrophoresis, the highest-resolution separations are achieved when two or more separation principles are applied one after the other in orthogonal dimensions.

In liquid chromatography methods used in proteomics, the stationary phase is a porous matrix, usually in the form of packed beads that are supported on some form of column. The mobile phase, a solvent containing dissolved proteins or peptides, flows through the column under gravity or is forced through under high pressure. The rate at which any particular

(a)

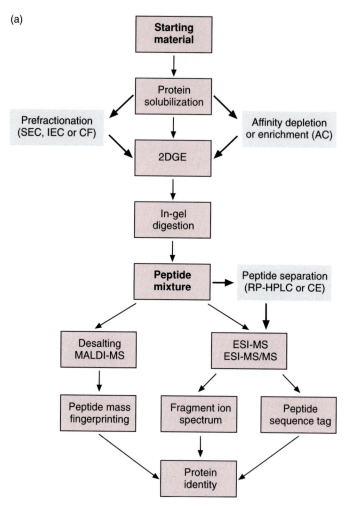

Figure 2.9 (continued on facing page)

(a) Liquid chromatography used in combination with 2DGE in standard proteomic analysis. Prior to 2DGE, the protein sample may be subject to affinity chromatography (AC) to deplete abundant proteins or enrich for certain types of protein. Prefractionation may then be carried out by size exclusion chromatography (SEC), ion exchange chromatography (IEC) or chromatofocusing (CF) to select protein in a particular range or isoelectric points or molecular masses for separation by 2DGE. After 2DGE, spots are digested in the gel with trypsin. The resulting peptides may be desalted and transferred to a MALDI mass spectrometer, or separated by microcapillary electrophoresis (CE) or microcapillary reversed-phase HPLC (RP-HPLC) before injection into the ESI mass spectrometer.

protein or peptide flows through the column depends on its affinity for the matrix, and matrices with different chemical and physical properties can be used to separate proteins or peptides according to different selective principles. These principles, and how they are applied, are discussed in the following sections.

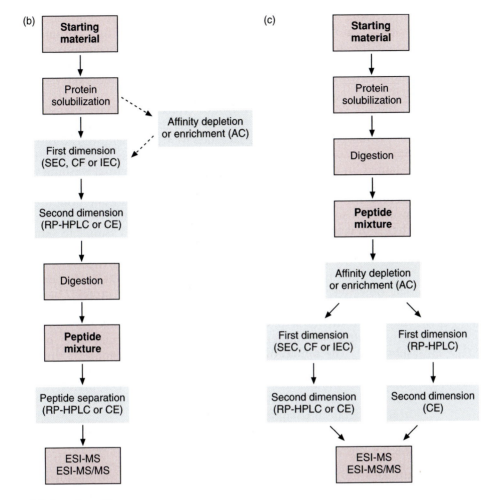

Figure 2.9 (continued)

Multidimensional liquid chromatography can be used instead of 2DGE for the separation of proteins and peptides. (b) Chromatography steps with different separative principles may be used as a direct replacement for 2DGE for the separation of proteins, with or without a prior affinity depletion or enrichment step. On-column digestion with trypsin is followed by a further round of RP-HPLC to feed individual peptide fractions into the mass spectrometer. (c) Multidimensional liquid-phase separations can also be applied directly to complex peptide mixtures. This strategy almost always involves an affinity depletion or enrichment step because of the very complex nature of the peptide mixture. Favored approaches include AC-SEC-RPHPLC-MS, AC-IEC-RPHPLC-MS and AC-RPHPLC-CE-MS. The analysis of proteins and peptides by mass spectrometry is discussed in Chapter 3.

2.5.2 Affinity chromatography

Affinity chromatography partitions proteins or peptides on the basis of their specific, ligand-binding affinity. The matrix on an affinity column contains ligands that are highly selective for particular proteins or classes of proteins. Beads containing antibodies, for example, can be used to isolate a single protein or peptide from a complex mixture, while beads coated with glutathione can be used to capture fusion proteins containing glutathione-*S*-transferase (GST) affinity tags. Similarly, immobilized metal-affinity chromatography (IMAC) is a form of affinity chromatography where the solid phase contains positively charged metal ions such as Fe^{3+} or Ga^{3+}. This can be used to selectively isolate phosphoproteins/peptides, proteins with oligo-histidine affinity tags and other negatively charged proteins.

Affinity chromatography methods typically involve a two-step elution procedure in which the first fraction emerging from the column comprises all the proteins or peptides that failed to interact with the affinity matrix, and the second fraction comprises all the proteins or peptides that were retained on the column. This is achieved by sequential washing with two solutions, the first of which flushes out all the unbound proteins and the second of which causes the bound proteins to dissociate from the affinity matrix. In some cases, it is the first fraction that is required, e.g. where their aim is to remove an abundant protein from a sample to simplify the analysis of the remaining proteins (affinity depletion). In most cases, however, the aim is to isolate the second fraction, which contains the proteins that bind selectively to the affinity matrix (affinity purification). The objective may be to isolate a single, specific protein, or to isolate fusion proteins bearing a particular affinity tag. Alternatively, the target may be a structural or functional class of proteins (e.g. phosphoproteins/peptides, or proteins that bind to a particular drug or enzyme substrate). The application of affinity chromatography to the study of phosphoproteins and other post-translational variants is discussed in Chapter 8. Another major application of affinity chromatography is the isolation of proteins that interact to form a complex, a subject discussed in more detail in Chapter 7.

2.5.3 Ion exchange chromatography

Unlike affinity chromatography, the other forms of chromatography used in proteomics are nonselective for particular classes of proteins, i.e. they are used to profile the sample rather than target individual components. Ion exchange chromatography (IEX, IEC) separates proteins or peptides according to their charge. It is based on the reversible adsorption of solute molecules to a solid phase that contains charged chemical groups. Cationic or anionic resins may be used (*Table 2.1*) and these attract molecules of opposite charge in the solvent. Instead of a two-step elution procedure, gradient elution is achieved by washing the column with

Table 2.1 Functional groups used on ion exchangers.

Anion exchangers	Functional group
Diethylaminoethyl (DEAE)	$-O-CH_2-CH_2-N^+H(CH_2CH_3)_2$
Quaternary aminoethyl (QAE)	$-O-CH_2-CH_2-N^+(C_2H_5)_2-CH_2CHOH-CH_3$
Quaternary ammonium (Q)	$-O-CH_2-CHOH-CH_2-O-CH_2-CHOH-CH_2-N^+(CH_3)_3$

Cation exchangers	Functional group
Carboxymethyl (CM)	$-O-CH_2-COO^-$
Sulfopropyl (SP)	$-O-CH_2-CHOH-CH_2-O-CH_2-CH_2-CH_2SO_3^-$
Methylsulfonate (S)	$-O-CH_2-CHOH-CH_2-O-CH_2-CHOH-CH_2SO_3^-$

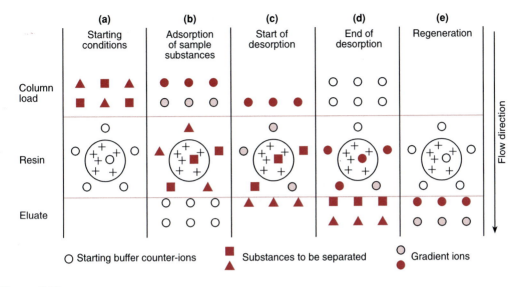

Figure 2.10

The principle of ion exchange chromatography. (a) Initially, the ion exchange resin is bound by simple counter-ions (ions with opposite charge to the resin) present in the equilibration buffer. (b) When the sample is added to the column, molecules in the sample with opposite charge to the resin displace the equilibration buffer ions and absorb to the column. (c) The first elution buffer displaces those components of the sample that are bound most weakly. (d) As the ionic strength of the elution buffer increases (or as the pH changes), more strongly associated solute ions are displaced. (e) After all solute ions have been displaced, the column is regenerated with equilibration buffer.

buffers of gradually increasing ionic strength or pH (*Figure 2.10*). The output of such a procedure is a chromatogram, where the *x*-axis displays elution time and the *y*-axis shows absorption peaks that correspond to individual components of the sample (*Figure 2.11*). The resolution of a chromatographic separation is expressed as the peak capacity, i.e. the number of peaks that can be resolved from the baseline over the full elution spectrum. The number of peaks on the chromatogram reveals the complexity of the sample, while quantitative data may be obtained by comparing peak areas.

A similar technique, chromatofocusing (CF), involves the use of an ion exchange column adjusted to one pH with a buffer adjusted to a second pH. This generates a pH gradient along the column, which can be used to elute proteins in order of their isoelectric points. Focusing effects taking place during the procedure produce sharp peaks and help to concentrate individual fractions.

2.5.4 Reversed-phase chromatography

Like ion exchange chromatography, reversed-phase (RP) chromatography involves the reversible adsorption of proteins or peptides to the stationary phase matrix, and multiple fractions are produced by gradient elution. In this case, however, the proteins and peptides are separated according

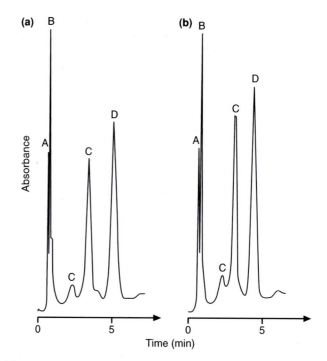

Figure 2.11

Chromatograms showing the results of separations of protein mixtures by ion exchange chromatography. The lettered peaks correspond to different proteins (A = ovalbumin, B = conalbumin, C = cytochrome c, D = lysozyme). The first separation (a) was performed at pH 5.85, while the second (b) was performed at pH 6.5. It is evident that operation conditions such as pH and temperature have a significant effect on the output. Courtesy of Rebecca Carrier and Julie Bordonaro, Rensselaer Polytechnic Institute.

to their hydrophobicity, and the reversed-phase resin consists of hydrophobic ligands, such as C_4 to C_{18} alkyl groups (*Figure 2.12*). In proteomics, reversed phase separations usually are carried out using high performance liquid chromatography (RP-HPLC) in which the mobile

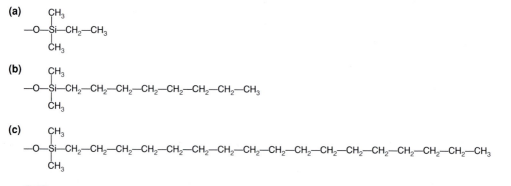

Figure 2.12

Some commonly used n-alkyl hydrocarbon ligands on reversed-phase resins. (a) Two-carbon capping group; (b) octyl (C_8) ligand; (c) octadecyl (C_{18}) ligand.

phase is forced through the column under high pressure. Although the separative principle is hydrophobicity, RP-HPLC results in a quasi-mass-dependent separation because retention tends to increase with molecular mass. Gradient elution is achieved by gradually increasing the amount of an organic modifier in the elution buffer, which disrupts the weakest hydrophobic interactions first (*Figure 2.13*). Of all the chromatography techniques used in proteomics, RP-HPLC is the most powerful method and has the highest resolution (a peak capacity of up to 100 components in practice). It is widely used for the separation of peptides following tryptic digestion and HPLC columns are often linked directly to electrospray ionization mass spectrometers to facilitate fully automatic peptide separation and analysis by LC-MS or LC-MS/MS (Chapter 3). Hydrophobic interaction chromatography is a similar technique, which also separates proteins on the basis of their hydrophobic properties, although using different resin compositions (C_2–C_8 alkyl groups, or aryl ligands) and more polar elution buffers. Similarly, hydrophilic interaction chromatography uses a polar solid phase to separate proteins on the basis of their hydrophilic properties.

2.5.5 Size exclusion chromatography

Size exclusion chromatography (also known as gel filtration chromatography) is a profiling technique used to separate proteins according to their size. The column is packed with inert beads made of a porous compound such as agarose. Small proteins can enter the pores in the beads and so they take longer to find their way through the column than larger

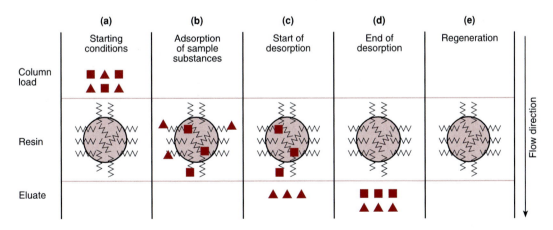

Figure 2.13

The principle of reversed-phase chromatography. (a) Initially, the reversed-phase resin is unoccupied. (b) When the sample is added to the column, most of the molecules in the sample bind to the resin because of the nature of the sample loading buffer. (c) The first elution buffer displaces those components of the sample that are bound most weakly to the hydrophobic resin. (d) As the level of organic modifier (e.g. acetonitrile) in the elution buffer increases, more strongly associated solute molecules are displaced. (e) After all the sample molecules have been displaced, the column is regenerated.

proteins, which do not fit in the pores and find a quicker path by moving through the gaps between beads. This separative principle is known as molecular exclusion and does not require any chemical interaction between the solutes and the stationary phase. Commercial preparations of size exclusion chromatography beads, e.g. Sepharose, have different-sized pores suitable for the optimal separation of protein or peptide mixtures over different size ranges.

2.6 Multidimensional liquid chromatography

2.6.1 Comparison of multidimensional liquid chromatography and 2DGE

As discussed above, liquid chromatography is often used either upstream or downstream of 2DGE to prefractionate samples and to separate tryptic peptides prepared from individual gel spots. However, the flexibility of LC methods in terms of combining different separative principles makes multidimensional chromatography an attractive technology to replace 2DGE all together. Many of the limitations of 2DGE are circumvented by LC systems. For example, the HPLC columns allow the loading of large sample volumes, which can be concentrated on the column making low-abundance proteins easier to detect. Many of the proteins that are difficult to analyze by 2DGE (e.g. membrane proteins, very basic proteins) can be separated easily using appropriate resins. Proteins separated in the liquid phase do not need to be stained in order to be detected. Perhaps most importantly, the fact that LC methods can separate peptides as well as proteins and the ability to couple LC columns directly to the mass spectrometer means that the entire analytical process from sample preparation to peptide mass profiling can be automated.

The disadvantages of LC methods are that the visual aspects of protein separation by 2DGE are lost, including the pI and molecular mass data that can be determined from the positions of spots on the gel (these data can be used in database searches). LC is also a serial analysis technique, while multiple gels containing related samples can be run at the same time. However, direct quantitative comparisons between samples can be carried out by labeling one of the samples with mass-coded tags, which can be identified in the mass spectrometer. These methods are described more fully in Chapter 4, and with respect to post-translational modifications, in Chapter 8.

2.6.2 Strategies for multidimensional liquid chromatography in proteomics

The sequential application of different chromatographic techniques exploiting different physical or chemical separative principles can provide sufficient resolution for the analysis of very complex protein or peptide mixtures. For example, the sequential use of ion-exchange chromatography (which separates proteins by charge) and RP-HPLC (which separates proteins approximately in a mass-dependent fashion) can achieve the same resolution as 2DGE, with added advantages of automation, increased sensitivity and better representation of membrane proteins. However, it is necessary to consider the practical limitations of such multidimensional chromatography techniques. The first issue to address is the compatibility of the buffers and solvents used in different steps of each procedure. In the example discussed above, the elution buffer used in the first-dimension ion exchange step would have to be a suitable solvent for RP-HPLC, and the elution buffer for the second-dimension RP-HPLC step would need to be compatible with the solvents used in the sample preparation stage for mass spectrometry. Otherwise, many of the advantages of speed, resolution and automation would be lost as the fractions were taken off-line to be cleaned up and prepared.

Fortunately, the solvents and buffers described above are indeed compatible, and ion exchange followed by RP-HPLC-MS has been used by several investigators to analyze the proteomes of organisms ranging from yeast to humans. The compatibility of RP-HPLC with the solvents used in MALDI-MS and ESI-MS (Chapter 3) means that HPLC is almost universally used as the final separation method in multidimensional chromatography (capillary electrophoresis can be used instead; see *Box 2.1*). All of the other profiling methods (size exclusion chromatography, ion exchange chromatography and chromatofocusing) have been used as a first-dimension separation method in combination with HPLC, sometimes with a prior affinity chromatography step resulting in a tri-dimensional separation strategy.

Initially, multidimensional chromatography was achieved by a discontinuous process in which fractions were collected from the ion exchange or gel filtration column and then manually injected into the HPLC column (Gygi *et al.*, Further Reading; *Figure 2.14*). Although labor intensive, the advantage of a discontinuous multidimensional system is the absence of time constraints. The fractions eluting from the first column can be stored off-line indefinitely, and fed one-by-one into the HPLC column, which is directly coupled to the mass spectrometer. A further advantage is that large sample volumes can be applied to the first column in order to obtain sufficient amounts of low-abundance proteins for analysis in the second dimension.

The need for manual sample injection can be circumvented by equipping the first column with an automatic fraction collection system and a column-switching valve. Fractions are then collected from the first column across the elution range, and the switching valve can bring the RP-HPLC column in line to receive the fractions sequentially. Alternatively, some researchers have developed apparatus comprising a single ion exchange system coupled, via an appropriate set of switching valves, to multiple HPLC columns arranged in parallel (*Figure 2.15*). In this scheme, fractions emerging from the ion exchange system are directed sequentially to the multiple HPLC columns, and the cycle is repeated when the first column has been regenerated (see Opitek *et al.*, Further Reading).

A third strategy for multidimensional chromatography separations is the use of biphasic columns, in which the distal part of the column is filled with reversed-phase resin and the proximal part with another type of matrix. As long as the elution solvents for each type of resin do not interfere with each other, this allows the stepped elution of fractions from the first resin and the gradient elution of second dimension fractions from the second. This technique was pioneered by Link and colleagues (see Further Reading) as *direct analysis of large protein complexes* (DALPC) and was modified by Yates and colleagues into a system called *multidimensional*

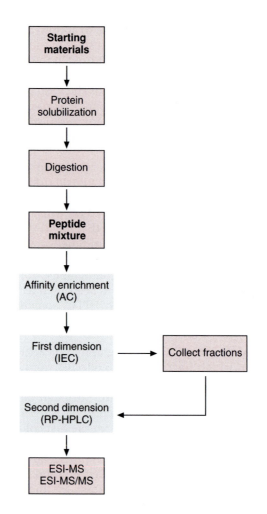

Figure 2.14

Discontinuous multidimensional chromatography for peptide separation, following the example of Gygi *et al.* (see Further Reading). In this experiment, proteins from two different yeast samples were labeled with mass-coded biotin affinity tags that reacted specifically with cysteine residues (this labeling strategy is not shown in detail; it is used for comparative protein quantitation between samples and further details can be found in Chapter 4, p. 79). The proteins from each sample were digested with trypsin and mixed together to produce a single peptide pool. Affinity chromatography was then used to select peptides carrying the affinity tag, reducing the complexity of the mixture about tenfold. However, since most proteins contain at least one cysteine residue, the remaining population of peptides still provided coverage of about 90% of the yeast proteome. The recovered peptides were separated by ion exchange chromatography using a strong cation exchange resin. Thirty individual samples were collected off-line, and four of these were subjected to second-dimension separation by RP-HPLC.

protein identification technology (MudPIT) (see Washburn *et al.*, Further Reading). As shown in *Figure 2.16*, peptide mixtures loaded onto the ion exchange resin are eluted using a stepped gradient of salt, resulting in the release of first-dimension fractions into the reversed-phase resin.

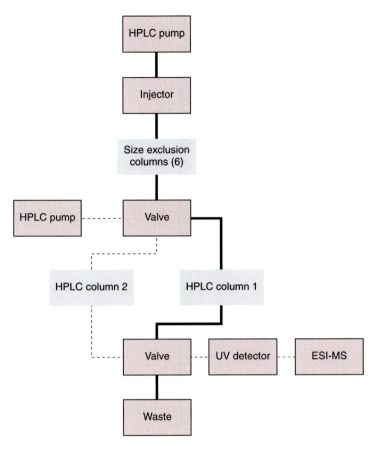

Figure 2.15

Continuous multidimensional chromatography with column-switching. In this example, simplified from Opiteck *et al.* (see Further Reading) two HPLC columns working in parallel receive alternating eluates from a bank of six size exclusion columns in series. After sample injection and separation by size exclusion chromatography, eluate from the size exclusion columns is directed to HPLC column 1 using a four-port valve (thick line). While the peptides are trapped in this column, HPLC column 2 is eluted and the sample is directed to the detector and fraction collector (broken line). After flushing and equilibrating column 2, the valves are reversed allowing column 2 to be loaded with the next fraction from the size exclusion separation, while column 1 is eluted. This cycle continues until the fractions from the size-exclusion separation are exhausted.

Second-dimension fractions are then eluted from the reversed-phase resin into the mass spectrometer using a gradient of acetonitrile. This process, and the subsequent regeneration step, does not interfere with the ion exchange chromatography step, and after regeneration another fraction is released from the ion exchange resin by increasing the salt concentration. When this method was applied to the yeast proteome, over 5000 peptides could be assigned to a total of 1484 yeast proteins, representing about one-quarter of the yeast proteome. The sample appeared to be representative of all classes of proteins, including those usually under-represented in 2DGE experiments.

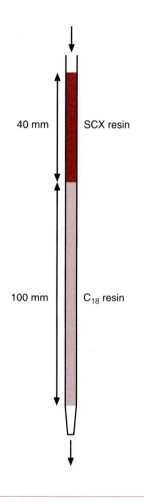

40 mm   SCX resin

100 mm   C$_{18}$ resin

Figure 2.16

Continuous multidimensional chromatography using a biphasic column. In this example, simplified from the MudPIT method developed by Yates and colleagues (see Washburn *et al.*, Further Reading) a 140 mm × 0.1 mm fused silica capillary is packed at the distal end with 5-μm C$_{18}$ (reversed phase) particles and at the proximal end with 5-μm strong cation exchange (SCX) particles. After introduction of the sample (top arrow) fractions are eluted from the SCX resin with a stepped salt gradient. After each salt step elution, the ion exchange fraction flows into the reversed phase material and is eluted using a gradient of acetonitrile (bottom arrow). Reversed phase elution and re-equilibration does not affect the SCX resin. This cycle is repeated until the SCX resin is exhausted.

While it is arguable whether multidimensional chromatography will ever displace 2DGE as the principal separations technology platform in proteomics, it is clear that it is a useful technique both alone and in combination with electrophoresis for protein and peptide separation. The combined advantages of sensitivity, representation, resolution and perhaps most importantly the potential to automate LC-MS and LC-MS/MS procedures may offset the disadvantages of losing the visual data provided by 2DGE. The use of mass spectrometry to identify proteins separated by 2DGE and/or LC methods is discussed in the next chapter.

Further reading

Gorg, A., Obermaier, C., Boguth, G., et al. (2000) The current state of two-dimensional electrophoresis with immobilized pH gradients. *Electrophoresis* **21**: 1037–1053.

Gygi, S.P., Rist, B., Gerber, S.A., Turecek, F., Gelb, M.H. and Aebersold, R. (1999) Quantitative analysis of complex protein mixtures using isotope-coded affinity tags. *Nature Biotechnol* **17**: 994–999.

Hames, B.D. and Rickwood, D. (1990) *Gel Electrophoresis of Proteins: A Practical Approach*. IRC Press, Oxford.

Herbert, B.R., Harry, J.L., Packer, N.H. et al. (2001) What place for poly-acrylamide in proteomics? *Trends Biotechnol* **19**: S3–S9.

Lecchi, P., Gupte, A.R., Perez, R.E., Stockert, L.V. and Abramson, F.P. (2003) Size-exclusion chromatography in multidimensional separation schemes for proteome analysis. *J Biochem Biophys Methods* **56**: 141–152.

Lee, W.C. and Lee, K.H. (2004) Applications of affinity chromatography in proteomics. *Anal Biochem* **324**: 1–10.

Lesney, M.S. (2001) Pathways to the proteome: from 2DE to HPLC. *Modern Drug Discovery* pp. 33–39.

Lilley, K.S., Razzaq, A. and Dupree, P. (2001) Two-dimensional gel electrophoresis: recent advances in sample preparation, detection and quantitation. *Curr Opin Chem Biol* **6**: 46–50.

Link, A.J. (2002) Multidimensional peptide separations in proteomics. *Trends Biotechnol* **20**: S8–S13.

Nägele, E., Vollmer, M., Hörth, P. and Vad, C. (2004) 2D-LC/MS techniques for the identification of proteins in highly complex mixtures. *Expert Rev. Proteomics* **1**: 37–46.

O'Farrell, P.H. (1975) High-resolution two-dimensional electrophoresis of proteins. *J Biol Chem* **250**: 4007–4021.

Opiteck, G.J., Ramirez, S.M., Jorgenson, J.W. and Moseley, M.A (1998) Comprehensive two-dimensional high-performance liquid chromatography for the isolation of overexpressed proteins and proteome mapping. *Anal Biochem* **258**: 349–361.

Rabilloud, T. (2002) Two-dimensional gel electrophoresis in proteomics: old, old fashioned, but still it climbs up the mountains. *Proteomics* **2**: 3–10.

Wang, H. and Hanash, S. (2003) Multi-dimensional liquid phase-based separations in proteomics. *J Chromatog B* **787**: 11–18.

Washburn, M., Wolters, D. and Yates, J. (2001) Large-scale analysis of the yeast proteome by multidimensional protein identification technology. *Nature Biotechnol* **19**: 242–247.

Wehr, T. (2002) Multidimensional liquid chromatography in proteomic studies. *LCGC* **20**: 954–962.

Internet resources

SWISS-2DPAGE, Two-dimensional polyacrylamide gel electrophoresis database.
http://us.expasy.org/ch2d/
WORLD-2DPAGE, Index to 2-D PAGE databases and services.
http://us.expasy.org/ch2d/2d-index.html
Useful overviews and resources for electrophoresis, chromatography and other separation methods
http://www.rpi.edu/dept/chem-eng/Biotech-Environ/CHROMO/chromintro.html
http://www.accessexcellence.org/LC/SS/chromatography_background.html
http://ntri.tamuk.edu/hplc/hplc.html
http://elchem.kaist.ac.kr/vt/chem-ed/scidex.htm
http://www.aber.ac.uk/parasitology/Proteome/Tut_2D.html

Strategies for protein identification

3

3.1   Introduction

The techniques described in Chapter 2 allow protein mixtures to be separated into their components but do not allow those components to be identified. Indeed, the individual fractions produced by such methods are almost always anonymous. Each spot on a 2D-gel and each fraction emerging from an HPLC column looks very much like any other. In the case of 2DGE, even differences in spot size and distribution provide only vague clues about protein identity, i.e. apparent molecular mass and pI. The next stage in proteomic analysis is therefore to characterize the fractions and thus determine which proteins are actually present.

In some cases, the aim is simply to catalog as many proteins as possible in the sample and produce a comprehensive proteome map. First-generation proteome maps have been assembled for some microbes since these organisms have relatively small proteomes. However, proteomic technology is not yet advanced enough to allow the systematic identification of every single protein in the cell. Problems of sensitivity, resolution and representation, and the sheer amount of work involved, make this an unrealistic, although no less desirable, goal.

More commonly, a small number of proteins is selected for careful analysis and identification, especially if those proteins are abundant in one sample but not in another. Alternatively, it may be desirable to investigate proteins that have undergone particular forms of post-translational modification, or to study proteins that interact with each other in complexes. We discuss these matters in later chapters, but first we must consider the basic problem of how to identify and characterize proteins in the first place. Although several technologies have been developed for protein identification on a small scale, there is no doubt that contemporary proteomic analysis would be impossible without recent advances in mass spectrometry, which allow hundreds or even thousands of samples to be processed and characterized in a single day.

3.2   Protein identification with antibodies

Proteins can often be characterized using probes – typically antibodies – that recognize structural features known as epitopes. Some epitopes may be entirely unique, therefore allowing unambiguous protein identification, while others are representative of particular classes of proteins, e.g. phosphoproteins or glycoproteins. Protein analysis techniques based on recognition by antibodies are many and varied, including affinity chromatography (Chapter 2), immunoblotting and enzyme-linked immunoassays (Chapter 4), co-immunoprecipitation (Chapter 7) and the development of antibody arrays (Chapter 9). Antibodies are very powerful for the isolation and identification of individual proteins but they are difficult to use on a proteomic scale. The first limitation is the fact that different antibodies are required to identify each protein. For example, a panel of antibodies could be used to identify all the different proteins in the proteome but this would require as many antibodies as there were target proteins, including specific antibodies for different post-translational variants of the same protein. This is difficult to achieve even for the simplest cellular proteomes, and in any case could only be applied to those organisms with complete genome sequences and/or abundant cDNA sequence resources (such resources would be necessary to express proteins systematically for antibody production).

Even if these difficulties could be overcome, a further problem arises in that thousands of different assays would need to be carried out in parallel to detect all the components of the proteome. This very principle is being explored with the development of analytical protein chips containing arrays of antibodies and similar capture agents. Thus far, however, antibody chips typically contain fewer than 100 different antibodies, and even these have demonstrated considerable problems in terms of sensitivity and specificity. This reflects the fact that proteins differ considerably in their chemical and physical properties, making it difficult to establish a set of conditions under which all antibodies would bind to their targets. The development and use of protein chips is discussed in Chapter 9.

For the reasons stated above, current methods for high-throughput protein identification cannot be based on the parallel use of specific detection reagents. Instead, annotation is achieved by the determination of protein *sequences* using reagents that can be applied to all proteins regardless of their structure or physical and chemical properties.

3.3 Determining protein sequences by chemical degradation

3.3.1 Complete hydrolysis

Proteins can be completely broken down into their constituent amino acids by boiling in highly concentrated hydrochloric acid for 24–72 hours. The amino acids can then be labeled with an agent such as ninhydrin (*Figure 3.1*) or fluorescamine (*Figure 3.2*), separated by HPLC (Chapter 2) and detected as they elute from the column using a panel of standard amino acids as a reference. The sensitivity of fluorescamine labeling is such that as little as 1 ng of an amino acid can be detected, allowing the analysis of very small quantities of purified protein. The acidic and polar amino acids are eluted first (i.e. Asp, Thr, Ser and Glu) while the basic amino acids are eluted last (i.e. Lys, His and Arg). In each case, the height of the absorption peak is proportional to the number of times that particular amino acid occurs in the protein.

While this method shows the amino acid composition of a protein, it does not reveal the sequence because all the peptide bonds in the protein are broken. There are algorithms such as AACompIdent, which attempt to predict protein sequences on the basis of amino acid compositions by searching protein sequence databases for entries that would give a similar composition profile. Such correlative search methods are only useful where there are significant existing sequence data, so they have been most

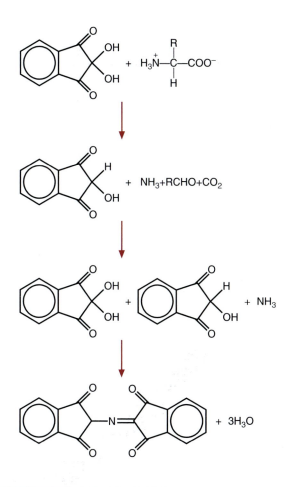

Figure 3.1

Chemical structure of ninhydrin, which reacts with the primary amine groups of amino acids as shown.

widely used in the microbial proteome projects. As we shall see below, protein identification by mass spectrometry is another approach that involves correlative searching but it can also determine protein sequences *de novo* (without reference to known sequences). Complete hydrolysis experiments do not allow *de novo* sequencing, but further evidence for

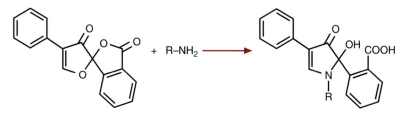

Figure 3.2

Chemical structure of fluorescamine, which reacts with the primary amine groups of amino acids as shown.

protein identification can be obtained by taking into account properties such as apparent molecular mass and pI, or by derivatizing the N-terminal and C-terminal amino acids allowing the first and last residues to be identified positively. For example, the N-terminal amino acid can be modified by dansyl chloride or 9-fluorenylmethyl chloroformate, resulting in a predictable shift in the position of the corresponding fraction. Even with terminal residue identification, however, it may be very difficult to identify the protein with confidence. Annotations are much more reliable if at least some sections of contiguous sequence can be determined directly, and this is a prerequisite for the *de novo* sequencing of proteins.

3.3.2   Protein sequencing by Edman degradation

In order to sequence a protein chemically, a method is required to remove amino acids selectively and progressively from one end of the molecule by breaking only the terminal peptide bond. Each amino acid can then be identified by HPLC as discussed above. There are several methods for sequencing proteins from either the N-terminal or C-terminal ends using broad-specificity exopeptidases, but the most widely used method is Edman degradation, which was developed and automated by Pehr Edman between 1960 and 1967. Edman degradation involves labeling the N-terminal amino acid of a protein or peptide with phenyl isothiocyanate (*Figure 3.3*). Mild acid hydrolysis then results in the cleavage of the peptide bond immediately adjacent to this modified residue, but leaves the rest of the protein intact. The terminal amino acid (or rather its phenylhydrodantoin derivative) can then be identified by chromatography, and the procedure is repeated on the next residue and the next, thus building up a longer sequence (*Figure 3.4*).

With automation, Edman degradation can sequence a small peptide (ten residues) in about 24 hours and a larger peptide (30–40 residues) in 3 days. It is not suitable for sequencing proteins larger than 50 residues in a single run because each cycle of degradation is less than 100% efficient. This means that after a large number of cycles there is a mixed population of molecules in the analyte rather than a pure sample, so single rounds of Edman degradation produce multiple peaks. The problem is addressed by cleaving large proteins into peptides, using either chemical reagents or specific endoproteases. For example, trypsin is an endoprotease that cleaves specifically at the C-terminal side of the basic amino acid residues lysine and arginine as long as the next residue is not proline. Since both lysine and arginine are common amino acids, a protein of ~500 residues might contain 20–50 sites and would be broken into an equivalent number of peptides each less than 25 residues in length. The determination of these individual sequences would allow the entire sequence of the protein to be built up as a series of fragments. However, without further

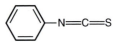

Figure 3.3

The chemical structure of phenyl isothiocyanate.

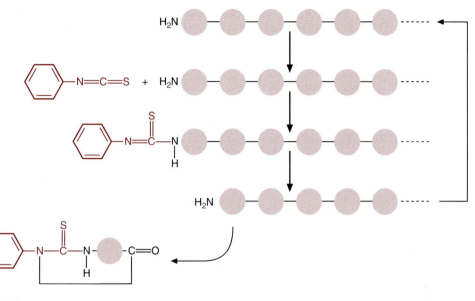

Figure 3.4

Edman degradation. The N-terminal amino acid of a peptide is derivatized with phenyl isothiocyanate (shown in red). Then, under acidic conditions, the adjacent peptide bond is cleaved and the terminal amino acid is released as a cyclic derivative that can be identified by HPLC. The peptide is now one residue shorter and the cycle begins again.

information there is no way to assemble the fragments in the correct order. This information can be obtained in two ways:

- Overlapping fragments can be sequenced following digestion of the protein with a reagent with different specificity to trypsin (*Figure 3.5*). It is important to choose a reagent that cuts frequently because a reagent with a very long and specific recognition site would not generate enough informative peptides (*Table 3.1*).

Digestion with trypsin	**Digestion with Glu-C (alkaline)**
Leu-Asp-Glu-Trp-Gly-Val-Ile-Lys	Trp-Gly-Val-Ile-Lys-Ala-Val-Ile-Leu-Ser-Glu
Ala-Val-Ile-Leu-Ser-Glu-Ile-Lys	Ile-Lys-His-Thr-Val-Glu
His-Thr-Val-Glu-Val-Arg	

Sequence deduced

Leu-Asp-Glu-Trp-Gly-Val-Ile-Lys|Ala-Val-Ile-Leu-Ser-Glu-Ile-Lys|His-Thr-Val-Glu-Val-Arg

Trp-Gly-Val-Ile-Lys-Ala-Val-Ile-Leu-Ser-Glu |Ile-Lys-His-Thr-Val-Glu

Figure 3.5

Protein sequences can be obtained by Edman sequencing of overlapping peptides generated with proteases of differing specificities.

Table 3.1 Cleavage of proteins into peptides using chemical and enzymatic reagents. The cleavage properties of all the endoproteases except Asp-N are dependent on the residue after the cleavage site not being proline

Reagent	Cleavage properties
Chemical agents	
70% formic acid	Asp-↓-Pro
Cyanogen bromide in 70% formic acid	Met-↓
2-nitro-5-thiocyanobenzoate, pH 9	↓-Cys
Hydroxylamine, pH 9	Asn-↓-Gly
Iodobenzoic acid in 50% acetic acid	Trp-↓
Endoproteases	
Trypsin	Arg/Lys-↓
Lys-C	Lys-↓
Arg-C	Arg-↓
Glu-C (bicarbonate)	Glu-↓
Glu-C (phosphate)	Asp/Glu-↓
Asp-N	↓-Asp
Chymotrypsin	Phe/Tyr/Trp/Leu/Met -↓ (also Ile/Val-↓)

• The solved amino acid sequences of the peptides can be used to design degenerate PCR primers, which can be used to isolate a corresponding genomic or cDNA sequence. This can then be translated to predict the full-length protein sequence.

3.3.3   Edman degradation in proteomics

In the mid 1980s, a technique was developed for the transfer of proteins separated by two-dimensional gel electrophoresis onto polyvinyldifluoride (PVDF) membranes. This provided a direct link between high-throughput protein separation techniques and emerging protein identification methods, since membrane-bound proteins could be digested with trypsin *in situ*, and the resulting peptides could be separated and analyzed by Edman degradation (*Figure 3.6*). Unfortunately, even with improved membranes and efficient digestion and processing methods, the technique was still laborious because of the length of time taken to complete a single Edman chemistry cycle. Furthermore, many proteins are blocked to Edman chemistry because the α-amino group of the N-terminal amino acid is modified and therefore does not react with phenyl isothiocyanate. Because of these intrinsic limitations, it was realized that proteins could never be sequenced on the same scale as DNA without a completely new approach. Towards the end of the 1980s, developments in mass spectrometry provided the necessary technological breakthrough. Despite the impact of mass spectrometry, Edman degradation remains the most convenient method for determining the N-terminal sequence of a protein. It is also extremely sensitive, in that robust sequences can routinely be obtained from as little as 0.5–1 pmol of pure protein, with some groups achieving sensitivities in the several hundred fmol range.

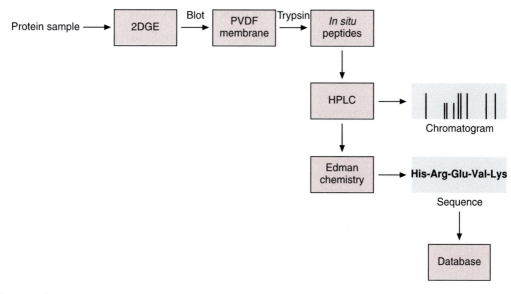

Figure 3.6

Early pipeline for protein identification using Edman degradation.

3.4 Mass spectrometry in proteomics – basic principles and instrumentation

3.4.1 Overview

A mass spectrometer is an instrument that can measure the mass/charge ratio (m/z) of ions in a vacuum. From these data, molecular masses can be determined with a high degree of accuracy, allowing the molecular composition of a given sample or analyte to be determined. In proteomics, the analyte is usually a collection of peptides derived from a protein sample by digestion with trypsin or a similar reagent. Two types of analysis can be carried out:

- *The analysis of intact peptide ions.* This allows the masses of intact peptides to be calculated, and these masses can be used to identify proteins in a sample by correlative database searching.
- *The analysis of fragmented ions.* This allows the masses of peptide fragments to be determined, which can be used in correlative database searching or to derive *de novo* sequences. In the latter case, the derived sequences can be used as standard queries in similarity search algorithms based on BLAST and FASTA (Chapter 5).

Mass spectrometers have three principal components: a source of ions, a mass analyzer and an ion detector. The function of the ionization source is to convert the analyte into gas phase ions in a vacuum. The ions are then accelerated in an electric field towards the analyzer, which separates them according to their m/z ratios on their way to the detector. The function of the detector is to record the impact of individual ions.

3.4.2 The importance of intact peptide ions

The analysis of proteins and other macromolecules by mass spectrometry has always been frustrated by the difficulty in producing intact gas phase ions. Generally, larger molecules are broken up by the volatization and ionization process, producing a collection of random fragments. While the fragments derived from a single peptide can be very informative, non-selective fragmentation of the 50 or so tryptic peptides that constitute a typical protein produces a mass spectrum that is far too difficult to interpret. This began to change in the 1990s with the development of so-called soft-ionization methods that achieve the ionization of peptides and other large molecules without significant fragmentation. Two such methods have been widely adopted in proteomics (*Figure 3.7*):

- *MALDI (matrix-assisted laser desorption/ionization)*. The analyte is mixed with a large excess of an aromatic 'matrix compound' that can absorb energy from the laser used with the mass spectrometer. For example, the matrix compound α-cyano-4-hydroxycinnamic acid can absorb the energy from a nitrogen UV laser (337 nm). The analyte and matrix are dissolved in an organic solvent and placed on a metallic probe or multiple-sample target. The solvent evaporates leaving matrix crystals in which the analyte is embedded. The target is placed in the vacuum chamber of the mass spectrometer and a high voltage is applied. At the same time, the crystals are targeted with a short laser pulse. The laser energy is absorbed by the crystals and emitted (desorbed) as heat, resulting in rapid sublimation that converts the analyte into gas phase ions. These accelerate away from the target through the analyzer towards the detector. MALDI is used predominantly for the analysis of simple peptide mixtures, such as the peptides derived from a single spot from a 2D-gel.
- *ESI (electrospray ionization)*. The analyte is dissolved and forced through a narrow needle held at a high voltage. A fine spray of charged droplets emerges from the needle and is directed into the vacuum chamber of

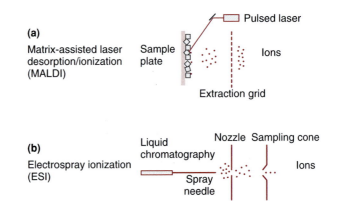

(a)

Matrix-assisted laser desorption/ionization (MALDI)

Sample plate

Pulsed laser

Ions

Extraction grid

(b)

Electrospray ionization (ESI)

Liquid chromatography

Nozzle Sampling cone

Spray needle

Ions

Figure 3.7

Soft ionization methods in proteomics. (a) MALDI involves heating crystals of analyte on a sample plate using laser pulses. (b) ESI involves forcing the sample through a narrow spray needle resulting in a fine spray of ions.

the mass spectrometer through a small orifice. As they enter the mass spectrometer, the droplets are dried using a stream of inert gas, resulting in gas-phase ions that are accelerated through the analyzer towards the detector. Because ESI produces gas-phase ions from solution, it is readily integrated with upstream protein separation by liquid-phase methods, particularly capillary electrophoresis and liquid chromatography (LC). Whereas MALDI-MS is used to analyze simple peptide mixtures, LC-ESI-MS is more suited to the analysis of complex samples.

3.4.3 Instrumentation

There are four basic types of mass analyzer used in proteomics, each with its own strengths and weaknesses in terms of accuracy, sensitivity and resolution. These can be used alone or in combination to generate different types of data. Conceptually the simplest instruments are the triple quadrupole (TQ) and time of flight (TOF) analyzers. The more sophisticated instruments are the ion trap and Fourier transform ion cyclotron resonance (FT-ICS) analyzers.

A quadrupole is a set of four parallel metal rods, opposite pairs of which are electrically connected so that a voltage can be applied across the space between them. Triple quadrupole mass spectrometers have three such devices arranged in series. Each quadrupole can be operated in RF-only mode (RF referring to radio frequency), which allows ions of any m/z ratio to pass through, or in scanning mode, where a potential difference is applied and the instrument acts as a mass filter. In the latter case, ions of a selected m/z ratio are allowed through to the detector whereas all others are deflected from their linear flight path and are eliminated from subsequent analysis. By varying the voltage over time, ions with different m/z ratios can be selectively allowed through to the detector and a mass spectrum of the analyte can be obtained.

Triple quadrupole (TQ) instruments can be set either for the analysis of intact peptides or their fragment ions (*Figure 3.8*). In the former case, the instrument is operated in standard MS mode where only one of the

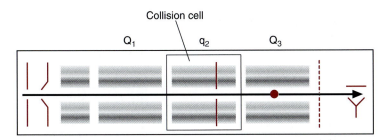

Collision cell

Q_1 q_2 Q_3

Figure 3.8

Layout of a triple quadrupole mass spectrometer, in which ions are selected by varying the electric fields between four rods. In this diagram, the mass spectrometer is running in product scan mode, where ions are selected in the first quadruple (Q1), q2 is used as a collision cell to induce fragmentation, and the resulting fragment ions are scanned in Q3.

quadrupoles is used for scanning, the others remaining in RF mode. In the latter case, the first quadrupole scans the ion stream and directs ions of a selected m/z ratio into the second quadrupole, which operates in RF-only mode and acts as a collision cell. That is, fragmentation of the intact peptide ions is induced by colliding them with a stream of inert gas such as argon, a process known as collision-induced dissociation (CID). The third quadrupole then scans the stream of ion fragments emerging from the collision cell to generate a CID spectrum, i.e. a mass spectrum of the fragments derived from one specific peptide. When the analysis is complete, the first quadrupole directs a different intact peptide ion into the collision cell and the fragmentation and analysis process is repeated. The use of two analyzers in series to separate intact ions and then their fragments is described as tandem mass spectrometry (MS/MS) or product ion scanning. Several other operational modes are also available in TQ instruments, including neutral loss scan mode and precursor ion scanning. These are often used to distinguish between phosphorylated and nonphosphorylated versions of the same protein and are discussed in Chapter 8.

Unlike quadrupole instruments, no electric field is required to separate ions in a time of flight (TOF) analyzer. Instead, this instrument exploits the fact that in any mixture of ions carrying the same charge, heavy ions will take longer to travel down a field-free flight tube than lighter ones (*Figure 3.9*). TOF analyzers have, until recently, been used almost exclusively with MALDI ion sources for the analysis of intact peptide ions (MALDI-TOF-MS). This is because the MALDI process tends to produce singly charged peptide ions, and under these conditions the time of flight of any ion is inversely proportional to the square root of its molecular mass. More recently, MALDI sources have been coupled to tandem TOF-TOF or hybrid quadrupole-TOF analyzers separated by a collision cell, allowing the analysis of CID spectra from MALDI-produced precursor ions with much higher sensitivity than is possible with the TQ and single TOF instruments. Today's MALDI instruments incorporating tandem TOF or hybrid analyzers are extremely sensitive and can be loaded with up to 384 samples simultaneously, for high-throughput analysis.

Fragment analysis can also be carried out in a standard MALDI-TOF instrument by exploiting a phenomenon known as post-source decay (PSD). This is achieved by increasing the laser power to about twice the level used to obtain a normal mass spectrum, resulting in multiple collisions between the peptides and the matrix compound during ionization.

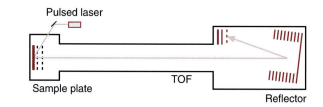

Figure 3.9

Layout of a MALDI-TOF mass spectrometer (reflector mode), in which ions are separated by virtue of the time taken to travel down a field-free flight tube to the detector.

This causes delayed fragmentation in a large proportion of the peptides and the fragmented ions can be separated from the intact peptides using ion gates and mirrors (reflectrons).

Both ESI and MALDI sources have also been coupled to ion trap analyzers, which consist of a chamber surrounded by a ring electrode and two end-cap electrodes (*Figure 3.10*). Unlike the quadrupole and TOF analyzers, which separate ions in space, the ion trap separates ions in time. The voltage applied to the ring electrode determines which ions remain in the trap. Ions above the threshold *m/z* ratio remain in the trap while others are ejected through small holes in the distal end-cap electrode. A mass spectrum of intact peptides can be obtained by gradually increasing the voltage in the ring electrode so that ions of progressively increasing *m/z* ratios are ejected over time. Alternatively, the trapped ions can be fragmented by injecting a stream of helium gas, and the resulting fragments can be ejected by ramping the voltage of the ring electrode to generate a CID spectrum. Multiple rounds of analysis can be carried out because one of the fragment ions from the first analysis can be retained in the trap and subject to further collision. Up to three rounds of fragmentation are routinely used, particularly for the analysis of glycoproteins, and in one experiment 12 rounds of fragmentation were reported.

The FT-ICR analyzer is the most complex and difficult to operate, but has by far the highest resolution, mass accuracy and sensitivity. The operating principle is that ions in a magnetic field will orbit at a frequency that is related to the ion's mass (*m*), charge (*z*) and the strength of the magnetic field (*B*). This is called the cyclotron frequency (f_c). The relationship can be described by the following equation:

$$m/z = B/2\pi f_c$$

Therefore, all ions with the same *m/z* value will orbit with the same cyclotron frequency in a uniform magnetic field, and this collection of ions is known as an ion packet.

Orbiting ions of a particular *m/z* value are then excited by an applied radio frequency field, which causes the cyclotron radius to expand. If the frequency of the applied field is the same as the cyclotron frequency of the ions, the ions absorb energy thus increasing their velocity (and the orbital radius) but keeping a constant cyclotron frequency. As the selected ions cycle between the two electrodes, electrons are attracted first to one plate and then the other, with the same frequency as the cycling ions (i.e. in resonance with the cyclotron frequency). This movement of electrons

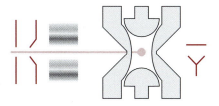

Figure 3.10

Layout of an ion-trap mass spectrometer, in which ions are constrained within a chamber surrounded by ring electrodes.

is detected as an image current on a detector. The image current is then converted, by Fourier transformation, into a series of component frequencies and amplitudes of the individual ions. Finally, the cyclotron frequency values are converted into *m/z* values to produce the mass spectrum. Of the four instruments, this has the greatest sensitivity, accuracy and also the broadest dynamic range but it is also the most expensive and the most complex in terms of operational requirements. Its use in proteomics has therefore been much more limited compared to the other instruments.

3.5 Protein identification using data from mass spectrometry

3.5.1 Peptide mapping (peptide mass fingerprinting)

Peptide mapping or peptide mass fingerprinting (PMF) refers to the identification of proteins using data from intact peptide masses (*Figure 3.11*). The principle of the technique is that each protein can be uniquely identified by the masses of its constituent peptides, this unique signature being known as the peptide mass fingerprint. Algorithms allowing database searching on the basis of peptide mass data were developed simultaneously by several groups in the early 1990s and have been implemented in a number of software packages, many of which are available over the Internet (*Table 3.2*). PMF involves the following steps:

- The sample of interest should comprise a single protein or a simple mixture, e.g. an individual spot from a 2D-gel or a single LC fraction.

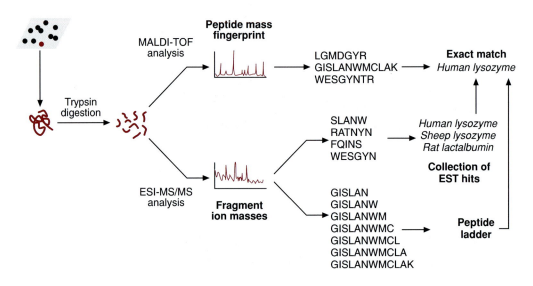

Figure 3.11

Protein identification by mass spectrometry. In a typical strategy, digested peptides are analyzed by MALDI-TOF MS in order to determine the masses of intact peptides. These masses can be used in correlative database searches to identify exact matches. If this approach fails, ESI-MS/MS analysis can be used to generate peptide fragment ions. These can be used to search less robust data sources (e.g. EST databases) and to produce *de novo* peptide sequences.

Table 3.2 Computer programs, most available over the Internet, that can be used to interpret or analyze MS data.

Program	Applications	Source	URL
CIDentify	Search	Immunex	http://www.immunex.com
Mascot	PMF, Tag, MS/MS	Matrix Science Ltd.	http://www.matrixscience.com
MassSearch	PMF	ETH	http://cbrg.inf.ethz.ch/Server/MassSearch.html
Mowse	PMF	Human Genome Mapping Project	http://www.hgmp.mrc.ac.uk/Bioinformatics/Webapp/mowse
MS BLAST	Search	EMBL	http://dove.embl-heidelberg.de/Blast2/msblast.html
MS-FIT	PMF	UCSF	http:/prospector.ucsf.edu
MS-Seq	Tag	UCSF	http:/prospector.ucsf.edu
MS-Tag	MS/MS	UCSF	http:/prospector.ucsf.edu
PepFrag	MS/MS	Rockefeller University	http://prowl.rockefeller.edu/PROWL/prowl.html
PepMAPPER	PMF	UMIST	http://wolf.bms.umist.ac.uk/mapper
PepSea	PMF, Tag	Protana	http://195.41.108.38/PepSeaIntro.html
PeptIdent	PMF	ExPASy	http://www.expasy.ch/tools/peptident.html
PeptideSearch	PMF,Tag	EMBL	http://www.narrador.embl-heidelberg.de/GroupPages/PageLink/peptidesearchpage.html
ProFound	PMF	Rockefeller University/Proteometrics	http://prowl.rockefeller.edu/PROWL/prowl.html
Sequest	MS/MS	Scripps Research Institute	http://fields.scripps.edu/sequest
Sonars MS/MS	MS/MS	Proteometrics	http://www.proteometrics.com
TagIdent	Tag	ExPASy	http://www.expasy.ch/tools/tagident.html

Under 'Applications' the following abbreviations indicate the programs can be used to search databases with peptide mass fingerprint data (PMF), to search data-bases with peptide tags from manually interpreted MS/MS data (Tag), or to search databases with uninterpreted MS/MS data (MS/MS). CIDentify and MS-BLAST are similarly seach algorithms based on FASTA and BLAST respectively which are specially adapted to use short peptides as the search query.

The sample is digested with a specific cleavage reagent, usually trypsin (*Table 3.1*).

- The masses of the peptides are determined, e.g. by MALDI-TOF-MS.
- The experimenter chooses one or more protein sequence databases to be used for correlative searching. Examples include the SWISS-PROT and TrEMBL protein databases (Chapter 1).
- The algorithm carries out a virtual digest of each protein in the sequence database using the same cleavage specificity as trypsin (or whichever other reagent has been used experimentally) and then calculates theoretical peptide masses for each protein.
- The algorithm attempts to correlate the theoretical peptide masses with the experimentally determined ones.
- Proteins in the database are ranked in order of best correlation, usually with a significance threshold based on a minimum number of peptides matched.

3.5.2 Advantages and limitations of peptide mass fingerprinting

The masses of intact peptides are extremely discriminatory, making the PMF technique very robust as a means of protein identification. However, because PMF relies on correlative searching, the likelihood of finding a matching protein depends on both the quality of the experimental data and the availability of sequence information for the organism from which the experimental sample was obtained. Data attributes that need to be considered for reliable protein identification include the quality and relative intensity of the peaks in the mass spectrum, the mass accuracy of the instrument, the coverage of the protein and possible interfering factors such as post-translational modifications and mis-cleavages (*Box 3.1*). These factors influence the likelihood that a match is genuine rather than spurious, a probability often expressed as a MOWSE score (from one of the original algorithms developed for PMF – MOlecular Weight SEarch). PMF is best suited to those organisms for which large amounts of genomic, cDNA and protein sequence data are available, and particularly for species with completed genome sequences.

Even in species with abundant sequence data, there are potential pitfalls in PMF analysis. Many protein sequences are modified after translation, e.g. by trimming or cleavage, or the removal of inteins (Chapter 8). Even if there is perfect correspondence between a cDNA sequence and a protein sequence, there remain many other reasons for the absence of a correlation between experimentally derived masses and those predicted from database entries (*Box 3.1*). Because protein identification by PMF depends entirely on the accurate correlation of determined and predicted masses, even small unanticipated differences in mass can prevent the detection of matching proteins. This is why PMF is carried out using peptides rather than whole proteins, since these provide greater scope for database correlation. For example, in the case of a protein that contains 50 tryptic peptides, matches between only two or three of these and a corresponding database entry might be sufficient to identify the protein.

The confidence attributed to PMF searching can also be increased by using so-called orthogonal datasets, e.g. data obtained from the digestion of the same protein with two different proteases (either separately or in combination), data obtained from the digestion of the same protein in a native

BOX 3.1

Peptide mass fingerprinting – possible causes of incorrect protein identification

There may be an error in the sequence database, causing the algorithm to generate an incorrect predicted mass for one or more peptides.

The mass spectrometer may not be functioning optimally, resulting in an inaccurate experimental mass determination. Calibration of the instrument is extremely important since small differences in mass tolerance can make a great deal of difference to the quality of the resulting matches. Many investigators use internal calibration standards in every sample, e.g. autolysis products (the peptides derived from trypsin when it is digested by other molecules of trypsin).

The protein might exist as two or more polymorphic variants, and the version stored in the sequence database might not be the same as the version found in the sample. For example, single nucleotide polymorphisms (SNPs) represent an abundant form of genetic variation that may contribute as many as 50 000 single amino acid differences in the human proteome.

Differences in mass may be caused by post-translational modifications occurring *in vivo*. Many of the algorithms used to correlate predicted and determined masses can build in anticipated mass changes brought about by known modifications such as phosphorylation. This is discussed in more detail in Chapter 8.

Differences in mass may be caused by non-specific modifications occurring during protein extraction, separation or processing. For example, many chemical modifications occur as a result of gel staining in 2DGE experiments (see *Box 4.1*). In some cases, it may be a good idea to carry out deliberate modifications. For example, the cysteine residues in denatured proteins may be modified universally with iodoacetamide to prevent sporadic modifications that could complicate the interpretation of mass spectra. The use of affinity mass tags for protein quantitation in mass spectrometry is also a form of deliberate modification and is discussed in Chapter 4.

There may have been nonspecific cleavage of the protein. Even highly specific cleavage reagents such as trypsin occasionally cut at nonspecific sites and ignore genuine sites. The presence of multiple adjacent or clustered lysine and arginine residues, for example, can prevent trypsin cleavage reactions reaching completion. However, while such ragged ends only complicate PMF analysis they can be useful in the interpretation of MS/MS spectra (see Section 3.5.3).

The presence of multiple proteins in the analyte may make the mass spectrum too difficult to interpret. In some cases, this can be due to external contamination. For example, it is easy for the laboratory staff to contaminate protein samples with minute amounts of keratin from shed hair and skin cells.

state and following some form of chemical modification or substitution, or partial sequence data from Edman degradation or PSD experiments.

3.5.3 Fragment ion analysis

Where peptide mass fingerprinting fails to identify any proteins matching those present in a given sample, the CID spectrum of one or more individual peptides may provide important additional information. The data can be used in two ways (*Figure 3.11*). First, the uninterpreted fragment ion masses can be used in correlative database searching to identify proteins whose peptides would likely yield similar CID spectra under the same fragmentation conditions. In probability-based matching, virtual CID spectra are derived from the peptides of all protein sequences in the database and these are compared with the observed data to derive a list of potential matches. In cross-correlation, it is the degree of overlap between the observed and predicted peaks that determines the best potential match. Several algorithms, such as Sequest (*Table 3.2*), are available for database searching with uninterpreted data. Second, the peaks of the mass spectrum can be interpreted, either manually or automatically, to derive partial *de novo* peptide sequences that can be used as standard database search queries. The advantage of both these approaches is that correlative searching is not limited to databases of full protein sequences. Both uninterpreted fragment ion masses and the short peptide sequences derived from interpreted spectra can be used to search through the less robust but much more abundant EST data. ESTs are expressed sequence tags, short sequence signatures derived by the random, single-pass sequencing of cDNA libraries. Millions of such sequences have been obtained and deposited in public databases, and when translated they represent a rich source of information about proteins. However, ESTs cannot be searched in peptide mass fingerprinting because that technique relies on the presence of sequences corresponding to several intact peptides. ESTs are generally too short (100–300 bp) to contain more than one intact peptide.

The interpretation of CID data is complex because fragmentation produces a diverse collection of thousands of different ions. The most informative fragments are those in which breakage has occurred along the polypeptide backbone, because these represent strings of contiguous and intact amino acids (*Figure 3.12*). If the charge remains on the N-terminal fragment, it is known as a *b*-series ion whereas if it remains on the C-terminal fragment, it is known as a *y*-series ion. There may also be multiple breakages producing internal fragments of several contiguous amino acids as well as immonium ions representing single amino acids. Interpretation generally involves the arrangement of *b*- or *y*-series ions in order of increasing mass. The differences in mass between consecutive ions in either series should correspond to the masses of individual amino acids (*Box 3.2*), and this can be used to derive a short sequence or peptide tag. Tags can also be derived from ragged termini generated adventitiously or by limited exopeptidase digestion, followed by MALDI-TOF-MS. Algorithms for database searching using peptide tags include MS-Seq and TagIdent (*Table 3.2*).

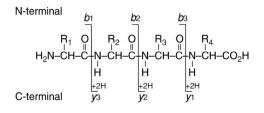

Figure 3.12

Fragment ion nomenclature for the most common positive N- and C-terminal ions.

3.5.4 Determining protein sequences *de novo* by mass spectrometry

While correlative search methods based on peptide mass fingerprints, peptide tags or uninterpreted CID spectra rely on sequence databases, it is also possible to use mass spectrometry for *de novo* sequence determination. This can be achieved by the complete interpretation of CID spectra, i.e. the arrangement of all *b*- or *y*-series ions to identify the amino acid differences at each step, or by the MALDI-TOF analysis of comprehensive peptide ladders generated by chemical or enzymatic degradation.

The complete interpretation of fragment ion spectra can be very difficult without some form of labeling to identify either the *b*- or *y*-series fragments. A useful approach is to divide the sample into two aliquots, attach a specific mass label to either the N- or C-terminus of the intact peptide in one of the aliquots, and then compare the mass spectra to identify the modified and unmodified forms. For example, methyl esterification of the C-terminus of a peptide adds 14 mass units. The comparison of mass spectra from treated and untreated samples therefore allows the *y*-series of ions to be identified by the specific mass displacement (*Figure 3.13a*). Unfortunately, this reaction also esterifies acidic side chains, so the analysis becomes more complex for peptides containing Asp and Glu residues. An alternative strategy is to carry out trypsin digestion in a buffer in which half the water contains a heavy isotope of oxygen (^{18}O). Trypsin incorporates an oxygen atom from water into the carboxyl group of the newly generated C-terminus of each peptide. Therefore, if the above buffer is used, each *y*-series fragment will be present as a mixture of two derivatives differing by two mass units, and will be represented on the mass

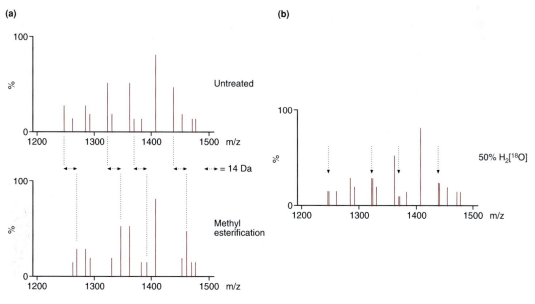

Figure 3.13

Identification of *b*-series ions in CID mass spectra. The mass spectra show characteristic mass shifts for (a) methyl esterification and (b) ^{18}O carboxyl group.

spectrum as a doublet (*Figure 3.13b*). A disadvantage of this approach is that the intensity of the signal for each *y*-series ion is also reduced by 50%. Derivatization of the tryptic peptide fragments can also improve the efficiency of fragmentation in MALDI PSD experiments, resulting in more sequence coverage. For example, Keough and colleagues (see Further Reading) describe how sulfonic acid-derivatized peptides fragmented more

BOX 3.2

Ladder sequencing by mass spectrometry

The *de novo* sequencing of peptides by mass spectrometry relies on the assembly of nested sets of N-terminal or C-terminal peptides (or peptide fragments) differing in length by a single residue. The differences in mass between consecutive members of a series can be compared with a standard table of amino acid residue masses to work out the sequence (*Table 3.3*). The residue mass table is shown below. Note that two pairs of residues – glutamine and lysine, leucine and isoleucine – have very similar or identical masses. In the case of glutamine and lysine there is a slight difference (128.13 and 128.17, respectively) which is very difficult to detect in fragment ion spectra but can be established quite easily when Edman chemistry is used because the side chain of lysine is modified. Other difficulties with CID spectra include the fact that two adjacent glycine residues (mass = 57) could be mistaken for a single asparagine residue (mass = 114) if the ion series was incomplete, whereas the complete ladder produced by conventional sequencing removes this ambiguity. Leucine and isoleucine have identical masses and can be distinguished only by inspection of the corresponding cDNA sequence.

Table 3.3   Residue and immonium ion masses of the 20 common amino acids[a]

Amino acid	Abbreviations – 3 letter (single letter)	Residue mass[b]	Immonium ion mass[b]
Alanine	Ala (A)	71	44
Asparagine	Asn (N)	114	87
Aspartate	Asp (D)	115	88
Arginine	Arg (R)	156	129, 112, 100, 87, 70, 43[c]
Cysteine	Cys (C)	103	76
Glutamine	Gin (Q)	128	101 (w/o 84)
Glutamate	Glu (E)	129	102
Glycine	Gly (G)	57	30
Histidine	His (H)	137	110
Isoleucine	Ile (I)	113	86
Leucine	Leu (L)	113	86
Lysine	Lys (K)	128	101, 84, 129[c]
Methionine	Met (M)	131	104
Phenylalanine	Phe (F)	147	120
Proline	Pro (P)	97	70 (w/o 112, 100 and 87)
Serine	Ser (S)	87	60
Threonine	Thr (T)	101	74
Tryptophan	Trp (W)	186	159
Tyrosine	Tyr (Y)	163	136
Valine	Val (V)	99	72

[a]The values were obtained from Jardine (1990 *Methods Enzymol*, **193**: 441–455).
[b]All masses are given as interger values and underlining indicates more abundant ions (Carr and Annan, 1997 *Current Protocols in Molecular Biology*, pp. 10.12.1–10.21.27); w/o = without.
[c]Arginine and lysine both exhibit multiple immonium ions, and these are listed.

extensively and up to 28 times more efficiently than the corresponding native peptides.

The alternative *de novo* sequencing approaches provide a good example of how Edman degradation and mass spectrometry can be used together to generate sequence information. Edman chemistry is used to derive a nested set of intact N-terminal peptides and these are then analyzed by MALDI-TOF-MS to identify mass differences corresponding to specific amino acids and therefore derive the sequence. Unlike MS/MS approaches, the Edman-based methods discriminate easily between the amino acids glutamine and lysine (*Box 3.2*). While Edman chemistry is limited to the generation of N-terminal peptides, both N-terminal and C-terminal peptide ladders can be produced by the limiting use of exopeptidases, with the resulting analyte again being subjected to MALDI-TOF-MS for sequencing.

Further reading

Aebersold, R. and Mann, M. (2003) Mass spectrometry-based proteomics. *Nature* **422**: 198–207.

Beavis, R.C. and Fenyo, D. (2000) Database searching with mass-spectrometric information. *Proteomics: A Trends Guide* **1**: 22–27.

Chakravarti, D.N., Chakravarti, B. and Moutsatsos, I. (2002) Informatic tools for proteome profiling. *Computational Proteomics* **32**: S4–S15.

Choudhary, J.S., Blackstock, W.P., Creasy, D.M. and Cottrell, J.S. (2001) Interrogating the human genome using uninterpreted mass spectrometry data. *Proteomics* **1**: 651–667.

Choudhary, J.S., Blackstock, W.P., Creasy, D.M. and Cottrell, J.S. (2001) Matching peptide mass spectra to EST and genomic DNA databases. *Trends Biotechnol* **19**: S17–S22.

Fenyo, D. (2000) Identifying the proteome: software tools. *Curr Opin Biotechnol* **11**: 391–395.

Griffen, T.J., Goodlet, D.R. and Aebersold, R. (2001) Advances in proteome analysis by mass spectrometry. *Curr Opin Biotechnol* **12**: 607–612.

Keough, T., Lacey, M.P. and Strife, R.J. (2001) Atmospheric pressure matrix-assisted laser desorption/ionization ion trap mass spectrometry of sulfonic acid derivatized tryptic peptides. *Rapid Commun Mass Spec* **15**: 2227–2239.

Mann, M. and Pandey, A. (2001) Use of mass spectrometry-derived data to annotate nucleotide and protein sequence databases. *Trends Biochem Sci* **26**: 54–61.

Mann, M., Hendrickson, R.C. and Pandey, A. (2001) Analysis of proteins and proteomes by mass spectrometry. *Annu Rev Biochem* **70**: 437–473.

Qian, W.-J., Camp, D.J. II and Smith, R.D. (2004) High-throughput proteomics using Fourier transform ion cyclotron resonance mass spectrometry. *Expert Rev. Proteomics* **1**: 87–95.

Internet resources

ExPasy proteomics tools, a selection of analysis tools and other resources for mass spectrometry http://us.expasy.org/tools/#proteome

Strategies for protein quantitation

4.1 Introduction

The objective in many proteomics experiments is to identify proteins whose abundance differs across two or more related samples. For example, the proteome varies according to cell type, developmental stage and the cell state (e.g. stage of the cell cycle) and also responds to changes in the environment. There are also proteomic changes associated with disease, e.g. a comparison of normal skin and squamous cell carcinoma might reveal a set of proteins unique to the disease. Once identified, these proteins could be useful as disease markers and might even represent potential new therapeutic targets. Unfortunately, there are very few proteins that show such unambiguous on/off changes. More often, the difference between samples is one of degree. Therefore, the accurate quantitation of proteins is a vital component of proteomics.

There are several well-established methods for the quantitation of individual proteins, either in solution or using a solid phase assay, which are based on the use of labeled antibodies (*Box 4.1*). The adaptation of such

---

BOX 4.1

Quantitation of individual proteins

Individual proteins can be quantitated using immunoassays in which specific antibodies are used as labeled probes. The western blot is a quick way to compare the abundances of gel-separated proteins. In this technique, proteins separated by gel electrophoresis, with different samples represented in different lanes, are blotted onto a sheet of polymeric material (usually nitrocellulose, nylon or polyvinylidenedifluoride) where they are immobilized. A general stain can be applied to reveal all the protein bands, e.g. Ponceau S, silver nitrate, India ink, colloidal gold or Amido black, but particular proteins are detected by flooding the sheet with a solution containing a specific antibody. The antibody may be conjugated to its own radioactive, fluorescent or enzymatic label or a secondary antibody may be used that recognizes the primary antibody and therefore amplifies the signal. This allows very small amounts of protein to be detected.

Very accurate quantitation of individual proteins in solution can be achieved using a solid phase immunoassay in which a capture antibody specific for the target protein is immobilized on a polymeric sheet or plastic dish. A drop of solution (e.g. serum, cell lysate, etc.) containing the target protein is added to the sheet and antigen–antibody complexes are allowed to form. The solution is washed away and the target protein is detected with a second antibody that recognizes a different epitope to the capture antibody. As with the western blot, this detection antibody may be labeled or it may be recognized in a further reaction with a secondary antibody. The most popular version of this technique is the enzyme-linked immunosorbent assay (ELISA) in which the detection antibody carries an enzyme that converts a colorless substrate into a colored compound, or a nonfluorescent substrate into a fluorescent compound.

assays for proteomic-scale analysis is difficult because even if antibodies could be found to bind to every protein in the proteome, the signal intensity for each antigen–antibody interaction would depend not only on the abundance of the target protein but also on the strength of the antigen–antibody binding (i.e. the affinity of the antibody). Despite these technical hurdles, some analytical protein chips have been manufactured that are arrayed with up to 100 antibodies, and these are described in Chapter 9. Generally, the most successful chips contain a small number of well-characterized antibodies. The more complex the chip, the greater the problems with sensitivity and specificity, and the less useful the resulting quantitative data.

At the current time, protein quantitation in proteomics relies primarily on the use of general labeling or staining, or on the selective labeling or staining of particular classes of proteins. There are various methods for measuring the total amount of protein in a solution (*Box 4.2*). However, what is required in proteomics is a selection of methods for comparing the abundances of thousands of proteins in parallel across multiple samples. The chosen strategy depends largely on how the protein samples are prepared and fractionated, and can be divided into two broad categories: those based on the image analysis of 2D-gels, and those based on differential labeling of samples for separation by liquid chromatography followed by mass spectrometry.

4.2   Quantitative proteomics with standard 2D gels

4.2.1   Image acquisition from 2D gels

The abundance of different proteins on a 2D-gel is determined by the shape, size and intensity of the corresponding spots. Therefore, protein quantitation requires the conversion of an analog gel image into digital

BOX 4.2

Measuring total protein concentrations in a solution

There are several methods for determining the total concentration of proteins in solution, each of which exploits properties that are general to all proteins. One widely used method is the measurement of UV absorbance. This is a nondestructive method, allowing the proteins to be recovered for further analysis. Therefore it is used not only for quantitation but also to detect protein and peptide fractions eluting from HPLC columns. The UV light is absorbed by aromatic amino acid residues (tyrosine and tryptophan) as well as by peptide bonds. It cannot be used in gels because polyacrylamide and proteins absorb UV light over the same range of wavelengths.

Other protein assay methods are colorimetric or fluorimetric and are based on covalent or noncovalent dye binding or chemical reactions. The Bradford assay measures the degree of binding to Coomassie brilliant blue dye, which changes color from brown to blue in the presence of proteins. Other protein-binding agents are fluorescent and more sensitive, e.g. OPA (o-phthaldialdehyde), fluorescamine and NanoOrange. The Lowry assay and the related BCA (bicinchoninic acid) assay each use the reduction of copper ions that occurs in the presence of proteins to chelate a colorless substrate and produce a colored complex that can be detected using a spectrophotometer.

data, resulting in a catalog of individual spots listed as x/y positions, shape parameters and quantitative values (integrated spot intensities). It then becomes possible to carry out objective comparisons of equivalent spots on different gels and thus to determine whether a particular protein is more or less abundant in one sample compared to another. It can be diffi-cult to reproduce the exact conditions for protein separation in 2DGE so the identification of corresponding spots even on 2D-gels containing the same original sample can be a challenge. Very robust methods are there-fore required for the analysis of gels representing different samples where many of the spots may differ in abundance and where some spots may be present on one gel and absent on another.

The first stage in protein quantitation is image acquisition, and the method used depends on how the proteins were labeled or stained. Radioactively labeled proteins are detected by X-ray film or phosphor-imaging. The X-ray film may be scanned by a CCD (charge-coupled device) camera or a densitometer, whereas phosphorimagers come with their own scanning devices. A charge-coupled device is simply a solid-state electrical component that is divided into a series of light-sensitive areas or photo-sites. Each photosite is composed of a material that emits electrons when struck by a photon of light. The image from a CCD camera is therefore gen-erated by a microprocessor that counts the electrons at each photosite. A densitometer is a scanning device that works on similar principles, i.e. light reflected from or transmitted through the surface of a film is detected by a photodiode, which therefore records the density of the light and dark areas on the image. Coomassie-stained and silver-stained gels may also be scanned with a CCD camera or densitometer, while gels stained with the fluorescent SYPRO agents or gels containing fluorescently labeled proteins may be scanned using a CCD camera or a fluorescence imager.

The quality of the digital data depends critically on the resolution of the scanned image, which can be considered both in terms of spatial reso-lution (expressed as pixels per unit length or area) and densitometric resolution (i.e. the range of gray values that can be interpreted). However, the densitometric resolution also depends on the labeling or staining method employed. Silver staining has been the major nonradioactive detection method used for separated proteins because it is 10–100 times more sensitive than Coomassie brilliant blue staining. However, silver stains do not detect glycoproteins very efficiently and the most sensitive detection methods lead to the chemical modification of cysteine residues, therefore interfering with downstream analysis by mass spectrometry. In terms of comparative protein quantitation, the major disadvantage of silver staining is its narrow linear range (about one order of magnitude). This means that it is possible to determine accurately whether one protein is twice as abundant as another (or more importantly, if one protein is twice as abundant in one sample compared to another) but that it is not possible to compare accurately protein abundance if there is a tenfold or greater difference. The newer SYPRO reagents, particularly SYPRO Ruby, are at least as sensitive as silver staining but share none of its disadvan-tages. That is, they detect glycoproteins efficiently, they do not cause any covalent modifications to the proteins and they have an extensive linear range (over three orders of magnitude) which means they can be used to compare protein abundances very effectively. The different ways for detecting proteins in 2D-gels are summarized in *Box 4.3.*

BOX 4.3

Detecting proteins *in situ* in gels

The *in situ* detection of proteins within gels can be achieved by labeling the proteins prior to electrophoresis or staining the proteins after electrophoresis. In both cases, it is important to make the procedure as sensitive as possible without interfering with downstream analysis by mass spectrometry (Chapter 3).

Prelabeling with organic fluorophores
A number of different organic molecules can be covalently attached to proteins prior to electrophoretic separation, allowing the direct detection and quantification of labeled proteins within 2D-gels. Methods utilizing well-characterized fluorophores such as fluorescamine and fluorescein isothiocyanate have been available since the 1970s but for proteomic analysis such methods have a number of drawbacks including the altered solubility and/or mobility of labeled proteins and the variable sensitivity of labeling depending on the number of functional groups available for modification. The use of two different fluorophores, e.g. propyl-Cy3 and methyl-Cy5, to label different protein samples allows the direct visualization of differential protein abundances on a single gel (see main text).

Coomassie brilliant blue
Coomassie brilliant blue is an organic dye that is commonly used to stain proteins in polyacrylamide gels. There are many variations on the staining protocol but staining is generally carried out using the dye in a mixture of concentrated acid with ethanol or methanol. This produces a colloidal suspension that stains proteins strongly with low background. Although widely used for general protein analysis, Coomassie brilliant blue and related organic dyes lack the sensitivity for proteomic analysis having a detection limit of about 10–30 ng. Depending on the exact make-up of the stain, the dye can also modify glutamic acid side chains, which can complicate the interpretation of mass spectrometry data (although algorithms can be added to analysis software to account for this).

Silver staining
Silver staining is one of the most popular techniques for staining proteins in polyacrylamide gels and many different protocols have been used. The best methods are about 10 times more sensitive than Coomassie staining but are incompatible with downstream mass spectrometry analysis. This is because silver stains can modify cysteine residues and alkylate-exposed amino groups. Other disadvantages of silver staining include the poor linear dynamic range, which makes quantitative analysis problematical, and the fact that certain types of protein, including many glycoproteins, stain rather poorly.

Reverse stains
Both Coomassie and silver-staining methods involve a protein-fixing step which reduces the recovery of protein from the gel for subsequent analytical steps. Reverse stains, which stain the gel rather than the proteins and generate a negative image, were developed to enhance the recovery of proteins from such gels. Many different formulations have been used, the most popular based on metal salts such as copper chloride or zinc chloride.

SYPRO stains
A number of fluorophores are known to bind noncovalently to proteins, which makes them particularly compatible with downstream mass spectrometry analysis. These stains generally demonstrate little fluorescence in aqueous solution but fluoresce strongly when associated with SDS–protein complexes, and therefore produce a very low background in stained gels. The most versatile of these molecules are the SYPRO dyes (SYPRO Orange, SYPRO Red, SYPRO

Ruby and SYPRO Tangerine) available from Molecular Probes Inc. These agents are very sensitive and show a broad linear dynamic range. SYPRO Ruby, for example, matches the sensitivity of the best silver-staining techniques but has a superior linear dynamic range (extending over three orders of magnitude) and stains proteins that do not show up well with silver stains, e.g. many glycoproteins. The staining protocol is also simple and rapid, unlike Coomassie and silver-staining techniques which each require a lengthy destaining step. The only disadvantage of SYPRO dyes is their cost (e.g. SYPRO Ruby costs approximately $200 per liter). However, similar compounds such as ruthenium II tris (bathophenanthroline disulfonate) can be synthesized in the laboratory and appear to work just as well.

4.2.2   Spot detection, quantitation and comparison

Spots on protein gels are not uniform in shape, size or density. Some spots appear as discrete entities while others overlap to a greater or lesser degree. The edges of some spots are clearly defined while those of others may be blurred. Small spots may appear as shoulders on larger ones, or several spots may be joined together in a line. The densitometric landscape within different spots (i.e. the distribution of gray values) is not always consistent. These variations may be compounded by nonspecific changes in the gel background.

The human eye can generally tell what is a spot and what is not a spot on a 2D gel but humans are too subjective in their judgment to define spots rigorously. Machines can apply a fixed set of rules and parameters to the definition of individual spots and therefore interpret spot patterns more objectively. However, getting machines to see the spots in the same way that we do can be extremely challenging. Normally, the first stage in automated spot detection is digital image enhancement, which helps to clear the background and improve the contrast of the image to make the spot boundaries easier to delineate. Smoothing is used to eliminate noise caused by variable background and the background is then subtracted from the rest of the image. The contrast in the subtracted image is enhanced by reassigning gray values from the mid range to make the pixels either darker or lighter. In many cases, edge detection filters are used that aim to identify regions of the image in which there is a sharp change in pixel intensity.

Once a processed image is available, a number of different algorithms can be applied to detect and quantitate individual spots. These must take all the possible variations in spot morphology into account and calculate the integrated spot intensities, which are essentially absolute values that represent protein abundances. The algorithms generally use either Gaussian fitting (which assumes the gray values in the spot have a normal distribution along both the x- and y-axes) or Laplacian of Gaussian (LOG) spot detection methods. Other algorithms are based on the watershed transformation method in which a grayscale image is converted into a topographical surface with darker sections representing peaks and lighter sections representing troughs. The idea is then to 'flood' the image from the minima, which divides the image into catchment basins representing individual spots and watershed lines representing divisions (*Plate 2a*). In practice, the indiscriminate flooding of gel images in this manner leads to oversegmentation due to background variation in pixel intensity. To avoid this outcome, flooding can be initiated from a previously defined set of markers, which avoids any oversegmentation (*Plate 2b*). Another method worth mentioning is line analysis in which the computer focuses on individual vertical scan lines to identify density peaks. The density peaks in adjacent scan lines can be assembled into chains and these represent the centers of spots.

Once the 2D-gel has been reduced to a series of digital data representing spot intensities, the comparison of different gels is a simple process of comparing data values and determining whether the abundance of a given protein differs significantly, according to some predefined threshold, among two or more samples. A prerequisite for this type of analysis is the identification of equivalent spots on different gels, which may be challenging because gel-running conditions cannot be reproduced exactly. This may be due to several factors:

- Differences in sample preparation.
- Differences in gel composition. This can be minimized by preparing several gels from the same mixture at the same time, or by using commercially available precast gels.
- Variations in running conditions. As discussed in Chapter 2, this is a significant problem for isoelectric focusing (IEF) gels with carrier ampholytes, particularly nonequilibrium gels, but it also applies to a lesser degree to immobilized pH gradient gels. The problems can be addressed to some extent by running several gels in parallel, but this is not always possible.
- Minor variations within each gel that lead to regional differences in protein mobility. Again this is a major problem with carrier ampholyte IEF gels but also applies to others.

In the absence of gels, or images thereof, showing perfect spot-to-spot correspondence, it becomes necessary to force equivalent gels into register, a process known as gel matching. This process makes use of landmarks, i.e. spots that are present on both gels (or a whole series of gels) and can be used as a common frame of reference. Gel-matching algorithms then apply image transformation procedures such as stretching, skewing and rotating, at both local and global levels, to bring multiple gel images into register and make them comparable. This can be thought of as a procedure in which several equivalent gels are stacked above each other and a pin is used to pierce the center of the first landmark spot through all the stacked gels. Further pins are inserted through other landmarks. When the gels are held in position by a number of pins, bendy wires can be inserted to link equivalent spots that are not perfectly in register (*Figure 4.1*). In some gels, a given spot may be absent, but with a number of matched landmarks surrounding the space, the algorithm can assign a zero value to the spot with reasonable confidence. As an alternative to matching gels at the spot level, other algorithms perform essentially the same task at the pixel level. An extension to the use of landmarks is a gel-matching method known as propagation. In this approach, the algorithm begins at a known landmark and then maps the nearby spots and returns a list of x/y displacement values. Other gels are scrutinized for spots at the same displacements relative to the landmark and matches are identified. These matches can then be used as new landmarks for recursive searching.

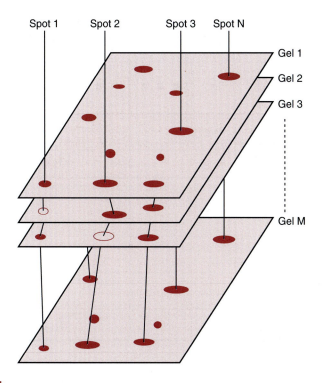

Figure 4.1

Principle of spot matching to identify corresponding spots on multiple gels. Empty circles represent absent spots.

The end result of spot detection, quantitation and gel matching should be a table of spot values (x/y coordinates, shape parameters and integrated spot intensities) arranged as a $N \times M$ matrix where N represents all the different spots that have been identified and M represents all the gels (*Figure 4.2*). M should be divided into groups based on the experimental conditions. For example, M_1–M_{15} might represent five control gels, five from experimental condition 1 and five from experimental condition 2 (perhaps different stages of a disease or different time points after drug administration). The quantitative values must be normalized for any differences in the overall signal intensities on the gels (e.g. due to different exposure times) and then various statistical methods can be used to identify protein spots whose abundance varies over the experimental conditions. Recent developments in proteomic gel-imaging technology allow matched gels to be overlain in false color so that protein spots with differential abundance over two or more gels can be visually identified. This is analogous to the use of difference gel electrophoresis as a separation method, as discussed below.

4.3 Multiplexed proteomics

Multiplexed proteomics is the use of fluorescent stains or probes with different excitation and emission spectra to detect different groups of proteins simultaneously on the same gel. This helps to reduce the number

Gel / Spot	Gel 1	Gel 2	■ ■ ■	■ ■ ■	Gel M-1	Gel M
Spot 1	$I_{1,1}$	$I_{1,2}$			$I_{1,M-1}$	$I_{1,M}$
Spot 2	$I_{2,1}$	$I_{2,2}$			$I_{2,M-1}$	$I_{2,M}$
■ ■ ■ ■						
Spot N	$I_{N,1}$	$I_{N,2}$			$I_{N,M-1}$	$I_{N,M}$

Control group — Experimental group

Figure 4.2

A generic data analysis matrix containing integrated spot densities. N is the number of spots (rows) and M is the number of gels (columns).

of gels that are required to compare different conditions and, at least in theory, obviates the need for gel matching to identify corresponding proteins. Gel matching is necessary because the staining methods discussed above are intrinsically limited to a single-color display. The use of different fluorescent labels for the multiplex analysis of DNA arrays is routine (Chapter 1) and the sample principles are now being applied in proteomics.

4.3.1 Difference gel electrophoresis

Comparative expression profiles on DNA arrays are often obtained by labeling mRNA populations from two sources with different fluorophores. These populations are mixed and applied to the array simultaneously and the array is scanned using two filters to detect the signals from each of the probes (see Chapter 1). As in other array experiments, the signal intensities from each probe show the relative abundance of each transcript in each sample. The real power of the method, however, comes from the comparison of signal intensities at each feature on the array. These signals can be rendered in false color and combined by the software included in the analysis package to provide a composite image that immediately identifies differentially expressed genes.

Difference gel electrophoresis (DIGE) is the analogous strategy in proteomics. Different protein samples, e.g. healthy *vs.* disease or stimulated *vs.* unstimulated, are labeled on lysine side chains with succinimidyl esters of propyl-Cy3 and methyl-Cy5, two fluorophores that emit light at different wavelengths. The protein samples are mixed prior to separation and loaded onto the 2D gel together. After electrophoresis, the gel is scanned using a CCD camera or fluorescence reader fitted with two different filters and two sets of data are obtained. The images from each filter can be pseudocolored and combined, immediately revealing the spots representing proteins with differential abundance (*Plate 3*). The use of further labels, e.g. Cy2, can allow even more samples to be run concurrently. Because the samples run together, all differences in gel preparation, running conditions and local gel structure are eliminated which considerably simplifies the downstream analysis.

The advantages of DIGE in terms of data analysis are undeniable, but the technique also has its drawbacks in that the fluorescent labels used are less sensitive than both SYPRO dyes and silver staining. This primarily reflects the fact that only a small proportion of the proteins in each sample can be labeled otherwise solubility is lost and the proteins precipitate during electrophoresis. A further consequence of partial labeling is that the bulky fluorescent conjugate retards the proteins during the SDS-PAGE separation so the gels must be post-stained, e.g. with Coomassie brilliant blue, to identify the 'true' protein spot to be excised for downstream analysis by mass spectrometry. Registration errors between the labeled and unlabeled protein populations is minimized during isoelectric focusing because the fluorescent conjugates are charge-matched. Accurate protein quantitation may also be difficult because proteins differ in their labeling efficiency, solubility when conjugated to the label, and the extent to which they might exhibit quenching (a phenomenon in which there is energy transfer between two fluorophores that are close together on the same molecule thus preventing the emission of light). Therefore bright spots and dim spots may represent abundant and scarce proteins, or may represent proteins that are present at approximately the same level but show differential labeling efficiency or quenching.

4.3.2 Parallel analysis with multiple dyes

The sensitivity of standard gels can be combined with the convenience of multiplex fluorescence in a new area of multiplexed proteomics in which the same SYPRO reagent is used to stain and compare protein spots on different gels, but the gels can also be stained with additional reagents that identify specific classes of proteins. These proteins can be used as landmarks for gel matching but more importantly the technique can be used to identify subsets of proteins in the proteome that share specific functional attributes. A number of stains have been developed by companies such as Molecular Probes Inc. that recognize various structurally or functionally related proteins, e.g. glycoproteins and phosphoproteins (these are discussed in more detail in Chapter 8), oligo-histidine tagged proteins, calcium-binding proteins and even proteins that have the capability to bind or metabolize particular drugs (see Chapter 7). For example, penicillin analogs have been produced carrying BODIPY dyes, which are relatively nonpolar and have a neutral chromophore and therefore do not interfere with the structure or chemical behavior of the antibiotic. These so-called BOCILLIN reagents can efficiently identify penicillin-binding proteins on a 2D-gel with SYPRO Ruby used as a general counterstain. Similarly, BODIPY dyes have been used to generate analogs of the cysteine protease inhibitor *trans*-epoxysuccinyl-Lleucylamido(4-guanidino) butane, therefore allowing cysteine proteases to be identified and changes in their expression levels following different types of cell treatment to be investigated.

4.4   Quantitative proteomics with mass spectrometry

Protein quantitation at the mass spectrometry stage makes it possible to use in-line liquid-phase separation methods such as multidimensional chromatography and capillary electrophoresis (Chapter 2). Quantitation can be carried out by comparing peptide ion currents but this is inherently inaccurate and is biased by instrument design. Instead, quantitation is often based on the use stable isotopes, although as discussed below isotopes are not required for all such methods. An important distinction between gel-based and MS-based methods for protein quantitation is that the former involves working with proteins while the latter involves working with peptides. The general approach is to label alternative samples with equivalent reagents, one of which contains a heavy isotope and one of which contains a light isotope. The samples are mixed, separated into fractions, and analyzed by mass spectrometry. The ratio of the two isotopic variants can be determined from the heights of the peaks in the mass spectra and used to identify proteins with differential abundance. Several variants of the approach can be used which are discussed below and summarized in *Figure 4.3*. While these MS methods are more reproducible

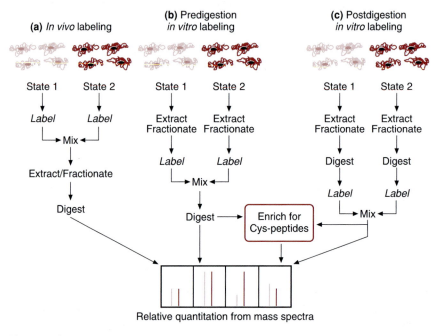

Figure 4.3

Overview of MS-based strategies for quantitative proteomics. Depending on the point at which the label is introduced, most procedures are classified as (a) *in vivo* labeling, (b) predigestion labeling *in vitro*, or (c) postdigestion labeling *in vitro*. Reprinted from Current Opinion in Chemical Biology, Vol. 7, Sechi and Oda, 'Quantitative Proteomics using mass spectrometry', pp 70–77, ©2003, with permission from Elsevier.

and sensitive than gel-based methods for protein quantitation, it should be noted that only gel-based methods provide the visual perspective of the proteome that may be important, e.g. to gain insight into the occurrence of isoforms and post-translational variants.

4.4.1 ICAT reagents

One of the first developments in quantitative mass spectrometry was a class of reagents known as isotope-coded affinity tags (ICATs). These are biotinylated derivatives of iodoacetamide, a reagent that reacts with the cysteine side chains of denatured proteins. Two versions of the reagent are used, one normal or light form and one heavy or deuterated form in which a hydrogen atom is replaced by deuterium. The heavy and light forms are used to label different protein samples and then the proteins are combined and digested with trypsin. The biotin allows cysteine-containing peptides to be isolated from the complex peptide mixture through affinity to streptavidin, therefore considerably simplifying the number of different peptides entering the mass spectrometer (*Figure 4.4*).

Variants on this theme include a cleavable ICAT reagent, which allows the biotin to be removed before mass spectrometry, and the use of heavy and light forms of acrylamide which also react with cysteine side chains. The cleavable ICAT is advantageous because the presence of fragmented ions derived from biotin can introduce complications into the mass spectra obtained for labeled peptides. A disadvantage of all the above

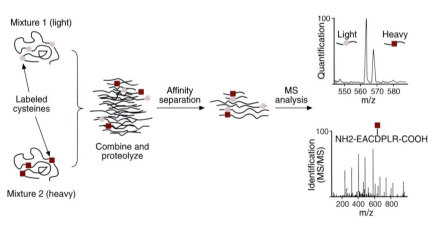

Figure 4.4

The ICAT reagent strategy for protein quantitation. Two protein mixtures representing two different cell states are treated with the isotopically light (pink) or heavy (red) ICAT reagents, respectively. The labeled protein mixtures are then combined and proteolyzed; tagged peptides are selectively isolated and analyzed by MS. The relative abundance is determined by the ratio of signal intensities of the tagged peptide pairs. The CID spectra are recorded and searched against large protein sequence databases to identify the protein. Therefore, in a single operation, the relative abundance and sequence of a peptide are determined. Reprinted from Current Opinion in Biotechnology, Vol. 14, Tao and Aebersold, 'Advances in quantitative proteomics via stable isotope tagging and mass spectrometry', pp 110–118, ©2003, with permission from Elsevier.

methods, however, is that proteins that do not contain cysteine cannot be quantified. This represents about 10% of all proteins.

4.4.2 Nonselective labeling of peptides after digestion

An alternative to the ICAT labeling of proteins that is not selective for cysteine-containing peptides is to label the peptides after digestion. As discussed in Chapter 3, when trypsin cleaves a protein and generates a peptide with a new C-terminus, it introduces an oxygen atom derived from a molecule of water into the carboxyl group of the peptide. This can be exploited for the identification of y-series ions in fragment ion spectra (see p. 66) but it can also be used to differentially label peptides derived

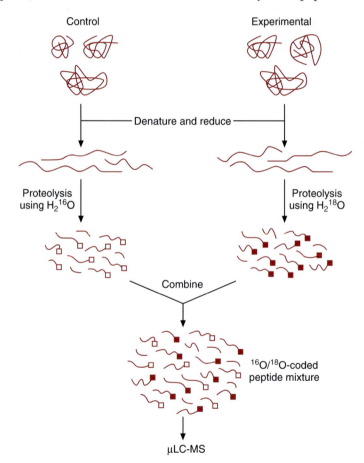

Figure 4.5

Enzymatic stable isotope coding of proteomes. For enzymatic labeling, proteins from two distinct proteomes are proteolytically digested in aqueous buffer containing either normal water (H$_2$^{16}O; white squares) or isotopically labeled water (H$_2$^{18}O; red squares). This encoding strategy effectively labels every C terminus produced during digestion. The samples are combined at the peptide level and then analyzed by microcapillary LC-MS. Reprinted from Current Opinion in Biotechnology, Vol. 14, Goshe and Smith, 'Stable isotope-coded proteomic mass spectrometry', pp 101–109, ©2003, with permission from Elsevier.

from alternative protein samples if normal water is used in one buffer and water substituted with heavy oxygen (^{18}O) is used in the other (*Figure 4.5*). The abundance of the peptides can then be compared, since they will appear as doublets separated by two mass units.

Alternative strategies include the chemical modification of the C-terminus, N-terminus or exposed lysine side chains of tryptic peptides using isotope-coded reagents. For example, a method has been described in which isolated spots from 2D-gels are digested with Asp/GluC protease and the resulting peptides are labeled at the N-termini with 1-nicotinoyl-oxysuccinimide (H_4NicNHS) or its heavy derivative D_4NicNHS (where the hydrogen at position 4 is replaced with deuterium). A hybrid of ICAT and postdigestion labeling strategies involves the use of a solid-phase ICAT reagent to capture cysteine-containing peptides from a complex mixture onto small plastic beads. The reagent has a photolabile linker arm so that isotope-tagged peptides can be released from the beads by exposure to light. These various coding strategies are summarized in *Table 4.1*

Table 4.1 Differential labeling methods used to quantify proteins in different samples by mass spectrometry

Method	Principle	Comments
Predigestion labeling, can also be applied after digestion		
ICAT, iodoacetamide	Deuterated iodoacetamide reacts with cysteine residues and carries biotin tag for affinity purification	Purification of cysteine peptides simplifies analysis but presence of biotin complicates it. Restricted to cysteine-containing proteins
Cleavable ICAT	As above, but contains acid-cleavable or photolabile linker	Biotin can be removed. Restricted to cysteine-containing proteins
ICAT, acrylamide	Deuterated acrylamide reacts with cysteine residues	Restricted to cysteine-containing proteins
Post-digestion labeling		
Esterification	Esterification of carboxyl groups by deuterated methanol	Can be inefficient
MCAT	Modification of lysine side chains with O-methylisourea	Inexpensive because stable isotopes are not used
N-acetoxysuccinimide	Derivitization of N-terminus and lysine side chains with deuterated N-acetoxysuccinimide	Can be inefficient
Proteolysis	Proteolysis in presence of ^{18}O incorporates label into C-terminal carboxyl group of peptides	Theoretically labels all peptides but there is incomplete incorporation

4.4.3 Isotope tagging *in vivo*

In another group of methods, cells treated under different conditions are grown in media containing either normal or heavy isotopes of nitrogen, carbon or hydrogen. A useful approach is the use of labeled amino acids (stable-isotope labeling with amino acids in cell culture, SILAC). The cells can then be harvested, combined, and the proteins extracted for separation, tryptic digestion and analysis by mass spectrometry. Equivalent

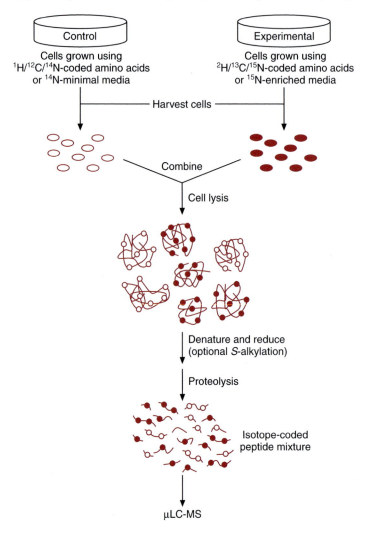

Figure 4.6

Metabolic stable isotope coding of proteomes. For metabolic labeling, cells from two distinct cultures are grown on media supplemented with either normal amino acids (^{1}H/^{12}C/^{14}N) or ^{14}N-minimal media (white spheres) or stable isotope amino acids (^{2}H/^{13}C^{15}N) or ^{15}N-enriched media (red spheres). These mass tags are incorporated into proteins during translation, thus providing complete proteome coverage. An equivalent number of cells for each sample is combined and processed for microcapillary LC-MS analysis. Reprinted from Current Opinion in Biotechnology, Vol. 14, Goshe and Smith, 'Stable isotope-coded proteomic mass spectrometry', pp 101–109, ©2003, with permission from Elsevier.

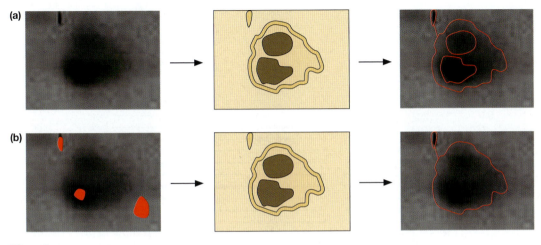

Plate 2

The watershed method for contour finding on 2D-gel images. (a) Any graytone image can be considered as a topographic surface. If flooded from its minima without allowing water from different sources to merge, the image is partitioned into catchment basins and watershed lines, but in practice this leads to over-segmentation. (b) Therefore, markers (red shapes) are used to initiate flooding, and this reduces over-segmentation considerably. Adapted from images by Dr Serge Beucher, CMM/Ecole de Mines de Paris.

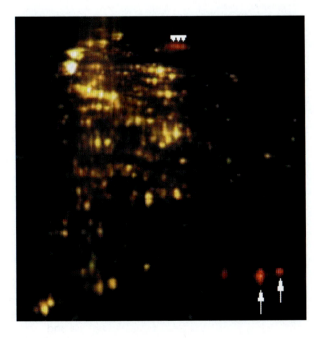

Plate 3

2D DIGE overlay image of Cy3- (green) and Cy5- (red) labeled test-spiked *Erwinia carotovora* proteins. The protein test spikes were three conalbumin isoforms (arrowheads) and two myoglobin isoforms (arrows). Spots that are of equal intensity between the two channels appear yellow in the overlay image. As spike proteins were eight times more abundant in the Cy5 channel, they appear as red spots in the overlay. The gel is oriented with the acidic end to the left. Reprinted from Current Opinion in Chemical Biology, Vol. 6, Lilley et al. 'Two-dimensional gel electrophoresis: recent advances in sample preparation, detection and quantitation', pp 46–50, ©2002, with permission from Elsevier.

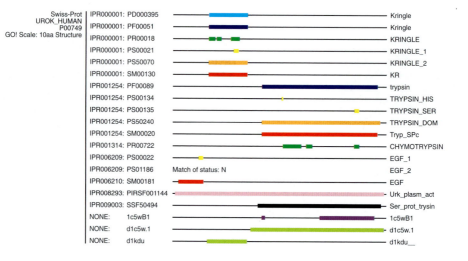

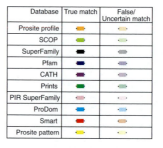

Plate 4

InterPro analysis of human urokinase-like plasminogen activator. Different colored bars represent matches to patterns and profiles in Prosite, SuperFamily, Prints, iProClass (PIR SuperFamily), ProDom, Smart and the structural databases CATH and SCOP.

peptides from each sample will differ in mass by a single mass unit and can easily be identified as doublets in mass spectra. The relative amounts of the two peptides can be determined on the basis of the relative heights of the two peaks.

The advantage of this metabolic labeling approach is that the label is introduced early in the experiment, therefore eliminating variation arising from sample preparation and purification losses (*Figure 4.6*). However, it can only be used for the analysis of live cells that can be maintained in a controlled environment. It is not useful, for example, for tissue explants, biopsies, body fluids or cells that are difficult to maintain in culture.

The *in vivo* tagging of proteins was used by Washburn and colleagues (see Further Reading) for the identification of yeast proteins expressed when yeast cells were switched from minimal to enriched medium. They grew yeast in N^{14} minimal medium or N^{15} enriched medium, separated the proteins by multidimensional HPLC (see Chapter 2) and then analyzed the fractions by tandem mass spectrometry. Over 800 differentially expressed proteins were thus identified.

4.4.4 Mass-coded abundance tags

A final strategy involves the use of mass-coded abundance tags (MCATs), chemical adducts with a specific mass which avoid the need for stable isotopes. In the MCAT method, proteins from one sample are labeled with O-methylisourea and those from the other sample are not labeled at all. This differs from the other methods described above where both samples are labeled but with different isotopes. This method is simple and inexpensive, but less accurate than those involving isotopes.

Further reading

Goshe, M.B. and Smith, R.D. (2003) Stable isotope-coded proteomic mass spectrometry. *Curr Opin Biotechnol* **14**: 101–109.

Gygi, S.P., Rist, B., Gerber, S.A., Turecek, F., Gelb, M.H. and Aebersold, R. (1999) Quantitative analysis of complex protein mixtures using isotope coded affinity tags. *Nature Biotechnol* **17**: 994–999.

Patton, W. (2000) Making blind robots see: the synergy between fluorescent dyes and imaging devices in automated proteomics. *BioTechniques* **28**: 944–957.

Patton, W. (2000) A thousand points of light; the application of fluorescence detection technologies to two-dimensional gel electrophoresis and proteomics. *Electrophoresis* **21**: 1123–1144.

Patton, W.F. and Beecham, J.M. (2001) Rainbow's end: the quest for multiplexed fluorescence quantitative analysis in proteomics. *Curr Opin Chem Biol* **6**: 63–69.

Rabilloud, T. (2002) Two-dimensional gel electrophoresis in proteomics: old, old fashioned, but still it climbs up the mountains. *Proteomics* **2**: 3–10.

Sechi, S. and Oda, Y. (2003) Quantitative proteomics using mass spectrometry. *Curr Opin Chem Biol* **7**: 70–77.

Tao, W.A. and Aebersold, R. (2003) Advances in quantitative proteomics via stable isotope tagging and mass spectrometry. *Curr Opin Biotechnol* **14**: 110–118.

Van den Bergh, G., Arckens, L. (2004) Fluorescent two-dimensional difference gel electrophoresis unveils the potential of gel-based proteomics. *Curr Opin Biotech* **15**: 38–43.

Washburn, M., Wolters, D. and Yates, J. (2001) Large-scale analysis of the yeast proteome by multidimensional protein identification technology. *Nature Biotechnol* **19**: 242–247.

Proteomics and the analysis of protein sequences

5

5.1 Introduction

One of the most widely used strategies in proteomics is correlative database searching. As discussed in Chapter 3, this involves searching the sequence databases for proteins containing peptides that match experimental data obtained by mass spectrometry, and when successful it results in definitive protein identification. However, sequence analysis can provide a great deal more information than simple identification. By comparing the sequence of a protein to all the other sequences that are stored in the databases, a researcher can find information about protein structure, interactions, biochemical activity and evolution, and even a potential role in disease. Indeed, in the current post-genomics era, database searching based on protein sequence similarity often provides the first leads in the elucidation of protein function.

Many thousands of protein sequences have been entered into databases, either following *de novo* sequence determination or (much more commonly) by the translation of nucleotide sequences. The three primary nucleotide sequence databases – GenBank, EMBL and DDBJ, see Chapter 1 – each contain nucleotide sequence translations where appropriate, and there are also the dedicated protein sequence databases SWISS-PROT and TrEMBL (p. 18). The number of stored sequences is growing at a phenomenal rate, reflecting the success of the genome projects, which result in thousands of new sequences being deposited every day. As discussed briefly in Chapter 1, the function of a protein is dependent on its three-dimensional structure, since this specifies the protein's shape, charge distribution and the juxtaposition of key amino acid residues, and therefore dictates how the protein interacts with other molecules. The three-dimensional structure depends in turn on how the chain of amino acids folds in space, and this reflects the length of the sequence, the particular amino acids that are present and their order, and whether those amino acids are post-translationally modified in any way. The gene encoding a given protein therefore contributes to the protein's functional properties by specifying the amino acid sequence and the potential for modification, although it cannot define post-translational modifications precisely.

Given the intimate relationship between sequence and function, it is not surprising that proteins with similar sequences generally have similar structures and functions. Such proteins can be grouped into families based on sequence similarity. This similar sequence/similar function paradigm lies at the center of bioinformatics and allows us to make structural and functional predictions based on a protein sequence.

5.2 Protein families and evolutionary relationships

5.2.1 Evolutionary relationships between proteins

Proteins that show a significant degree of sequence similarity are unlikely to have originated independently and are therefore said to be homologous, i.e. they have arisen by divergence from a common ancestor.* Often, different sequences in a protein family show similarities over their entire lengths, which indicates the sequences have diverged by the accumulation of point mutations alone (*Figure 5.1*). In such cases, the degree of relatedness often corresponds to the level of functional conservation. If two protein sequences are very similar, they might represent homologous molecules that carry out identical functions in different species, and which have accumulated mutations due to speciation. Such proteins, which are known as orthologs, include for example the human and mouse β-globin proteins (*Figure 5.1*). A lower degree of relatedness might indicate that the proteins are homologous but have diverged in functional terms. Such proteins are known as paralogs, and they arise by gene duplication and divergence within a genome. Human myoglobin and β-globin are paralogs, as are mouse myoglobin and β-globin. However, paralogous relationships are not restricted to within species since the human myoglobin and mouse β-globin proteins could also be classed as paralogs (*Figure 5.1*).

In other cases, proteins are not related over their entire lengths but show partial alignments corresponding to individual domains. This reflects the modular nature of proteins and the fact that different functions can be carried out by different protein domains. Such proteins have not diverged simply by the accumulation of point mutations, but also by more complex events such as recombination between genes and gene segments leading to the shuffling and rearrangement of exons. Human proteins involved in

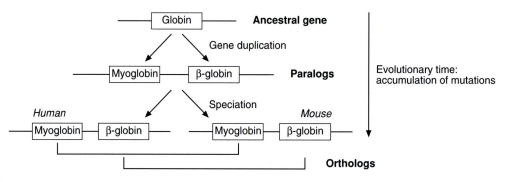

Figure 5.1

Evolution by the accumulation of point mutations alone leads to large families of proteins related to each other along their entire primary sequences. Proteins that have arisen by gene duplication within a species are known as paralogs, while equivalent proteins in different species are known as orthologs.

* This means that two proteins are either homologous or not, i.e. homology is an absolute term. In the same way that it is impossible to be 65% pregnant it is impossible for two sequences to show 65% homology. For the quantitation of the degree of relationship between two sequences, the terms identity or similarity should be used instead (see Section 5.3).

the blood-clotting cascade provide a useful example of this process (*Figure 5.2*). Tissue plasminogen activator (TPA) contains four types of domain: a fibronectin type II domain (fnII), an epidermal growth factor (EGF) domain, two kringle domains and the serine protease domain. These domains are shared with a number of other hemostatic proteins, but the organization is different in each case. For example, the fnII domain in TPA is adjacent to the EGF domain, whereas in factor XII, the fnII domain is sandwiched between two EGF domains. In contrast, urokinase lacks a fnII domain and is therefore not activated by fibronectin, but it does contain an EGF domain and a kringle domain. These types of relationship indicate that the protein domain, rather than the whole protein, is the unit of evolution.

5.2.2 Predicting function from sequence

Functional predictions based on protein sequences vary in their usefulness according to the degree of sequence similarity. Orthologous sequences are usually very good predictors, especially in closely related species. For example, if a protein sequence was determined for a relatively uncharacterized mammal, such as the polar bear, and that sequence was nearly identical to human β-globin, one could predict the function of that protein at the biochemical, cellular and biological levels with reasonable accuracy (*Box 5.1*). Paralogous sequences are less reliable, but usually allow at least the biochemical function of a protein to be predicted. A protein with a globin-like sequence, for example, that was not strongly related to any known globin, is still likely to be an oxygen-carrier although a more detailed function would have to be established experimentally. For shuffled proteins, functions can be assigned to individual domains. In the case of TPA, for example, a combined biochemical function can be deduced from the functions of the individual domains: the presence of a fnII domain suggests it is a protein that interacts with fibrin, the serine protease domain shows that it cleaves other proteins and the EGF domain indicates

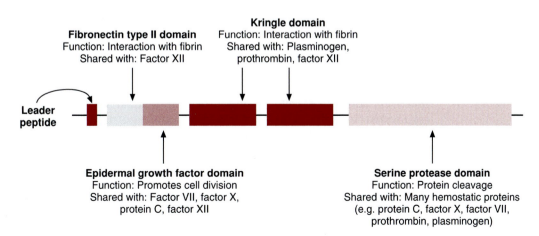

Figure 5.2

Human tissue plasminogen activator is a multidomain protein whose domains are widely shared within the family of hemostatic proteins.

BOX 5.1

The function of a protein

The high-throughput determination of protein function is dependent on the use of databases to store sequence, structural and functional information in a readily accessible form (Chapter 1). The increasing globalization of database resources made possible by the Internet means that a systematic nomenclature for protein function is required so that scientists all over the world can exchange information and understand what that information means. However, standardization is not easy to achieve because scientists work on different systems and organisms, and because the function of a protein can be described at three different levels:

- Molecular/biochemical function: e.g. phosphatase, DNA-binding protein.
- Cellular function: e.g. growth factor signaling pathway, amino acid metabolism, DNA synthesis.
- Biological function: e.g. control of bone growth, regulation of flower development.

Molecular and cellular functions are the easiest to standardize because they can be described very precisely (e.g. the reaction catalyzed by an enzyme) but a standard approach for the classification of biological function is more difficult to envisage. Another complication is that in bacteria and unicellular eukaryotes, the cellular and biological functions of a protein would be combined, whereas in multicellular organisms they could be separated. As an example, the table below shows the possible classifications for the human protein glucokinase.

> Molecular/biochemical function: kinase, substrate glucose
> Cellular function: glycolysis, glucose metabolism
> Biological function: expressed specifically in pancreatic β-cells and hepatocytes, primary regulator of glucose-controlled insulin secretion, loss of function mutations cause diabetes, gain of function mutations can cause hyperinsulinism

Several functional classification systems have been devised. One of the oldest and most established, but which only applies to enzymes, is the Enzyme Commission hierarchical system for enzyme classification. Other more general approaches are used in the Kyoto Encyclopedia of Genes and Genomes (http://www.genome.ad.jp/kegg/), and most recently, the Gene Ontology system (http://www.geneontology.org/). The latter is very flexible because it is not restricted to a hierarchical classification architecture and because molecular and biological functions can be assigned independently.

that TPA influences cell division. These individual functions are all required for its overall biological function in the regulation of blood clotting. As we shall see later, however, similar sequence does not guarantee a similar function as some very similar proteins can carry out quite distinct roles in the cell or body (p. 101).

5.3 Basic principles of protein sequence comparison

5.3.1 Identity and similarity between protein sequences

The basis of sequence comparison is the ability to align two sequences manually, or more often automatically, and compare them to determine the number of shared residues. The result is an alignment score, which represents the quality of the alignment and, at the same time, the close-ness of the evolutionary relationship. For nucleotide sequences, comparisons are always made on the basis of sequence identity, which is the percentage of identical residues in the alignment. For protein sequences, identity can be suitable for the comparison of very similar sequences but a more useful measure is sequence similarity, which takes into account conservative substitutions between chemically or physically similar amino acids (e.g. valine and isoleucine). When evolutionary changes occur in protein sequences, they tend to involve substitutions between amino acids with similar properties because such changes are less likely to affect the structure and function of the protein. Therefore, while sequence identity will reveal the total number of differences between two proteins, sequence similarity attaches less significance to those changes that substitute equivalent amino acids and much more significance to changes that are more likely to impact on the protein's structure and func-tion. Taylor's Venn diagram of amino acids, which clusters amino acids on the basis of conserved physical and chemical properties, is shown in *Figure 5.3*.

5.3.2 Substitution score matrices

The significance of different amino acid substitutions is incorporated into alignment scores by the use of a substitution score matrix. This is simply a table that attaches probabilities (or weights) to all the possible exchanges and applies this weighting when the alignment score is calculated. In the absence of substitution scores, an identity matrix is used: identical amino acids in an alignment are given the score 1 and nonidentical residues are given the score 0. A more realistic strategy is to weight the probabilities

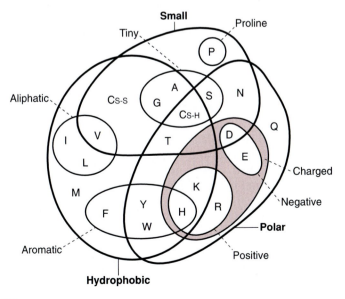

Figure 5.3

Taylor's Venn diagram of amino acid properties. (Cs-s, cysteine in a disulfide bond; Cs-H, free cysteine)

of each exchange by the minimum number of mutations necessary to convert one codon into another, since it is well known that pairs of codons interconvertible by a single base change often encode conservative amino acids. For example, the four codons encoding serine (UCX, where X is any nucleotide) can be changed by a single mutation in the first position to ACX, which encodes the similar amino acid threonine. In contrast, it takes at least two mutations and in many cases three to convert the proline codons (CCX) into the single codon encoding tryptophan (UGU). While better than the identity matrix, this genetic code matrix is theoretical and does not take data from real measurements of evolutionary changes into account.

The first empirical substitution matrices were devised by Margaret Dayhoff and colleagues in the 1970s and are sometimes called Dayhoff matrices or mutation data matrices because they were generated by studying alignments of very similar protein sequences and counting the frequencies with which each type of substitution occurred. Because such matrices are based on the tabulation of actual mutations (mutations that have been 'accepted' in an evolutionary sense) they are generally referred to as PAM matrices, with PAM meaning 'accepted point mutations'. The result was a set of relative mutability scores for each amino acid, based on a defined evolutionary unit of time measured in PAM units. One PAM represents the evolutionary time for one residue to change in a sequence of amino acids 100 residues long. The most widely used PAM matrix is the PAM_{250} matrix (*Figure 5.4*) which represents a much longer evolutionary time scale during which a sequence of 100 amino acids is expected to undergo 250 changes (i.e. an average of 2.5 mutations per residue). The PAM_{250} matrix gives high scores for very common substitutions (e.g. valine/isoleucine substitutions score 4) and low scores for rare ones (e.g. proline/tryptophan substitutions score –6). By applying this matrix to the two short sequences in *Figure 5.5*, which show almost no identity, a meaningful alignment is achieved in which the basic residues lysine and arginine are aligned, the hydrophobic residues leucine and valine are aligned, and the aspartic and glutamic acid residues are aligned. Note that the scores for alignments of identical amino acids, which are shown along the diagonal of the matrix, are not all the same. This reflects the fact that not all amino acids are equally common in proteins, and that some residues have a more important impact on protein structure than others and are therefore more highly conserved during evolution. For example, two aligned tryptophan residues score 17 because this is one of the rarest of the amino acids and it also plays a critical structural role in many proteins, while two aligned arginine residues score only 2 because this is quite likely to happen by chance when any two protein sequences are compared.

There are several different substitution matrices in common use, some of which are applied very generally while others are used for particular types of protein with special features (e.g. integral membrane proteins). The PAM series of matrices was derived by comparing the observed changes in closely related protein sequences and extrapolating those results to longer evolutionary distances. BLOSUM matrices, in contrast, are not based on an explicit evolutionary model, and are thought to outperform PAM matrices in many situations. The BLOSUM (BLOcks SUbstitution Matrix) matrices are based on amino acid substitutions

	C	S	T	P	A	G	N	D	E	Q	H	R	K	M	I	L	V	F	Y	W
C	12																			
S	0	2																		
T	-2	1	3																	
P	-1	1	0	6																
A	-2	1	1	1	2															
G	-3	1	0	-1	1	5														
N	-4	1	0	-1	0	0	2													
D	-5	0	0	-1	0	1	2	4												
E	5	0	0	-1	0	0	1	3	4											
Q	-5	-1	-1	0	0	-1	1	2	2	4										
H	-3	-1	-1	0	-1	-2	2	1	4	3	6									
R	-4	0	-1	0	-2	-3	0	-1	-1	1	2	6								
K	-5	0	0	-1	-1	-2	1	0	0	1	0	3	5							
M	-5	-2	-1	-2	-1	-3	-2	-3	-2	-1	-2	0	0	6						
I	-3	-1	0	-2	-1	-3	-2	-2	-2	-2	-2	-2	-2	2	5					
L	-6	-3	-2	-3	-2	-4	-3	-4	-3	-2	-2	-3	-3	4	2	6				
V	-2	-2	0	-1	0	-1	-2	-2	-2	-2	-2	-2	-2	2	4	2	4			
F	-4	-3	-3	-5	-4	-5	-4	-6	-5	-5	-2	-4	-5	0	1	2	-1	9		
Y	0	-3	-3	-5	-3	-5	-2	-4	-4	-4	0	-4	-4	-2	-1	-1	-2	7	10	
W	-8	-2	-5	-6	-6	-7	4	7	7	5	3	2	-3	-4	-5	-2	-6	0	0	17
	C	S	T	P	A	G	N	D	E	Q	H	R	K	M	I	L	V	F	Y	W

Figure 5.4

The PAM250 matrix.

observed in blocks of aligned sequences with a certain level of identity. For example, the $BLOSUM_{62}$ matrix uses aligned blocks showing 62% sequence identity. The higher the number next to BLOSUM, the closer the evolutionary relationship between sequences (the opposite of PAM). BLOSUM matrices are based on the local alignment of a much more diverse collection of sequences than PAM, but because the blocks contain sequences at all different evolutionary distances they may be biased towards highly conserved residues.

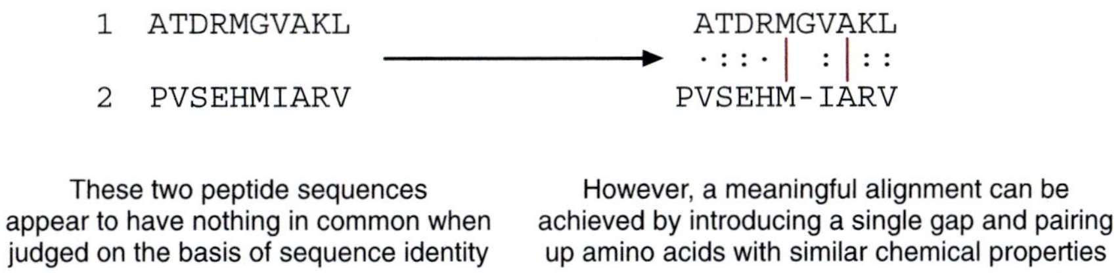

```
1   ATDRMGVAKL                          ATDRMGVAKL
                                        · : : ·  |   :  |  : :
2   PVSEHMIARV                          PVSEHM-IARV
```

These two peptide sequences appear to have nothing in common when judged on the basis of sequence identity

However, a meaningful alignment can be achieved by introducing a single gap and pairing up amino acids with similar chemical properties

Figure 5.5

Manual alignment of two short peptide sequences to demonstrate the use of amino acid substititution scores where there is little or no sequence identity. A meaningful alignment can still be achieved if conservative substitutions are allowed.

5.3.3   Pairwise similarity searching

The similarity between any two short sequences can be demonstrated by manual alignment as shown in *Figure 5.5*. Most of the amino acids in the top sequence have an equivalent in the bottom sequence, and in evolutionary terms we can presume that any changes between the sequences resulted from the accumulation of point mutations in the corresponding genes. However, one of the amino acids in the top sequence has no equivalent and a gap has been introduced into the bottom sequence to make the alignment more meaningful. We can presume that the gap arose due to a deletion in the bottom sequence or an insertion in the top sequence, although without further information from other protein sequences it is impossible to tell. For this reason, gaps are sometimes called indels.

Real protein sequences are much longer than those shown in *Figure 5.5*, and computer algorithms are required to find the best alignments. There are two algorithms in common use, known as the Needleman–Wunsch algorithm and the Smith–Waterman algorithm, and both use dynamic programming to achieve the best alignment scores. Although the algorithms work on similar principles, the Needleman–Wunsch algorithm looks for global similarity between sequences while the Smith–Waterman algorithm focuses on shorter regions of local similarity. The Smith–Waterman algorithm is the most useful for identifying partial sequence alignments such as those found in proteins that share a domain but are dissimilar in other respects. Both algorithms can be used to align sequences over their entire lengths.

In their simplest forms, dynamic programming algorithms find alignments containing the largest possible number of identical and similar amino acids by inserting gaps wherever necessary. The problem with this approach is that the indiscriminate use of gaps can make any two sequences match, no matter how dissimilar (*Figure 5.6*). Apart from making alignments meaningless, this does not reflect the true nature of evolution, where insertions and deletions occur much less frequently than substitutions. The problem is addressed by constraining the dynamic programming algorithms with gap penalties, which reduce the overall alignment score as more gaps are introduced. For example, the alignment of α-globin and β-globin is shown in *Figure 5.7*. A head-to-head alignment with no gaps provides a relatively low score (*Figure 5.7a*) whereas the indiscriminate insertion of gaps would produce a higher score but a meaningless alignment. A sensible gap penalty, which reduces the alignment

```
1   ATDPMGVAKLRHHDKYWKKRAIV                  These two peptide
                                             sequences are unrelated
2   PVATEEDMPMRGRVIAKDKYIHW
```

```
    AT--D-PM-G-V-AKLRHHDKY--WKKRAIV          But the indiscriminate insertion
    ||   | || | |  |||   |   |     |         gaps can force them to align
    PVATEEDMPMRGRVIAK----DKYIHW
```

Figure 5.6

Any two sequences can be made to align if enough gaps are introduced, which is why gap penalties are required to generate meaningful alignments.

(a) VLSPADKTNVKAAWGKVGAHAGEYGAEALERMFLSFPTT
     VHLTPEEKSAVTALWGKVNVDEVGGEALGRLLVVYPWTQ

     KTYFPHFDLSHGSAQVKGHGKKVADALTNAVAHVDDMPN
     RFFESFGDLSTPDAVMGNPKVKAHGKKVLGAFSDGLAHL

     ALSALSDLHAHKLRVDPVNFKLLSHCLLVTLAAHLPAEF
     DNLKGTFATLSELHCDKLHVDPENDRLLGNVLVCVLAHH

     TPAVHASLDKFLASVSTVLTSKYR
     FGKEFTPPVQAAYQKVVAGVANALAHKYH

(b) -VLSPADKTNVKAAWGKVGAHAGEYGAEALERMFLSFPT
     VHLTPEEKSAVTALWGKV--NVDEVGGEALGRLLVVYPW

     TKTYFPHF-DLSH-----GSAQVKGHGKKVADALTNAVA
     TQRFFESFGDLSTPDAVMGNPKVKAHGKKVLGAFSDGLA

     HVDDMPNALSALSDLHAHKLRVDPVNFKLLSHCLLVTLA
     HLDNLKGTFATLSELHCDKLHVDPENFRLLGNVLVCVLA

     AHLPAEFTPAVHASLDKFLASVSTVLTSKYR
     HHFGKEFTPPVQAAYQKVVAGVANALAHKYH

Figure 5.7

Alignment of two distantly related globin sequences (α-globin and β-globin) with only identical residues highlighted. (a) Head-to-head alignment results in a relatively small number of identical residues. (b) While the indiscriminate insertion of gaps would make the alignment meaningless, the introduction of a small number of gaps permits a better alignment where a greater number of identical residues are paired.

score as more gaps are introduced, produces the optimal alignment shown in *Figure 5.7b* in which there are three gaps.

While it is possible to apply a constant penalty regardless of gap length, most algorithms employ more complex penalty systems in which the penalty is proportional to the length of the gaps or in which there is an initial penalty for opening a gap and then a lower penalty for extending it (affine gap penalty). These are more likely to reflect true evolutionary mechanisms, since a protein is less likely to tolerate an insertion at a new site than it is to tolerate further insertions at a site where a previous insertion has already been shown to be compatible with biochemical function.

Dynamic programming algorithms are guaranteed to find the best alignment of two sequences for a given substitution matrix and gap penalty system but they are slow and resource-hungry. Therefore, if they are applied to large sequence databases, the searches could take many hours to perform. To allow more rapid searches, alternative methods have been developed which are not based on dynamic programming, and which are faster but less accurate. These have been important in the development of Internet-based database search facilities which otherwise could be rapidly saturated by researchers carrying out similarity searches.

The two principal algorithms are BLAST and FASTA. There are several variants of each algorithm that are adapted for different types of searches depending on the nature of the query sequence and the database, the most relevant for protein sequences being BLASTP, BLASTX, TBLASTN, FASTA and TFASTA (*Table 5.1*). Both BLAST and FASTA take into account the fact that high-scoring alignments are likely to contain short stretches of identical or near-identical letters, which are sometimes termed words. In the case of BLAST, the first step is to look for words of a certain fixed word length (W, which is usually equivalent to three amino acids) that score above a given threshold level, T, set by the user. In FASTA, this word length is two amino acids and there is no T value because the match must be perfect. Both programs then attempt to extend their matching segments to produce longer alignments, which in BLAST terminology are called high-scoring segment pairs. FASTA is slower than BLAST because the final stage of the alignment process involves alignment of the high-scoring regions using full dynamic programming.

5.3.4 The significance of sequence alignments

The significance of a sequence identity or sequence similarity score depends on the length of the sequence over which the alignment takes place. For example, a score of 100% sequence similarity suggests that two proteins are very closely related, but this is meaningless if the alignment is assessed over just three amino acid residues! A 60% similarity over 30 residues is much more worthy of attention, but 60% similarity over 300 residues would be more significant still.

The difference between chance similarity and alignments that have real biological significance is determined by the statistical analysis of search scores, particularly the calculation of p values and E values. The p value of a similarity score S is the probability that a score of at least S would have been obtained in a match between any two unrelated protein sequences of similar composition and length. Significant matches are therefore identified by low p values (e.g. $p = 0.01$), which indicate that it is very unlikely that the similarity score was obtained by chance, and probably indicates a real evolutionary relationship. The E value is related to p and is the expected frequency of similarity scores of at least S, would occur by chance. E increases in proportion to the size of the database that is searched, so even searches with low p values (e.g. $p = 0.0001$) might

Table 5.1 Variants of the BLAST and FASTA programs for similarity searching

Program	Query	Database
BLASTN	Nucleotide	Nucleotide
BLASTX	Translated nucleotide	Protein
BLASTP	Protein	Protein
TBLASTN	Protein	Translated nucleotide
FASTA	Nucleotide	Nucleotide
	or	
	Protein	Protein
TFASTA	Protein	Translated nucleotide

uncover some spurious matches in a database containing 100 000 sequences ($E = 0.001 \times 100\,000 = 10$).*

5.3.5 Multiple alignments

While pairwise alignments can be used to search for related proteins and provide identification and an initial classification of a newly determined protein sequence, the inter-relationships between members of a protein family are better illustrated by multiple alignments. This is because the conservation of any two amino acid residues between two protein sequences could occur by chance, i.e. the fortuitous absence of a mutation at that particular site, but if that same residue is found in five or ten proteins in the family, especially if the proteins are otherwise diverse, this suggests the residue may play a key functional role.

An example of a multiple alignment within the serine protease domains of some of the hemostatic proteins discussed earlier in the chapter is shown in *Figure 5.8*. This alignment shows that some residues are absolutely conserved, some positions are occupied only by very similar amino acid residues (those giving the highest substitution scores in the PAM$_{250}$ matrix) and others are more variable. The most highly conserved residues are those whose physical and chemical properties are absolutely essential to maintain protein function. For example, the histidine residue sixth from the right is part of the catalytic triad of the enzyme, and is essential for the protein's ability to cleave peptide bonds. As might be expected, it is conserved in all the sequences. Equally important is the

```
SecStructure    .....................bBBBBBb...-----.bBBBBBb.....bBBb.aaa.bba
THRB_HUMAN      LESYIDGRIVEGSDAEIGMSPWQVMLFRKSP----QELLCGASLISDRWVLTAAHCLLYP
THRB_BOVIN      FESYIEGRIVEGQDAEVGLSPWQVMLFRKSP----QELLCGASLISDRWVLTAAHCLLYP
THRB_MOUSE      LDSYIDGRIVEGWDAEKGIAPWQVMLFRKSP----QELLCGASLISDRWVLTAAHCILYP
THRB_RAT        LDSYIDGRIVEGWDAEKGIAPWQVMLFRKSP----QELLCGASLISDRWVLTAAHCILYP
LFC_TACTR       SDSPRSPFIWNGNSTEIGQWPWQAGISRWLADHNMWFLQCGGSLLNEKWIVTAAHCVTYS
FA9_RAT         EPINDFTRVVGGENAKPGQIPWQVILNGEIE------AFCGGAIINEKWIVTAAHCLK--
FA9_RABIT       QSSDDFTRIVGGENAKPGQFPWQVLLNGKVE------AFCGGSIINEKWVVTAAHCIK--
FA9_PIG         QSSDDFIRIVGGENAKPGQFPWQVLLNGKID------AFCGGSIINEKWVVTAAHCIEP-
FA7_BOVIN       NGSKPQGRIVGGHVCPKGECPWQAMLKLNGA------LLCGGTLVGPAWVVSAAHCFER-
FA7_MOUSE       NSSSRQGRIVGGNVCPKGECPWQAVLKINGL------LLCGAVLLDARWIVTAAHCFDN-
FA7_RABIT       GASNPQGRIVGGKVCPKGECPWQAALMNGST------LLCGGSLLDTHWVVSAAHCFDK-
PRTC_HUMAN      QEDQVDPRLIDGKMTRRGDSPWQVLLDSKK-----KLACGAVLIHPSWVLTAAHCMDE-
PRTC_RAT        EELELGPRIVNGTLTKQGDSPWQAILLDSKK-----KLACGGVLIHTSWVLTAAHCLES-
PRTC_MOUSE      DELEPDPRIVNGTLTKQGDSPWQAILLDSKK-----KLACGGVLIHTSWVLTAAHCVEG-
PSS8_HUMAN      CGVAPQARITGGSSAVAGQWPWQVSITYEGV------HVCGGSLVSEQWVLSAAHCFPS-
                     :   *          ***. :              **. ::    *:::*****.
```

Figure 5.8

Part of a multiple alignment of 15 serine protease sequences. Symbols at the bottom of each column indicate the degree of conservation at that residue position: * = completely conserved (same residue in each sequence), : = highly conserved (conserved residues in each sequence), . = partly conserved (predominantly conservative substitutions). Symbols at the top of each column indicate secondary structure predictions based on structural propensity (p. 118).

* Note that E can be calculated in different ways according to the search algorithm used. In this example, $E = Np$, where N is the number of sequences in the database. This is the calculation used by FASTA but other algorithms use different methods.

maintenance of the protein's tertiary structure, since this brings all the functionally critical residues into the correct relative spatial positions. In this respect there are two completely conserved cysteine residues, one adjacent to the aforementioned histidine residue and one just to the right of the sequence gap. These are conserved because they form a disulfide bridge, which is essential for holding two parts of the polypeptide backbone in the correct relative positions. There is also a conserved proline residue, proline having an unusual side chain which allows the formation of *cis*-peptide bonds, therefore influencing the way the polypeptide backbone folds. There are also highly conserved residues in the secondary structural elements, and we return to this subject in the next chapter.

There are several software packages that can be used for multiple sequence alignment, perhaps the most commonly used of which is ClustalW/X. These programs use progressive alignment strategies in which pairwise alignments are carried out first to assess the degree of similarity between each sequence and then to produce a dendrogram of these relationships, which is similar to a phylogenetic tree. The two most similar sequences are aligned first and the others are added in order of similarity. The advantage of this method is its speed, but a disadvantage is that information in distant sequence alignments that could improve the overall alignment is lost. In many cases, the multiple alignments have to be adjusted manually, e.g. to bring conserved cysteine residues into register when it is known that such residues are involved in disulfide bonds.

5.4   Finding more distant relationships

The standard similarity search algorithms discussed above are able to detect sequences showing 30% similarity with reasonable reliability. However, as sequences begin to diverge even further, the evolutionary relationships between proteins are more difficult to detect. We know proteins with very little sequence similarity are related because, as discussed in the following chapter, protein structure is much more strongly preserved in evolution than sequence. The globin family provides many examples of proteins that are structurally very similar, functionally conserved (they are all oxygen carriers) but are barely recognizable as homologs at the sequence level. Recently, new bioinformatic methods have been developed which help to probe these relationships more effectively. Some of these methods are discussed below.

5.4.1   PSI-BLAST

PSI-BLAST (position-specific iterated BLAST) is an extension of the basic pairwise search program and can identify three times as many related proteins as standard BLAST. The principle of PSI-BLAST is iterated database searching, where the results of a standard BLAST search are collected into a profile, which is then used for a second round of searching. The process can be repeated for a defined number of cycles as determined by the user, or it can be repeated indefinitely until no more hits are obtained. The theoretical basis of PSI-BLAST is outlined in *Figure 5.9*. Essentially, a given query sequence A will find any sequences that show a significant degree of similarity (B, C, D) but would be less likely to find sequences that are more distantly related (E, F, G). However, if B, C and D are used

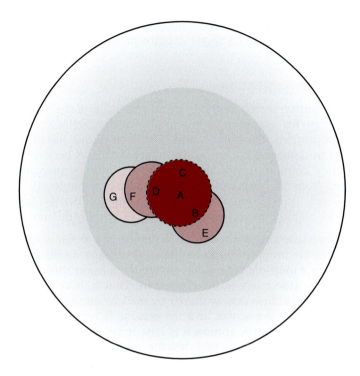

Figure 5.9

Theoretical basis of PSI-BLAST. The largest circle represents the whole of sequence space. The smaller gray circle represents all sequences that are homologous to the query sequence A, which is placed in the center of the diagram. The red inner circle with a broken circumference incorporates all sequences that will be identified when A is used as a query in a standard BLAST search. Sequences E, F and G, which are more distantly related to A, will not be identified in this initial search. However, sequence F would be identified if D was used as the query and sequence E would be identified if sequence B was used as the query. By combining A to D in a sequence profile, the next search should identify E and F. A further iteration would identify G, because the features of F would be included in the profile.

as the search queries, the threshold of detection would be extended to include E and F. Therefore a profile including sequences A—D should identify E and F. In the next iteration, a profile that includes all the sequences from A to F should identify G.

   While extending the power of standard BLAST searching, one problem with PSI-BLAST is its tendency to identify spurious matches. This often results from the incorporation of false-positive matches early in the process, which progressively contaminate further iterations with their own relatives. For example, if the original query sequence identifies a multi-domain protein which shares one domain (X) with the query sequence and a second unrelated domain (Y) the resulting profile will incorporate both domains. Further iterations will identify proteins containing the Y domain that are completely unrelated to domain X. Indeed this method, known as the Rosetta stone method, is sometimes used to functionally annotate bacterial genomes since multidomain proteins in one species are often represented by several single domain proteins in others (p. 137).

5.4.2 Pattern recognition

Pattern recognition search methods are an extension of the multiple alignment strategy for identifying structurally and functionally conserved elements of proteins. The information from such studies has been distilled and stored in databases known as secondary databases because the information they contain is not derived directly from sequencing, but is assimilated from the primary sequence databases (Chapter 1). There are many different ways of representing the information derived from multiple sequence alignments and different databases employ different methods.

- *Consensus sequences.* A consensus sequence is a single sequence that represents the most common amino acid residues found at any given position in a multiple alignment. Generally, a lower threshold is set to improve the stringency of the consensus. That is, if at any given position no single amino acid is shared by 60% or more of the sequences, then there is no consensus and the residue is represented by X. The major drawback of this approach is that it does not take into account conservative substitutions (e.g. leucine, isoleucine and valine) which would be informative. In addition, it biases the consensus in favor of any sequence family that predominates in the alignment. A consensus sequence for the last few residues of the protein alignment shown in *Figure 5.8*, for example, would be W–V–X–T–A–A–H–C. Note that the initial tryptophan and the last four residues are invariant, the valine and threonine are the consensus residues for the second and fourth positions because the alternative residues (isoleucine and serine, respectively) are in the minority. The big surprise is the X in the third position. This occurs because approximately half the residues are leucine and half are valine, i.e. there is no consensus. Due to these disadvantages, consensus sequences are rarely used in protein databases.
- *Sequence patterns.* Sequence patterns are like consensus sequences except that variation is allowed at each position and is shown within brackets. For example, the sequence pattern equivalent to the above consensus sequence would be W–[VI]–[LV]–[ST]–A–A–H–C. Sequence patterns are found in the PROSITE database (see *Table 5.2*), although the actual pattern for the above protein family would be shown as W–[LIVM]–[ST]–A–[STAG]–H–C, representing further variations found in other sequences that are not listed in *Figure 5.8*. Although variation is allowed, probabilities are not shown. Therefore, the fact that valine and isoleucine are equally represented at the second position but methionine is comparatively rare is not evident. The PROSITE sequence patterns are generally shorter than consensus sequences and can therefore be useful in assigning distant homologs to protein families when only the most conserved regions remain. However, their very shortness can lead to false assignments, even when common patterns such as those involved in post-translational modification are taken into account.
- *Motifs and blocks.* These are not individual sequences but multiply-aligned ungapped segments derived from the most highly conserved

Table 5.2 Secondary sequence databases containing sequences relating to protein domain families, and a selection of protein family classification databases whose data are based on those classifications

Database	Contents	URL
PROSITE	Sequence patterns associated with protein families and longer sequence profiles representing full protein domains.	http://ca.expasy.org/prosite
PRINTS, BLOCKS	Highly conserved regions in multiple alignments of protein families. These are called motifs in PRINTS and blocks in BLOCKS	http://bioinf.man.ac.uk/dbbrowser/PRINTS http://www.blocks.fhcrc.org
Pfam, SMART, ProDom	Collections of protein domains	http://www.sanger.ac.uk/Software/Pfam http://smart.embl-heidelberg.de/ http://prodes.toulouse.inra.fr/prodom/current/html/home.php
Superfamily	HMM library and genome assignments	http://supfam.org/SUPERFAMILY/
PROT-FAM	Protein sequence homology database	http://www.mips.biochem.mpg.de/desc/protfam/
ProClass and iProclass	Protein classifications based on PROSITE patterns and PIR superfamilies	http://pir.georgetown.edu/iproclass/ http://pir.georgetown.edu/gfserver/proclass.html
ProtoMap	Automatic hierarchical classification of all SWISS-PROT and TrEMBL sequences	http://protomap.cornell.edu/
SYSTERS	Protein families database	http://systers.molgen.mpg.de/
InterPro	A search facility that integrates the information from other secondary databases	http://www.ebi.ac.uk/interpro/

Individual URLs are shown but most of the above can be reached from the ExPASy website at http://www.expasy.ch/ or through direct links in search results from InterPro. (HMM, hidden Markov model.)

regions in protein families. They are found in two databases: PRINTS (where they are called motifs) and BLOCKS (where they are called, eponymously, blocks). In PRINTS, individual motifs from a single protein family are grouped together as fingerprints (*Figure 5.10*). Because the fingerprints are larger than PROSITE patterns and the search process uses an amino acid substitution matrix, relationships that are more distant can be identified in the PRINTS database than in PROSITE.

- *Domains*. A protein domain is an independent unit of structure or function which can often be found in the context of otherwise unrelated sequences. A number of databases have been established to catalog protein domains including ProDom, which lists the sequences of known protein domains created automatically by searching protein primary sequence databases. Other databases also contain elements of

Motif 1	Motif 2	Motif 3	Motif 4
GYVSALYDYDA	DELSFDKDDIISVLGR	EYDWWEARSL	KDGFIPKNYIEMK
YTAVALYDYQA	GDLSFHAGDRIEVVSR	EGDWWLANSL	YKGLFPENFTRHL
RWARALYDFEA	EEISFRKGDTIAVLKL	DGDWWYARSL	YKGLFPENFTRRL
PSAKALYDFDA	DELSFDPDDVITDIEM	EGYWWLAHSL	YKGLFPENFTRRL
EKVVAIYDYTK	DELGFRSGEVVEVLDS	EGNWWLAHSV	VTGYFPSMYLQKS

Figure 5.10

Example sequences of the four conserved motifs that define the SH3 domain, as shown in the PRINTS database. These represent the most conserved regions from the multiple alignment of many SH3 domains. Only five examples are shown, and many further examples can be found in the database itself.

protein domains. PROSITE, for example, lists sequence profiles corresponding to domain sequences, with weight matrices showing the likelihood of particular amino acids being found at each position. Pfam and SMART contain multiple domain alignments and hidden Markov models, which are among the statistically most sophisticated tools for representing protein domains as they can model the likelihood that a particular sequence belongs to a given domain family.

Each of the above secondary databases has its strengths and weaknesses, which can make the interpretation of results from different databases quite difficult. To resolve this problem, an integrated cross-referencing tool called InterPro has been developed which allows a query sequence to be screened against all of the databases and then extracts and presents the relevant information. An example InterPro search using the human urokinase-like plasminogen activator sequence is shown in *Plate 4*.

5.5 Pitfalls of functional annotation by similarity searching

Standard similarity searches, recursive methods and pattern or profile searching can all identify sequences which are more or less related to a particular query. However, these methods are not foolproof and all have the potential to come up with spurious matches or annotations. One of the most pressing dangers is database pollution. Databases contain errors, so annotating a new sequence on the basis of database information alone can sometimes serve only to reinforce and propagate misinformation. Some databases contain better-quality data than others, primarily reflecting the degree of manual curation. The SWISS-PROT database is actively managed and the data quality is very high, while the less-robust TrEMBL database contains translations of all the sequences in the EMBL nucleotide database but with lower-quality automatic annotations. The TrEMBL database is used to store protein sequences that are awaiting annotation and are not already deposited in SWISS-PROT.

Errors can also be introduced by the user if the similarity search algorithms are not understood properly. An example is the use of PSI-BLAST with an *E* value cutoff that is not stringent enough. This results in the incorporation of low-quality alignments in the profile used for the next round of searching. The bad seed can grow, resulting in a large collection of false positives that bear no relationship to the original query sequence.

As stated earlier in this chapter, another drawback to similarity searching is that sequence conservation does not always predict functional conservation. Although bioinformatics is based on the paradigm of similar sequence/similar function, this is only an axiom; the entire rationale of molecular evolution depends on the principle that sequences diverge and become functionally different. There are many examples of proteins that show strong sequence conservation but quite different functions. The enzyme lysozyme and the regulatory protein α-lactalbumin provide one example. There are also proteins that have entirely different sequences but perform essentially the same function, such as the diverse collection of mundane metabolic enzymes that have been recruited as crystallins in the lens of the vertebrate eye. It is also necessary to watch out for low-complexity sequences, i.e. sequences such as transmembrane domains that are present in many proteins with extremely diverse functions.

5.6   Alternative methods for functional annotation

In any genome project, a stubborn minority of sequences resists all forms of functional annotation by homology searching. In the case of the yeast genome project, for example, 30% of the predicted 6000 proteins were previously known and had been functionally characterized in experiments while another 30% could be assigned tentative functions, although in many cases only at the biochemical level, by homology searching. This left 30% of the proteins completely uncharacterized, the remaining 10% being regarded as unsafe predictions (questionable open reading frames) (see *Figure 1.2* p. 3). The anonymous proteins were placed into two categories:

- Hypothetical proteins, the products of orphan genes, which are predicted protein sequences that do not match any other sequence in the databases.
- Members of orphan families, i.e. predicted protein sequences with homologs in the databases, but the homologs themselves are of unknown function.

In some cases, expression-profiling experiments either at the mRNA level (Chapter 1) or at the protein level (Chapters 2–4) can help to provide some functional information about these proteins. Other strategies, including the investigation of protein structures and interactions, are discussed in Chapters 6 and 7.

Further reading

Attwood, T.K. and Parry-Smith, D.J. (1999) *Introduction to Bioinformatics.* Addison Wesley Longman, Harlow, UK.

Brenner, S.E. (1998) Practical database searching. *Bioinformatics: A Trends Guide* **5**: 9–12.

Davidson, D. and Baldock, R. (2001) Bioinformatics beyond sequence: mapping gene function in the embryo. *Nature Rev Genet* **2**: 409–417.

Eddy, S.R. (1998) Multiple-alignment and sequence searches. *Bioinformatics: A Trends Guide* **5**: 15–18.

Goodman, N. (2001) Biological data becomes computer literate: new advances in bioinformatics. *Curr Opin Biotechnol* **13**: 68–71.

Kanehisa, M. (1998) Databases of biological information. *Bioinformatics: A Trends Guide*, **5**: 24–26.

Lan, N., Montellione, G.T. and Gerstein, M. (2003) Ontologies for proteomics: towards a systematic definition of structure and function that scales to the genome level. *Curr Opin Chem Biol* **7**: 44–54.

Nagl, S.B. (2003) Function prediction from protein sequence. In: Orengo CA, Jones DT, Thornton JM (eds) *Advanced Text – Bioinformatics*. BIOS Scientific Publishers, Oxford, UK.

Orengo, C.A. (2003) Sequence comparison methods. In: Orengo CA, Jones DT, Thornton JM (eds) *Advanced Text – Bioinformatics*. BIOS Scientific Publishers, Oxford, UK.

Stein, L. (2001) Genome annotation: from sequence to biology. *Nature Reviews Genet* **2**: 493–503.

Valdar, W.S.J. and Jones, D.T. (2003) Amino acid residue conservation. In: Orengo CA, Jones DT, Thornton JM (eds) *Advanced Text – Bioinformatics*. BIOS Scientific Publishers, Oxford, UK.

Westhead, D.R., Parish, J.H. and Twyman, R.M. (2002) *Instant Notes in Bioinformatics*. BIOS Scientific Publishers, Oxford, UK.

Internet resources

National Center for Biotechnology Information homepage, a resource for public databases, bioinformatics tools and applications: http://www.ncbi.nlm.nih.gov/

The EMBL European Bioinformatics Institute outstation, a resource for biological databases and software: http://www.ebi.ac.uk/

The ExPASy (Expert Protein Analysis System) Molecular Biology Server, maintained by the Swiss Institute of Bioinformatics (SIB), provides links, databases and software resources for the analysis of protein sequences, structures and expression: http://www.expasy.ch/

BLAST and PSI-BLAST searches at NCBI: http://www.ncbi.nlm.nih.gov/BLAST

FASTA searches at EBI: http://www.ebi.ac.uk/fasta33/index.html

InterPro, integrated protein family databases, at EBI: http://www.ebi.ac.uk/interpro/

Kyoto Encyclopedia of Genes and Genomes: http://www.genome.ad.jp/kegg/

Gene Ontology Consortium database: http://www.geneontology.org/

Structural proteomics

6

6.1 Introduction

Proteins have evolved under selective pressure to carry out specific functions, and all of those functions depend, in one way or another, on interactions with other molecules. The way in which a protein interacts with the molecules in its environment depends critically on its three-dimensional structure or *fold* – the overall shape, the presence of clefts and cavities that complement particular ligands or substrates, the distribution of charges internally and over the surface, and the positioning of key amino acid residues. This book is not the place to find a detailed account of the principles of protein structure, although a brief overview is provided in *Box 6.1* and additional sources of information can be found in the Further Reading section. The important point here is that proteins with similar structures often have similar functions. Structures, like sequences, therefore have a predictive value in the assignment of protein functions.

In the past, structural analysis was only undertaken when the function of a protein was already well understood, but proteomics has revolutionized structural biology and brought it to the beginning of the investigative process. Structural proteomics* is concerned with the high-throughput determination of protein structures, with the ultimate aim of providing complete coverage of fold space. As is the case for proteomics in general, it has been realized that the protein universe is large but ultimately finite and with suitably large-scale approaches it can be studied and cataloged in a systematic fashion. In the future, hypothetical proteins (proteins whose functions are unknown and cannot be predicted by sequence comparisons) may have tentative functions assigned on the basis of structural analysis and structural comparison. Structural proteomics has demanded a revolution in the traditional methods for protein structure determination, and has also seen significant improvement in techniques for protein structure prediction. We discuss these methods and techniques in the first part of the chapter and then summarize the progress that has been made by structural proteomics initiatives around the world.

6.2 The value of protein structures in proteomics

6.2.1 Structure–function concordance

Both sequences and structures can be used to predict protein functions, but it is much easier to obtain sequences than structural data. At the end

---

* Structural proteomics is often termed 'structural genomics' in the current literature, but the reader should be careful when consulting earlier papers because the same term was originally used to refer to the physical phase of the genome projects, including the mapping of physical markers, the assembly of clone contigs, sequencing and gene annotation.

of 2002, the primary sequence databases contained over 22 million sequences, while the primary structural database, the Protein DataBank (PDB, http://www.rcsb.org), contained just over 20 000 structures. Many of the structures in the PDB are redundant, i.e. closely related proteins and even variants of the same protein created by point mutations, and there are fewer than 1000 unique folds. Therefore, sequence data exceeds structural data by over three orders of magnitude and would seem to be a much richer source of information than structures, so why bother with protein structures at all?

There are several reasons for using structures in addition to sequences for functional annotation, but perhaps the most important is that protein structures are far better conserved than sequences over evolutionary time. Proteins that show less than 10% sequence identity can have very similar structures, and structural comparisons can therefore reveal more distant evolutionary relationships than any of the sequence-based methods discussed in Chapter 5. This provides a valuable approach for the annotation of hypothetical proteins when sequence analysis is of no use, and it has been estimated that perhaps half of all hypothetical proteins could be assigned to protein families if their structures were available for comparison.

Let us consider two members of the globin superfamily: myoglobin and β-globin (a component of hemoglobin). These were among the first protein structures to be solved and they are strikingly similar, reflecting their evolutionary relationship and their conserved function as oxygen carriers (*Figure 6.1a*). Despite the obvious homology revealed by their structures, the sequences of human β-globin and myoglobin show only 26% identity (*Figure 6.1b*). There are likely to be thousands of hypothetical proteins with similar relationships to known proteins. Their sequences have diverged too far to be useful but their structures could identify previously unknown homologous relationships.

An example is the recent characterization of AdipoQ, a protein of originally unknown function that is secreted from adipocytes. Structural analysis of this protein showed a clear and unambiguous relationship to the tumor necrosis factor (TNF) family of chemokines and therefore suggested that AdipoQ is also a signaling protein. The structural relationship between AdipoQ and TNFα is shown in *Plate 5* along with a multiple sequence alignment of five superfamily members based on the conserved structures. Note that AdipoQ and TNFα show only 9% sequence identity, far below the level detectable by algorithms such as BLAST and FASTA, and similar to the level of conservation expected between completely unrelated proteins. Once the structures have been compared, however, it is easy to see the relationship between the proteins even at the sequence level, with several conserved residues at critical positions and ten aligned strings of amino acids that form β-strands.

The fact that apparently unrelated sequences can have similar structures indicates that the total number of protein folds should be much smaller than the total number of sequences. Additionally, since we know that the number of sequences is large but finite, it follows that the number of folds is also finite but not quite so large. Estimates as to the total number of protein folds in the structural universe vary from 4000–10 000, but it is clear that we have discovered only a fraction of them so far. The goal of structural proteomics is to find representative members of every protein fold

(a)

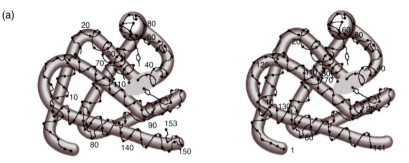

(b)

```
1      VLSPADKTNVKAAWGKVGAHAGEYGAEALERMFLSFPTTKTYFPHF----      46
       .||..:....|...||||.|....:|.|.|.|:|...|.|...|..|
1      GLSDGEWQLVLNVWGKVEADIPGHGQEVLIRLFKGHPETLEKFDKFKHLK     50


47     --DLSHGSAQVKGHGKKVADALTNAVAHVDDMPNALSALSDLHAHKLRVD    94
       |....|..:|.||..|..||...:..........:..|:..||.|.|.::
51     SEDEMKASEDLKKHGATVLTALGGILKKKGHHEAEIKPLAQSHATKHKI-   99


95     PVNF-KLLSHCLLVTLAAHLPAEFTPAVHASLDKFLASVSTVLTSKYR    141
       ||.:.:.:|.|::..|.:..|.:|.....:::|.|.......:.|.|:
100    PVKYLEFISECIIQVLQSKHPGDFGADAQGAMNKALELFRKDMASNYKELGFQG  153
```

Figure 6.1

(a) The three-dimensional structures of human myoglobin and β-globin are strongly conserved even though (b) the sequences are very different (26% identity, 39% similarity). The sequences were aligned using the EBI EMBOSS-Align program (http://www.ebi.ac.uk/emboss/align/). From Primrose and Twyman, 'Principles of Genome Analysis and Genomics' 3e, ©2002 Blackwell Publishing.

family, solve the structures and provide a template for comparison. This should allow the functional annotation of many hypothetical proteins even if sequence homology has dwindled to undetectable levels (*Figure 6.2*).

While structural comparisons and the identification of homologous relationships are perhaps the most useful applications of protein structures in proteomics, there are further benefits to the direct analysis of structures. First, structural analysis may reveal features of proteins that have obvious functional significance but which cannot be identified by studying the underlying sequence. Examples include the overall shape (which may reveal clefts and crevices that could function as ligand-binding pockets or active sites), the juxtaposition of particular amino acid side chains (which could reveal potential catalytic sites), the electrostatic composition of the surface (which may suggest possible interactions with other molecules) and the crystal packing of the protein (which may reveal possible interacting surfaces and biologically relevant multimeric assemblies). Additionally, the unexpected presence of a ligand, cofactor or substrate in a protein structure can provide the basis for a functional hypothesis. Some real examples from current structural proteomics initiatives are discussed later in the chapter. Finally, a direct application of structural proteomics is in the rational design of drugs, a topic we return to in Chapter 10.

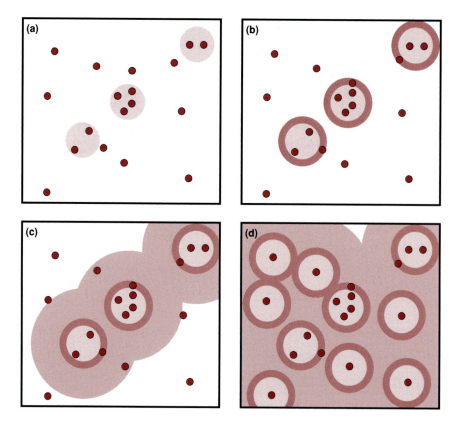

Figure 6.2

The goal of structural proteomics. Dots represent individual proteins. (a) In current sequence space, many proteins are orphans because their relationship to other proteins cannot be determined at the sequence level. Circles show proteins linked by sequence relationships. (b) Pattern and profile matching algorithms can extend the range of sequence analysis and discover new homologous relationships. (c) Known protein structures can extend these relationships even further, because structures are much more highly conserved than sequences. (d) Structural proteomics aims to solve enough structures so that all proteins can be related to other proteins.

6.2.2 Structure–function nonconcordance

Although protein structure is helpful in predicting functions, it should be emphasized that there is no simple, one-to-one relationship between structure and function. There are many examples of proteins with similar structures that have evolved to perform a myriad of different functions, such as the α/β hydrolase fold which is known to have at least six different enzymatic activities as well as turning up in a cell adhesion molecule (*Table 6.1*). This is similar to the situation discussed in Chapter 5, where proteins with conserved sequences were shown to carry out distinct functions. However, the problem of functional diversification is likely to be greater at the structural level because more distant evolutionary relationships can be identified.

Table 6.3 The universal genetic code. Amino acids are identified by their three-letter designation. Nonsense codons are identified by name. Note the dual functions of codons UAG and UGA. (Sec, selenocystenine; Pyr, pyrrolysine)

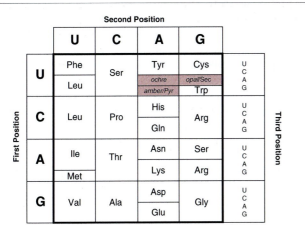

Table 6.1 Known functions associated with the a/b-hydrolase fold

Cholesterol esterase
Dienelactone hydrolase
Haloalkane dehalogenase
Neurotactin (cell adhesion molecule)
Non-heme chloroperoxidase
Serine carboxypeptidase
Triacylglycerol lipase

The fact that quite divergent sequences can adopt the same structure is useful for identifying distant evolutionary relationships, but it can also identify false relationships where functionally equivalent structures have evolved independently. Such structures are described as analogous rather than homologous, since they are not related by descent. Proteins can also be functionally analogous without any obvious homology. The enzyme glycosyl hydrolase, which is represented by at least seven distinct structures, provides a useful example (*Table 6.2*).

Table 6.2 Known structures associated with glycosyl hydrolase activity. (TIM, triose phosphate isomerase)

α/α toroid
Cellulase-like β/α-barrel
Concanavalin A-like two-layer β-sandwich
Double-psi β-barrel
Orthogonal α-bundle
Six-bladed β-propeller
TIM barrel

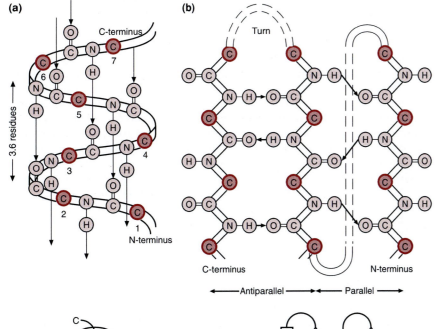

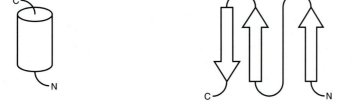

Figure 6.4

Common secondary structures in proteins: (a) the α-helix; (b) the β-sheet. Detailed molecular structures shown above; arrows show direction of hydrogen bonds. Topological structures shown below.

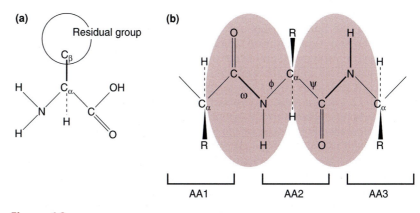

Figure 6.3

(a) General chemical structure of an amino acid. (b) Structure of the trans-peptide bond. (AA, amino acid.)

BOX 6.1

An overview of protein structure

Proteins are macromolecules composed of one or more polypeptides, each of which is a linear chain of amino acids. There are 20 standard amino acids specified by the genetic code plus at least two modified derivatives discovered thus far, selenocysteine and pyrrolysine, which are inserted in a context-dependent manner (see *Table 6.3*). Amino acids have a standard structure (*Figure 6.3a*) but chemically diverse residual groups or side chains, allowing the synthesis of proteins with a wide range of physicochemical properties (see *Figure 5.3* p. 88). Further diversity is generated by over 400 different types of post-translational modification (Chapter 8).

Primary structure
The sequence of amino acids in a polypeptide is known as the primary structure. The amino acids are joined together by peptide bonds, which usually adopt the *trans*-configuration such that the carbonyl oxygen and amide hydrogen of adjacent amino acids point away from each other (*Figure 6.3b*). The peptide bond itself is rigid, but the other bonds are quite flexible and allow the polypeptide backbone to fold in space. Exceptionally, proline residues have limited conformational freedom because the residual group is bonded to the main polypeptide backbone (indeed, strictly speaking, proline is an imino acid rather than an amino acid). Such residues are therefore also able to form *cis*-peptide bonds so the carbonyl oxygen and amide hydrogen of adjacent residues project in the same direction, although the *trans*-configuration is still preferred. This has a major influence on the folding of the peptide backbone and the substitution of proline residues with other amino acids inevitably has a significant effect on the overall structure. For this reason proline residues are often highly conserved in protein folds. Similarly, glycine residues are important because of their small residual group (a single hydrogen), which allows a much greater degree of flexibility than other residues. Cysteine residues are also highly conserved because they have the ability to form disulfide bridges, which help to stabilize the three-dimensional structure of individual polypeptide chains as well as joining discrete polypeptides together.

Secondary structure
Secondary structures in proteins are regular and repeating local configurations generated by intramolecular hydrogen bonds. These sometimes involve polar side chains (such as those of serine and threonine residues) but the polypeptide backbone itself is also polar because the NH group can act as a hydrogen donor while the C=O group can act as a hydrogen acceptor. The regular spacing of peptide bonds throughout the polypeptide chain allows regular, ordered structures to form. The two most common structures are the α-helix and the β-sheet (*Figure 6.4*). α-helices are usually right-handed and occur when hydrogen bonds form between peptide units four residues apart. This aligns the peptide bonds, giving the entire structure a significant dipole moment, but the bond angles are acute. α-helices vary in size from 4–40 residues, corresponding to 1–12 turns of helix. In contrast, β-sheets form from regions of the polypeptide chain where the bond angles are fully extended (these are known as β-strands). Several β-strands can align in parallel, antiparallel or mixed arrays, and hydrogen bonds form between peptide units in adjacent strands. Both α-helices and β-sheets may be joined together by linker regions that adopt their own secondary structures, and these are known as turns. For example, a β-turn is formed when a hydrogen bond forms between peptide units three residues apart. Where no hydrogen bonds are present, linker regions are known as loops. The core of a protein is often rich in secondary structures, because this allows energy-efficient packing, whereas loops are generally found on the surface where interactions can occur with the solvent.

Motifs (supersecondary structure)
Proteins are usually classified as being predominantly α-helical, predominantly β-sheet, mixed, and this often depends on the types of motifs that are present. A motif, at the seque level, is generally defined as a recognizable consensus sequence that represents a partic function (this applies to both nucleic acids and proteins). In structural biology, a motif group of secondary structures that are found connected together and perform a comm function. Simple examples include the helix-turn-helix, which is often found in DNA-bind proteins, the helix-loop-helix, which acts as a dimerization interface, and the coiled coil, wl is often found in fibrous proteins such as keratin. More complex examples, which con more secondary structures, include the globin fold (eight α-helices), the Greek key (a f strand antiparallel β-sheet) and the αβ-barrel (in which several β-α-β motifs roll up in cylinder).

Tertiary structure (fold)
The tertiary structure, or fold, of a polypeptide is its overall shape, reflecting the way secondary structures and motifs pack together to form compact domains. A domain ca regarded as a part of a polypeptide chain that can fold independently into a stable ter structure. Domains are also defined as units of protein function. A protein may contain a si domain, or multiple domains, and in the latter case the different domains can carry out dis biochemical functions in the context of the overall biological function of the protein. As st above, disulfide linkages between cysteine residues are often required to maintain ter structures.

Quaternary structure
Many proteins are single polypeptides, but others are composed of multiple polype subunits. The way these subunits assemble determines the protein's quaternary struc There is no functional difference between a multidomain protein and protein with se different polypeptide subunits, and many proteins can exist in both forms. For example, transcription factors are single polypeptides with DNA-binding and transcriptional activ domains, but others assemble from independent subunits. Indeed, the assembly of a scription factor from interacting subunits is the basis of the yeast two-hybrid system detecting binary protein interactions (see p. 147). Protein subunits may interact noncoval or may be joined together by inter-polypeptide disulfide bridges.

Protein folding
Like all physical and chemical reactions, protein folding is driven by the need to attain a of minimum thermodynamic free energy with respect to the surrounding solvent mole This ideal state is known as the native conformation of the protein and is generally the in which the protein is functional. For every native state there is an infinite number of tured conformations. Protein folding therefore cannot involve a random search throu these possible conformations, as this would take an infinite amount of time (the Lev paradox). In other words, protein folding must follow a defined pathway, perhaps by ing a framework of local secondary structures or perhaps by condensing around a s nucleation point. One of the major determinants of protein folding, at least in gl proteins, is hydrophobic collapse – the formation of a central core of hydrophobic re excluded from contact with the solvent. Experiments with some proteins have identified mediate folding states, such as the molten globule which lacks tertiary structure but is secondary structures, providing support for the framework and collapse models. Ho several small proteins have been shown to undergo single-step global folding, which with the nucleation model. It is also notable that many proteins cannot attain their states spontaneously, and require the assistance of specialized enzymes called mc chaperones that catalyze the latter stages of the folding process.

6.3 Techniques for solving protein structures

It is not yet possible to predict the tertiary structure of a protein *de novo* from its sequence without some form of pre-existing structural data (see below). Therefore, the only way to determine the structure of an otherwise uncharacterized protein with any degree of confidence is to solve it experimentally. The two major techniques that can be used for this purpose are X-ray crystallography (XRC) and nuclear magnetic resonance (NMR) spectroscopy. More than 98% of the structures in the PDB have been solved using one of these two methods, and most of the remaining 2% are theoretical models based on XRC or NMR structures. Fewer than 100 protein structures in total have been solved using other methods, which include neutron diffraction, electron diffraction and electron microscopy.

Both X-ray crystallography and NMR spectroscopy are notoriously demanding, and the precise experimental conditions must be determined empirically for each protein. The preparation of protein crystals for XRC is regarded almost as an art form, and many attempts to determine protein structures fail because suitable crystals are unavailable. In the case of NMR spectroscopy, which is carried out on proteins in solution, the proteins must be stable and soluble at high concentrations and must not aggregate or denature under these conditions. Each technique involves the collection and processing of large amounts of data and the painstaking assembly of a model or models that agree with these empirical results to generate atomic coordinates. Neither method, at a first glance, appears suitable for the type of high-throughput investigations undertaken in proteomics.

Like other analytical techniques, however, both XRC and NMR spectroscopy have benefited from advances in technology and the development of highly parallel assay formats that allow many different conditions to be tested simultaneously. Advances in bioinformatics, which allow structural data to be processed and modeled more quickly than ever before, have also made an invaluable contribution to the structural proteomics field. We discuss the principles of XRC and NMR spectroscopy below and summarize the recent advances that have brought structural biology into the proteomics era. We then briefly consider some additional methods that are used to investigate protein structure.

6.3.1 X-ray crystallography

X-ray crystallography exploits the fact that X-rays are scattered, or diffracted, in a predictable manner when they pass through a protein crystal. X-rays are diffracted when they encounter electrons, so the nature of the scattering depends on the number of electrons that are present in each atom and the organization of the atoms in space. Like other waves, diffracted X-rays can positively or negatively interfere with each other. Therefore, when protein molecules are regularly arranged in a crystal, the interaction between X-rays scattered in the same direction by equivalent atoms in different molecules generates a pattern of spots, known as reflections, on a detector (*Figure 6.5*). These diffraction patterns can be used to build a 3D image of the electron clouds of the molecule, which is known as an electron density map. The structural model of the protein is built within this map.

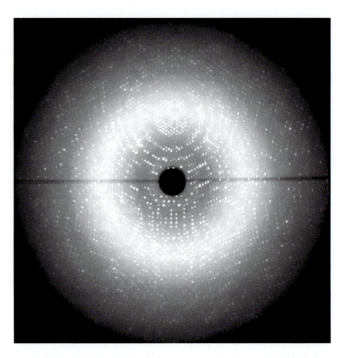

Figure 6.5

Pattern of reflections generated by a protein phosphatase crystal. Picture courtesy of Daniela Stock, MRC Laboratory of Molecular Biology, Cambridge.

Accurate structural determination requires a well-ordered crystal that diffracts X-rays strongly. This can be a significant bottleneck in structural determination because, as discussed above, protein crystals can be extremely difficult to grow. Hydrophobic proteins or proteins with hydrophobic domains are the most difficult to crystallize, and for this reason the PDB contains relatively few structures of complete membrane proteins, since these possess hydrophobic transmembrane domains. One of the major advances that has helped to increase the throughput of XRC is the development of automated crystallization workstations, which allow thousands of different parameters – e.g. different protein concentrations, salt concentrations, temperatures and pH – to be tried at the same time in order to identify the best crystallization condition. Smaller sample volumes can also be used, allowing crystallization studies with nonabundant proteins.

The next problem encountered in XRC is the calculation of an electron density map from the diffraction patterns. This process requires three pieces of information: the wavelength of the incident X-rays (which is already known), the amplitude of the scattered X-rays (which can be determined by the intensity of the reflections) and the phase of diffraction. Unfortunately, the phase cannot be determined from the pattern of reflections, and this has come to be known as the phase problem. Sometimes it is possible to 'borrow' phases from related solved structures already in the protein database, an approach known as molecular replacement. More usually, however, further experiments are carried out to determine the diffraction phases. The standard approach is to produce heavy atom-containing isomorphous crystals, i.e. crystals of the same overall structure incorporating heavier atoms that produce alternative diffraction patterns. This is done by soaking the crystals in a heavy metal salt solution so that heavy metal atoms diffuse into the spaces originally occupied by the solvent and bind to defined sites in the protein. Metal atoms diffract X-rays more strongly than the atoms normally found in proteins because they contain more electrons. By comparing the reflections generated by several different isomorphous crystals (a process termed multiple isomorphous replacement, MIR) the positions of the heavy atoms can be worked out and this allows the phase of diffraction in the unsubstituted crystal to be deduced. A complete description of each reflection – wavelength, amplitude and phase – is known as a structure factor.

More recently, this rather laborious process for determining structure factors has been superseded by methods that rely on the phenomenon of anomalous scattering. This occurs when heavy metal atoms in a protein crystal are struck by X-rays whose wavelength is close to their natural absorption edge, causing them to re-emit some of the energy as further X-rays. The magnitude of anomalous scattering varies with the wavelength of the incident X-rays, so one type of metal-containing crystal can be bombarded at several different wavelengths and different diffraction patterns obtained from which the phase of scattering can be calculated. This is the basis of techniques such as SIRAS (single isomorphous replacement with anomalous scattering) and MAD (multiple wavelength anomalous dispersion). A streamlined approach, which avoids the necessity for crystal soaking, is to express the protein in bacteria and incorporate a metal-substituted amino acid derivative, such as selenomethionine. In each case, the differences in the intensities of the reflections caused by anomalous scattering are very small. Therefore, synchrotron radiation sources are required, which produce high-intensity X-ray beams that can be tuned precisely. The availability of synchrotrons with robotized crystal-mounting and alignment systems, and beamlines and detectors of steadily increasing performance, has been instrumental in the acceleration of protein structure determination over the last few years.

Finally, a structural model is built into the electron density map. This requires one more crucial piece of information – the amino acid sequence – because carbon, oxygen and nitrogen atoms cannot be distinguished with certainty by X-ray diffraction so amino acid side chains are difficult to identify. The resulting model is a set of XYZ atomic coordinates, assigned to all atoms except hydrogens (XRC cannot resolve the positions of hydrogen atoms and where these are present in crystal structures they have been added by modeling after the structure was determined). The more data used to create the electron density map, the greater the degree of certainty about the atomic positions and the higher the resolution of the model. Even so, there may be areas of the protein for which atomic positions cannot be determined precisely. Each atom is assigned a so-called temperature factor, which is a measure of certainty. The higher the temperature factor, the lower the certainty. High temperature factors indicate either a degree of disorder (i.e. the particular atom was in different relative positions in different protein molecules within the crystal) or dynamism (i.e. the particular atom had the tendency to vibrate around its rest position).

The combination of high-throughput expression systems, highly parallel protein crystallization workstations, synchrotron radiation sources, data collection by MAD and improvements in the computer handling of diffraction data mean that the time from protein availability to high-resolution model has now been reduced from months or years to a matter of hours. In the best-reported case, a protein structure has been determined in 30 minutes. This is essential in structural proteomics initiatives, where progress from protein isolation to structural resolution can be viewed as a production pipeline fed with proteins at one end and yielding structures at the other.

6.3.2 Nuclear magnetic resonance spectroscopy

Nuclear magnetic resonance (NMR) is a phenomenon that occurs because some atomic nuclei have magnetic properties. In NMR spectroscopy these properties are utilized to obtain chemical information. Subatomic particles can be thought of as spinning on their axes, and in many atoms these spins balance each other out so that the nucleus itself has no overall spin. In hydrogen (^{1}H) and some naturally occurring isotopes of carbon and nitrogen (^{13}C, ^{15}N), the spins do not balance out and the nucleus possesses what is termed a magnetic moment. Quantum mechanics tells us that such nuclei can have one of two possible orientations, and under normal circumstances these orientations have the same energy. However, in an applied magnetic field, the energy levels split because in one orientation the magnetic moment of the nucleus is aligned with the magnetic field and in the other it is not (*Figure 6.6*). Where such energy separations exist, nuclei can be induced to jump from the lower-energy magnetic spin state to the less favorable higher-energy state when exposed to radio waves of a certain frequency. This absorption is called resonance because the frequency of the radio waves coincides with the frequency at which the nucleus spins. When the nuclei flip back to their original orientations, they emit radio waves that

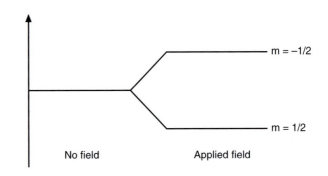

No field   Applied field

Figure 6.6

Energy levels in a nucleus with noninteger spin. In the absence of a magnetic field, the nucleus can exist in one of two orientations, each of which has the same energy. In an applied magnetic field, the energy levels split because in one orientation the magnetic moment of the nucleus is aligned with the field and in the other it is not. m is the magnetic quantum number.

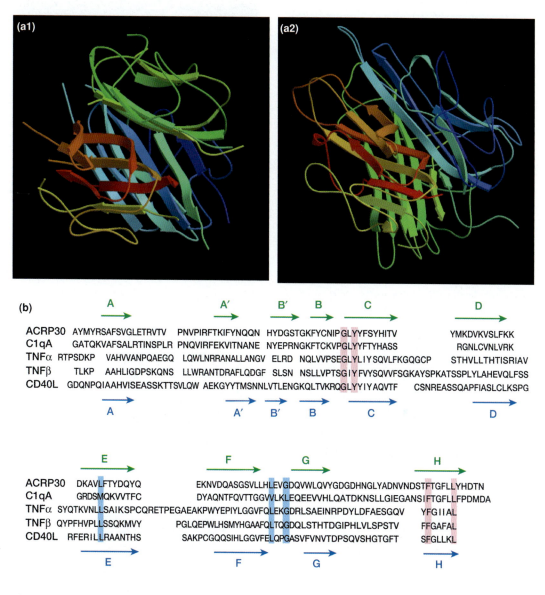

Plate 5

(a) A ribbon diagram comparison of AdipoQ and TNFα. The structural similarity is equivalent to that within the TNF family. (b) Structure-based sequence alignment between several members of the TNF family (CD40L, TNFα and TNFβ) and two members of the C1q family (C1qA and AdipoQ). Highly conserved residues (present in at least four of the proteins) are shaded, and arrows indicate β-strand regions in the proteins. There is little sequence similarity between AdipoQ and the TNF proteins (e.g. 9% identity between AdipoQ and TNFα) so BLAST searches would not identify a relationship. Modified from Current Opinion in Biotechnology, Vol. 11, Shapiro and Harris, 'Finding function through structural genomics', pp 31–35, ©2000, with permission from Elsevier. Images courtesy of Protein DataBank.

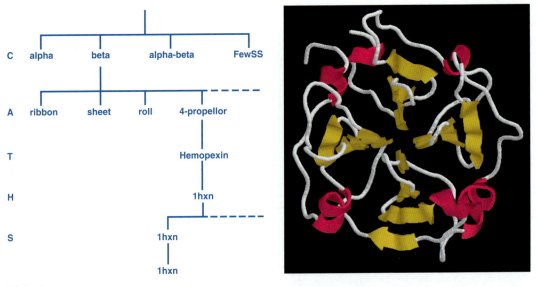

Plate 6

Structural classification of proteins using the CATH database. The protein shown is hemopexin, a protein rich in β-sheets with few α-helices. Courtesy of Christine Orengo.

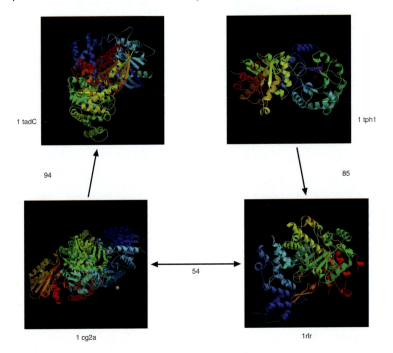

Plate 7

The Russian doll effect. Four proteins are shown that show continuous structural variation over fold space. Each of the proteins shares at least 74 structurally equivalent residues with its nearest neighbor, but the two extreme proteins show only 54 structurally equivalent residues when compared directly. Key: 1cg2A, carboxypeptidase G2; 1tadC, transducin-K; 1tph1, triose phosphate isomerase; 1rlr, ribonucleotide reductase protein R1. Courtesy of Protein DataBank. Reprinted by permission of Federation of the European Biochemical Societies from The role of protein structure in genomics, by Domingues *et al. FEBS Letters*, Vol 476, pp 98–102, ©2000.

can be measured. Protons (^{1}H) give the strongest signals, and this is the basis of protein structural analysis by NMR spectroscopy.

NMR spectroscopy is used to determine the structures of proteins in solution, and as discussed earlier this requires that the proteins are both highly soluble and stable. Solutions of approximately 1 mM are required and relatively large volumes (1–5 ml) are necessary. Structures can be determined by NMR spectroscopy because the magnetic resonance frequency of each nucleus is influenced by nearby electrons in bonded atoms, which generate their own magnetic fields. The external magnetic field strength must be increased to overcome this opposition, or shielding, and the degree of perturbation or chemical shift depends on the chemical environment of each nucleus. In this way it is possible to discriminate between hydrogen atoms in, for example, methyl and aromatic groups.

One-dimensional NMR experiments can detect chemical shifts and other shielding effects, such as spin–spin coupling, but are generally insufficient to characterize complex molecules like proteins. However, instead of using a single radio pulse, a sequence of pulses can be used separated by different time intervals. This gives a two-dimensional NMR spectrum with additional peaks indicating pairs of interacting nuclei. Three types of interactions can be measured by using different pulse sequences:

- COSY (correlation spectroscopy) detects sets of protons interacting through bonds, i.e. protons linked to adjacent bonded pairs of carbon or nitrogen atoms. This allows the experimenter to trace a network of protons linked to bonded atoms.
- TOCSY (total correlation spectroscopy) detects groups of protons interacting through a coupled network, not just those joined to adjacent bonded pairs of carbon or nitrogen atoms. TOCSY can often identify all the protons associated with a particular amino acid, but cannot spread to adjacent residues because there are no protons in the carbonyl portion of the peptide bond.
- NOESY (NOE spectroscopy) takes advantage of the nuclear Overhauser effect (NOE), i.e. signals produced by magnetic interactions between nuclei that are close together in space but not associated by bonds. This is most useful for determining protein structures because interactions can be identified between protons that are widely separated along the polypeptide backbone but close together in space due to the way in which the protein folds.

When these effects are taken into account, the result of NMR analysis is a set of distance constraints, which are estimated distances between particular pairs of atoms (either bonded or nonbonded). If enough distance constraints are calculated, the number of protein structures that fit the data becomes finite. Therefore, NMR analysis produces an ensemble of 10–50 models instead of a unique structure. Good NMR resonance depends on the protein molecule tumbling rapidly in the solvent, which limits the size of proteins that can be analyzed to those with fewer than 300 residues. More recently, the use of novel probes and high-frequency magnetic fields in the GHz range has allowed proteins up to 100 kDa in mass to be analyzed. Where proton NMR spectra are very crowded, analysis can be extended to other nuclei (e.g. ^{13}C and/or ^{15}N) to produce multidimensional and heteronuclear NMR spectra, which reduce data densities and help to eliminate ambiguities.

XRC tends to produce more accurate models than NMR although where both methods have been applied to the same protein there appears to be excellent agreement in the structures. This is probably because protein crystals have large water contents and thus exist in a similar state to solvated proteins. An important advantage of NMR is that it is possible to measure the dynamics of each residue with this method and it can therefore distinguish between regions of the protein that vibrate and those that are disordered. NMR also provides the positions of many hydrogen atoms, which is not possible with XRC.

6.3.3   Additional methods for structural analysis

While XRC and NMR spectroscopy are regarded as the gold standards for structural determination, various other methods have been used either to provide additional information about solved structures or to look at the structures of proteins that cannot be analyzed by XRC or NMR.

Circular dichroism spectrophotometry (CDS), for example, is a useful method for determining protein secondary structures. Circular dichroism (CD) is an optical phenomenon that occurs when molecules in solution are exposed to circularly polarized light. Asymmetric molecules such as proteins show different absorption spectra in left and right circularly polarized light, and this allows their secondary structures to be characterized. CDS using light between 160 and 240 nm generates distinct and characteristic spectra for proteins rich in α-helices and β-sheets respectively (*Figure 6.7*). Although CD spectrophotometry cannot determine protein tertiary structures, the technique is a useful complement to XRC and NMR spectroscopy in structural biology. Synchrotron radiation CD (SRCD) allows the rapid structural classification of large numbers of proteins.

Alternative methods that can be used to study tertiary structure include neutron diffraction and electron diffraction. Neutron diffraction is used much less frequently than X-ray diffraction because neutron sources are less

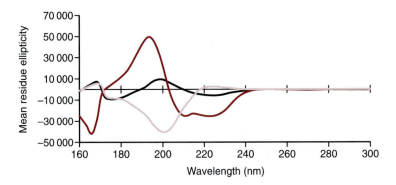

Figure 6.7

SRCD spectra of proteins representing primarily α-helical (myoglobin; red), β sheet (concanavalin A; black), and polyproline II helical (type VI collagen; pink) secondary structures, showing that substantial differences are present in the low-wavelength region. Reprinted from Current Opinion in Chemical Biology, Vol. 5, Wallace and Janes, 'Synchrotron radiation circular dichroism spectroscopy of proteins: secondary structure, fold recognition and structural genomics', pp 567–571, ©2001, with permission from Elsevier.

widely available and the flux of neutron beams is about ten orders of magnitude lower than that of X-ray beams. Neutrons are scattered by the nuclei of atoms in a protein crystal, rather than the electrons. The advantage of neutron scattering is that neutrons are scattered by hydrogen atoms, which cannot be 'seen' by X-rays. Neutron diffraction is therefore used to determine the positions of important hydrogen atoms, such as those in critical hydrogen bonds or catalytic sites. Electron diffraction is used to study proteins that crystallize or naturally assemble into two-dimensional arrays, but do not form orderly three-dimensional crystals. An example is tubulin, whose structure was solved by electron diffraction in 1998. This protein forms large flat sheets in the presence of zinc ions. Another advantage of electron microscopy is that single molecules can be analyzed in the same way as crystalline arrays, allowing the structures of large protein complexes to be determined without crystallization. The resolution is not usually as good as is possible with XRC, but since crystals are not required it is possible to work with small amounts of sample that are not completely pure. Although three-dimensional information is lost in an EM image, this can be reconstructed by repeating the analysis at many tilt angles. An interesting recent development is electron tomography, which can be used to study the structures of proteins and protein complexes inside the cell.

6.4 Techniques for modeling protein structure

Although the technology for solving protein structures has advanced significantly, it remains a labor-intensive and expensive process. An alternative, although somewhat less accurate, method for obtaining structural data is to predict protein structures using bioinformatic methods. At the current time, it is possible to predict secondary structures in hypothetical proteins quite accurately from first principles but tertiary structures require a template on which the model can be based.

6.4.1 Predicting protein secondary structures from sequence data

Secondary structure predictions are often known as three-state predictions because each residue in the sequence is categorized as helix (H), extended β-strand (E) or coil (C). Early methods for predicting secondary structures were based on the statistical likelihood of a particular amino acid residue appearing in a given type of structure. Some amino acids, such as glutamate, have a helical propensity (i.e. they are more likely to occur in α-helices than elsewhere in the protein) while others, such as valine, have a strand propensity (i.e. they are most abundant in β-strands and β-sheets). Some amino acids, such as leucine, are equally likely to appear in helices and strands. Glycine and proline residues, due to their unusual residual groups and the effects these have on the flexibility of the polypeptide backbone, are rarely found in secondary structures at all. Indeed they are often found at the ends of helices and strands and thus act as secondary structure breakers (*Table 6.4*). The appearance of a string of residues with helical or strand propensity strongly indicates the presence of such a structure in the protein. However, secondary structure predictions based on single proteins are unreliable because there are individual examples of all amino acids appearing in all types of secondary structure. Multiple alignments can remove much of this uncertainty by identifying conserved blocks of residues that favor the formation of helices or strands. Algorithms using neural networks to learn rules from such alignments have been employed successfully. Sophisticated structural prediction algorithms, such as PSI-PRED, use multiple alignments and also incorporate evolutionary and structural information from the databases in the form of sequence profiles to increase the accuracy of their predictions to over 75%. It should be noted that many of the incorrectly predicted residues occur at ambiguous positions, such as the ends of helices.

Accuracy in secondary structure predictions is generally expressed as the Q_3 score, which is the arithmetic mean of the correlation coefficients for helical, strand and coil predictions:

$$Q_3 = (C_h + C_s + C_c)/3$$

In the above equation, C_h is the correlation coefficient for helical predictions, C_s is the correlation coefficient for strand predictions and C_c is the correlation coefficient for coil predictions.

The helical correlation coefficient (C_h) is calculated as follows, and the same principles are used to calculate C_s and C_c:

$$C_h = \frac{ab - cd}{\sqrt{(a + c)\,(a + d)\,(b + c)\,(b + d)}}$$

In the above equation, a = number of residues assigned correctly as helix, b = number of residues assigned correctly as nonhelix, c = number

Table 6.4 Helical and strand propensities of the amino acids. A value of 1.0 signifies that the propensity of an amino acid for the particular secondary structure is equal to that of the average amino acid, values greater than one indicate a higher propensity than the average, and values less than one indicate a lower propensity than the average. The values are calculated by dividing the frequency with which the particular residue is observed in the relevant secondary structure by the frequency for all residues in that secondary structure

Amino acid	Helical (α) propensity	Strand (β) propensity
GLU	1.59	0.52
ALA	1.41	0.72
LEU	1.34	1.22
MET	1.30	1.14
GLN	1.27	0.98
LYS	1.23	0.69
ARG	1.21	0.84
HIS	1.05	0.80
VAL	0.90	1.87
ILE	1.09	1.67
TYR	0.74	1.45
CYS	0.66	1.40
TRP	1.02	1.35
PHE	1.16	1.33
THR	0.76	1.17
GLY	0.43	0.58
ASN	0.76	0.48
PRO	0.34	0.31
SER	0.57	0.96
ASP	0.99	0.39

of residues assigned incorrectly as helix and d = number of residues assigned incorrectly as nonhelix.

Another relatively simple way to predict the occurrence of α-helices in proteins is to construct a helical wheel, a diagram in which the positions of amino acids are plotted on a circle corresponding to the pitch of an ideal α-helix (*Figure 6.8*). In globular proteins, α-helices tend to exhibit the clustering of hydrophobic residues on one face of the helix and the clustering of polar residues on the other. However, the transmembrane domains of membrane-spanning proteins often contain α-helices composed predominantly of hydrophobic residues. Transmembrane helices can therefore be identified by scanning the protein sequence with a moving window of about 20 residues to identify highly hydrophobic segments.

6.4.2 Tertiary structure prediction by comparative modeling

The tertiary structure of a protein can be predicted from its sequence with reasonable accuracy if the structure of a closely related protein is available and can be used as a template. This approach is known as comparative modeling or homology modeling and generally works well if the two sequences show >30% identity over 80 or more residues.

The first step in comparative modeling is to find suitable templates, this is achieved by searching for homologous protein sequences and identifying those with solved structures. This is not always possible, and the main

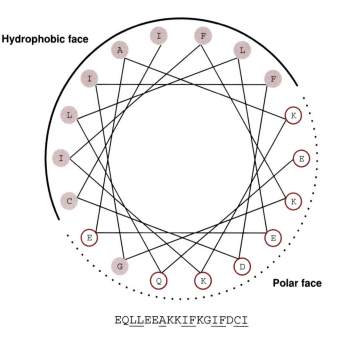

EQLLEEAKKIFKGIFDCI

Figure 6.8

This diagram shows a short amino acid sequence plotted in the form of a helical wheel. The hydrophobic amino acids are underlined in the sequence and shown shaded on the helical wheel. Glycine can be thought of as either hydrophobic or polar as it has no side chain.

limitation to comparative modeling as a structural prediction method is the lack of template structures. When a suitable template has been found, the sequences of the template protein(s) and query protein are aligned using an algorithm such as ClustalW/X (Chapter 5). Accurate alignment is critical for the accuracy in the resulting structural model. Therefore, better models are obtained with more closely related proteins. If the template and query protein are more than 70% identical, automatic alignment methods are suitable. As the percentage falls, so more human intervention becomes necessary. As discussed earlier, any residue known to be required for protein function (such as key residues in an active site) or to maintain structure (especially cysteine, glycine and proline residues; see *Box 6.1*) are likely to have conserved positions in the protein structure and should be aligned in the sequence. If multiple template structures are available, it is often appropriate to superimpose the structures and use the average atomic positions in the modeling template.

Although different software packages use slightly different methods, a common strategy is to identify residues in the template that are part of the protein's structural core and those forming surface loops. Generally, the positions of residues in the structural core are highly conserved because the core is rich in secondary structure. The loops are more variable and these often correspond to gaps in the sequence alignment, i.e. places where the template and query proteins have different numbers of residues. Structural prediction in the loop regions is therefore more difficult. A simple method is to use a so-called spare parts algorithm, which searches through databases of loop structures from other proteins. The query protein may not necessarily be related to any of the proteins in this database at any gross level, but particular loops of up to four residues in length may be analogous in sequence allowing their structures to be predicted. These structures are fitted into the model. The use of a spare parts algorithm may be combined with other methods that attempt to calculate the folding behavior of particular loops from first principles.

Once the path of the polypeptide backbone has been mapped, further algorithms are employed to predict the positions of the amino acid side chains. Where particular residues are conserved in the template and query sequence, the side chain positions can be based on those in the template. For nonconserved residues, algorithms are employed that attempt to fill space in the protein interior in the most energetically favorable manner. The initial model may be refined through the use of energy minimization software that makes minor adjustments to atomic positions to reduce the overall potential energy of the structure.

6.4.3 *Ab initio* prediction methods

The major disadvantage of comparative modeling methods is that only structures with suitable templates can be modeled. In contrast, *ab initio* methods aim to predict protein tertiary structures from first principles, i.e. in the absence of any structural information. A typical procedure would be to define a mathematical representation of a polypeptide chain and the surrounding solvent, define an energy function that accurately represents the physicochemical properties of proteins and use an algorithm to search for the chain conformation which possesses the minimum free energy.

The problem with *ab initio* methods is that even short polypeptide chains can fold into a potentially infinite number of different structures. If enough solvent molecules are incorporated into the model to make it realistic, the system becomes too complex to study without applying some knowledge of the behavior of known proteins. For this reason, *ab initio* methods are impractical as a method of structural prediction for polypeptides greater than about 200 residues. In the case of shorter polypeptides, recent results have been encouraging. For about a third of all polypeptides less than 150 residues in length that have been analyzed by such method, one of the resulting models was close enough to the true structure to identify it in the PDB. However, the resolution of each model was poor, and the practical applications of *ab initio* prediction remain limited.

6.4.4   Fold recognition (threading)

Although in theory a given polypeptide chain could adopt an almost infinite number of different conformations, good sense tells us that most of these would be energetically unfavorable and would never exist in nature. As discussed in *Box 6.1*, the way a protein chain folds – either by condensation around a nucleation site or through intermediate stages rich in secondary structure – also limits the total number of conformations that are possible. Finally, we know that the total number of protein folds in the structural universe is limited to a few thousand by the total number of sequences.

These observations and deductions suggest that searching the whole of conformational space looking for energy-efficient ways to fold a polypeptide chain is probably wasteful when only a few thousand energetically stable folds actually exist. Many hypothetical proteins are likely to have homologous structures in the PDB, but without sequence homology or empirical structural data such relationships cannot be recognized. Fold recognition (or threading) methods address this problem by detecting folds that can be used for structural modeling without homology at the sequence level.

The principle of fold recognition is the identification of folds that are compatible with a given query sequence, i.e. instead of sequences being used to predict folds, the folds are fitted to the sequence. This involves searching through a database of known protein structures, known as a fold library, scoring the folds and identifying candidates that fit the sequence, and aligning the query and best-scoring proteins. Once such a template has been identified, the remainder of the process is the same as comparative modeling. Fold recognition methods are generally based on both sequence similarity searches and structural information. For example, the 3D-PSSM method (three-dimensional position-specific scoring matrix) employs the PSI-BLAST algorithm to find sequences that are distantly related to the query protein and supplements this with secondary structure predictions (see above) and information concerning the tendency of hydrophobic amino acids to reside in the protein's structural core. Fold recognition methods are generally able to detect distantly related sequences but the accuracy of structural prediction is limited by errors in sequence alignment.

6.5   Comparing protein structures

Once the tertiary structure of a protein has been determined by X-ray crystallography or NMR spectroscopy, or modeled by comparative modeling techniques, it is deposited in the PDB and can be accessed by other researchers. As discussed at the beginning of the chapter, the key benefit of structural data in proteomics is the ability to compare protein structures and predict functions on the basis of conserved structural features. There are two requirements to fulfill this aim – an objective method for comparing protein structures and a system of structural classification that can be applied to all proteins, so that protein scientists in different parts of the world use the same descriptive language.

Several programs are available, many of which are free over the Internet, which convert PDB files into three-dimensional models (e.g. Rasmol, MolScript, Chime). Furthermore, a large number of algorithms have been written to allow protein structures to be compared. Generally, these work on one of two principles although some of the more recent programs employ elements of both. The first method is intermolecular comparison, where the structures of two proteins are superimposed and the algorithm attempts to minimize the distance between superimposed atoms (*Figure 6.9a*). The function used to measure the similarity between structures is generally the root mean square deviation (RMSD), which is the square root of the average squared distance between equivalent atoms (*Figure 6.9a*). The RMSD decreases as protein structures become more similar, and is zero if two identical structures are superimposed. Examples of such algorithms include Comp-3D and ProSup. The second method is intramolecular comparison, where the structures of two proteins are compared side by side, and the algorithm measures the internal distances between equivalent atoms within each structure and identifies alignments in which these internal distances are most closely matched (*Figure 6.9b*). An example of such an algorithm is DALI. Algorithms that employ both methods include COMPARER and VAST.

Similar methods are used to gauge the accuracy of structural models when the actual structures become available. When alignments are good, as is generally the case with comparative modeling, then very accurate models are possible. RMSDs of less than 1.0 Å represent very good predictions, since this is similar to the degrees of difference between two separate experimental determinations of the same protein structure. When the percentage sequence identity between template structures and target sequence exceeds 70% it is reasonable to expect that the model should be accurate to an RMSD of less than 2–3 Å even using completely automated methods. When the percentage identity drops below 40% then getting a good alignment, often with manual intervention, becomes more critical.

6.6   The structural classification of proteins

Functional annotation on the basis of protein structure requires a rigorous and standardized system for the classification of different structures. Several different hierarchical classification schemes have been established, which divide proteins first into general classes based on the proportion of various secondary structures they contain (predominantly α-helix, predominantly β-strand and mixed), then into successively more specialized groups based

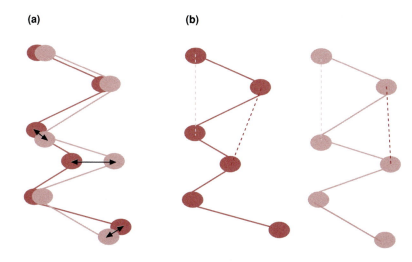

Figure 6.9

Comparison of protein structures, with circles representing Cα atoms of each amino acid residue and lines representing the path of the polypeptide backbone in space. (a) Intermolecular comparison involves the superposition of protein structures and the calculation of distances between equivalent atoms in the superimposed structures (shown as bi-directional arrows). These distances are used to calculate the root mean square deviation (RMSD), with the following formula

$$RMSD = \sqrt{\frac{1}{N}\Sigma_i d'^2_i}$$

where d_i is the distance between the ith pair of superimposed Cα atoms and N is the total number of atoms aligned. A small RMSD value computed over many residues is evidence of significantly conserved tertiary structure. (b) Intermolecular comparison involves side-by-side analysis based on comparative distances between equivalent atoms within each structure (shown as color-coded dotted lines).

on how those structures are arranged. These schemes are implemented in databases such as SCOP (Structural Classification of Proteins), CATH (Class, Architecture, Topology, Homologous superfamily) and FSSP (Fold classification based on Structure-Structure alignment of Proteins) with further examples listed in *Table 6.5*. An example SCOP classification, showing the structural classification hierarchy, is shown in *Plate 6*.

These databases differ in the way classifications are achieved. For example, the FSSP system is implemented through fully automated structural comparisons using the DALI program. CATH is semi-automatic, with comparisons carried out using the program SSAP, but the results of comparisons are manually curated. SCOP is a manual classification scheme and is based on evolutionary relationships as well as geometric criteria. Not surprisingly, the same protein may be classified differently when the alternative schemes are used. There is broad general agreement in the upper levels of the hierarchy, but problems are encountered when more detailed classifications are sought because this depends on the thresholds used to recognize fold groups in the different classification schemes.

Table 6.5 Internet resources for protein structural classification

Database	Location	Coverage (in January 2002)	Structure comparison algorithm	Type	Description	URL
3Dee	EBI, Cambridge, UK	7231 PDB entries	STAMP	Fully automatic – utilizes the SCOP classification	Multi-hierarchical classification of protein domains	http://jura.ebi.ac.uk:8080 3Dee/help/ help_intro.html
CAMPASS	Cambridge University, UK	4612 protein domains 1067 superfamilies	COMPARER	Mixture of SCOP superfamilies and those derived from the literature	**CAM**bridge database of **P**rotein **A**lignments organized as **S**tructural **S**uperfamilies. Contains a compilation of sequence alignments of proteins that belong to a superfamily	http://www-cryst.bio cam.ac.uk/~campass/
CATH	UCL, London, UK	13 938 PDB entries. 34 287 fully classified domains. 1386 superfamilies. 3 285 sequence families	SSAP	Semi-automatic. Some manual validation of homologous superfamilies required	CATH is a hierarchical classification of protein domain structures, which clusters proteins at four major levels, **C**lass, **A**rchitecture, **T**opology and **H**omologous superfamily	http://www.biochem. ucl.ac.uk/bsm/cath_new/
CE	SDSC, La Jolla, CA, USA	14 878 PDB entries. 28 687 chains	CE	Fully automatic. (Nearest neighbor)	Combinatorial **E**xtension of the optimal path Databases of pairwise alignments for all polypeptide chains, kept current within the PDB	http://cl.sdsc.edu/ce.html
DDD	EBI, Cambridge, UK	11 886 PDB entries 21 493 chains 35 492 domains	Dali	Fully automatic classification	**D**ali **D**omain **D**ictionary A structural classification of recurring protein domains. Domain boundaries are identified automatically by searching for topological recurrence in large, compact units from known protein structures	http://www2.ebi.ac.uk/ dali/domain/

Name	Location	Method	Contents	Classification	Description	URL
DHS	UCL, London, UK	SSAP, CORA	903 homologous superfamilies 22 295 domains	Fully automatic relies on CATH classification	Dictionary of Homologous Superfamilies Structural alignment of members of homologous superfamilies defined in the CATH database. Data are augmented with SWISS-PROT keywords and EC numbers	http://www.biochem.ucl.ac.uk/bsm/dhs
ENTREZ/ MMDB	NCBI, Bethesda MD, USA	VAST	~15 000 PDB entries ~35 000 chains ~50 000 domains	Fully automatic (Nearest neighbor)	MMDB contains pre-calculated pairwise comparison for each PDB structure. Integrated into ENTREZ	http://www.ncbi.nlm.nih.gov/Structure
FSSP	EBI, Cambridge UK	Dali	2977 sequence families 27 946 protein structures (chains)	Fully automatic (Nearest neighbor)	Fold classification based on Structure-Structure alignment of Proteins. Integrated sequence alignments	http://www.embl.ebi.ac.uk/dali/fssp/
HOMSTRAD	Cambridge University	COMPARER	2898 structures 864 families	Manual classification. Relying on SCOP, Pfam, PROSITE and SMART	(HOMologous STRucture Alignment Database) Database of annotated structural alignments for homologous families	http://www.cryst.boic.cam.ac.uk/~homstrad/
SCOP	LMB, MRC, Cambridge, UK	None	14 729 PDB entries 1007 superfamilies 35 685 domains 1699 families	Manual classification	A Structural Classification Of Proteins, Hierarchical classification of protein structure manually curated. The major levels in the classification are family, superfamily, fold and class	http://scop.mrc-lmb.cam.ac.uk/scop/

Additional problems that lead to confusion in the structural classification of proteins include the existence of so-called superfolds, such as the TIM barrel, which are found in many proteins with diverse tertiary structures and functions. It is necessary to distinguish between homologous structures (which are derived from a common evolutionary ancestor) and analogous structures (which evolved separately but have converged). Similarly, variations in the fold structure between diverse members of the same protein family can result in a failure to recognize homologous relationships. In its most extreme form, this can be seen as the Russian doll effect, which describes the continuous variation of structures between fold groups (*Plate 7*).

6.7 Structural proteomics: initiatives and results

Structural proteomics initiatives have been set up all over the world, some comprising dispersed laboratories working towards a common goal and some focused at particular centralized sites. In America, the National Institute of General Medical Sciences (NIGMS) has funded nine structural proteomics pilot centers, and several academic and industrial consortia have been established in America, Europe and Japan (see Further Reading). While the overall goal of structural proteomics is to provide representative structures for all protein families, various different approaches have been used to select an initial set of target proteins. Research has focused on microbes, which have smaller genomes (and thus smaller proteomes) than higher eukaryotes, but a fundamentally similar basic set of protein structures. Several groups have chosen thermophilic bacteria such as *Methanococcus jannaschii* for their pilot studies, on the basis that proteins from these organisms should be easy to express in *E. coli* in a form suitable for X-ray crystallography and/or NMR spectroscopy. A favorable strategy in model eukaryotes is to focus on proteins that are implicated in human diseases. Overall, the idea has been to choose structures that maximize the amount of information returned from the structural proteomics programs.

The progress of the structural proteomics projects is difficult to judge at present because the early years have been taken up largely by technology and infrastructure development. The overall aims can be summarized as shown in *Figure 6.10*. A common theme emerging from these projects is a 'funnel effect' in terms of the number of solved structures compared to the number of proteins chosen for analysis. This is due to the failure of a proportion of the target proteins at each stage of the analysis procedure (e.g. in the case of X-ray crystallography, the essential stages are: cloning, expression, solubilization, purification, crystallization, and structural determination). Despite an overall success rate that is probably no higher than 10% at present, a large number of structures have emerged from recently established and semi-automated production pipelines and the PDB is likely to expand quickly over the next few years as these structures are confirmed and deposited.

In principle, the value of the structural proteomics approach has been validated by the functional annotation of many of the initial hypothetical proteins chosen for structural analysis. For example, of the first ten proteins analyzed in the *Methanobacterium thermoautotrophicum* project, seven could be assigned a function due to structural similarity with known

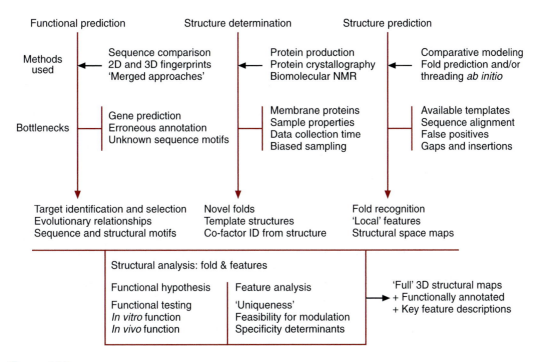

Figure 6.10

An overview of key factors impacting research programs in structural proteomics as well as their desired outcomes. Reprinted from Trends in Biotechnology, Vol. 20, Norin and Sundström, 'Structural proteomics: developments in structure-to-function predictions', pp 79–84, ©2002, with permission from Elsevier.

protein folds or other structural criteria, including the presence of bound ligands in the crystal (*Table 6.6*). The presence of a ligand or cofactor can often be helpful, and was instrumental in the functional annotation of *M. jannaschii* hypothetical protein MJ0577, the first structure to be generated in a structural proteomics initiative. In this example the crystal contained ATP, suggesting a role in ATP hydrolysis that was later confirmed by biochemical experiments. Therefore, even when the structure of a protein does not match any other in the database, structural analysis may still provide functional information that can be followed up with other experiments. Another interesting example is hypothetical protein TM0423, from *Thermotoga maritime*, which copurified and cocrystallized with a molecule of Tris buffer. In this case, the position of the buffer suggested that the protein would be able to bind to glycerol, and identified it as a glycerol hydrogenase.

While one goal of structural proteomics is to assign functions to hypothetical proteins on the basis of their relationship to known folds, another is to discover new folds and assemble a comprehensive directory of protein space. It appears that about 35% of the structures emerging from current structural proteomics initiatives contain novel folds, which confirms the hypothesis that protein space is finite and probably comprises at most a few thousand distinct structures. Every time a new fold is discovered, a little bit more of that protein space is filled. Furthermore, many of the new folds can be assigned functions because they bind particular ligands

Table 6.6 Some of the early structures determined by structural proteomics initiatives. (TIM, triose phosphate isomerase; eIF, eukaryotic initiation factor; FMN, flavin mononucleotide; NAD$^+$, nicotinamide adenine dinucleotide; PLP, pyridoxal phosphate.)

Target ID	Organisms	Technique	Fold family	Function
HI1434	H. influenzae	X-ray	Novel	Unknown
Maf	B. subtilis	X-ray	MJ0226-like	Nucleoside triphosphate binding
MJ0226	M. jannaschii	X-ray	Novel	Nucleoside triphosphate hydrolysis
MJ0541	M. jannaschii	X-ray	Unknown	Nicotinamide mononucleotide adenylyltransferase
MJ0577	M. jannaschii	X-ray	Adenine nucleotide-binding domain-like	ATP hydrolysis
MJ0882	M. jannaschii	X-ray	Rossmann fold	Unknown
MTH1048	M. thermoautotrophicum	NMR	Novel	Subunit in RNA polymerase II
MTH1175	M. thermoautotrophicum	NMR	Ribonuclease H-like	Unknown
MTH1184	M. thermoautotrophicum	NMR	Novel	Unknown
MTH0129	M. thermoautotrophicum	X-ray	TIM-barrel	Orotidine 5'-monophosphate decarboxylase
MTH0150	M. thermoautotrophicum	X-ray	Nucleotide binding	NAD$^+$ binding
MTH0152	M. thermoautotrophicum	X-ray	Novel	Ni^{2+} and FMN binding
MTH1615	M. thermoautotrophicum	NMR	Armadillo repeat	DNA binding, transcription factor
MTH1699	M. thermoautotrophicum	NMR	Ferredoxin-like	Transcription elongation factor
MTH0040	M. thermoautotrophicum	NMR	Three-helix bundle	Zn^{2+} binding, scaffold in RNA polymerase II
MTH0538	M. thermoautotrophicum	NMR	Rossmann fold	Mg^{2+} binding, putative ATPase
YbI036C	Yeast	X-ray	TIM barrel	PLP binding
Ycih	E. coli	NMR	eIF1-like	Translation initiation factor
YjgF	E. coli	X-ray	Bacillus chorismate mutase-like	Unknown
Yrdc	E. coli	X-ray	Novel	RNA binding

or have other properties, and this reveals new structure–function relationships that can be applied more widely. Sequence analysis and structural comparisons with these novel folds can identify previously unanticipated evolutionary relationships. At some point in the future, we may reach the stage where there is no such thing as an orphan gene or a hypothetical protein.

Further reading

Nature Structural Biology's *Structural Genomics Supplement Issue* (November 2000) contains a collection of informative reviews on structural genomics and can be accessed free on-line (see Internet resources below).

A further collection of very informative reviews about the organization of structural proteomics initiatives was published in Volume 73, Issue 2 of *Progress in Biophysics & Molecular Biology* (2000).

Aloy, P., Oliva, B., Querol, E., Aviles, F.X. and Russel, R.B. (2002) Structural similarity to link sequence space: new potential superfamilies and implications for structural genomics. *Protein Sci* **11**: 1101–1116.

Bork, P. and Koonin, E.V. (1998) Predicting functions from protein sequences – where are the bottlenecks? *Nature Genet* **18**: 313–318.

Brenner, S.E. (2001) A tour of structural genomics. *Nature Rev Genet* **2**: 801–809.

Burley, S.K. *et al.* (1999) Structural genomics: beyond the Human Genome Project. *Nature Genet* **23**: 151–157.

Campbell, I.D. (2002) Timeline: the march of structural biology. *Nature Rev Mol Cell Biol* **3**: 377–381.

Fiser, A. (2004) Protein structure modeling in the proteomics era. *Expert Rev. Proteomics* **1**: 97–110.

Heinemann, U. (2000) Structural genomics in Europe: slow start, strong finish? *Nature Struct Biol* **7**: 940–942.

Heinemann, U., Illing, G. and Oschkinat, H. (2001) High-throughput three-dimensional protein structure determination. *Curr Opin Biotechnol* **12**: 348–354.

Jones, D.T. (2000) Protein structure prediction in the postgenomic era. *Curr Opin Struct Biol* **10**: 371–379.

Lan, N., Montelione, G.T. and Gerstein, M. (2003) Ontologies for proteomics: towards a systematic definition of structure and function that scales to the genomic level. *Curr Opin Chem Biol* **7**: 44–54.

Lesley, S.A. *et al.* (2002) Structural genomics of the *Thermotoga maritima* proteome implemented in a high-throughput structure determination pipeline. *Proc Natl Acad Sci USA* **99**: 11664–11669.

Mittl, P.R.E. and Grutter, M.G. (2001) Structural genomics: opportunities and challenges. *Curr Opin Chem Biol* **5**: 402–408.

Murzin, A.G. (1998) How divergent evolution goes into proteins. *Curr Opin Struct Biol* **8**: 380–387.

Norin, M. and Sundstrom, M. (2002) Structural proteomics: development is structure-to-function predictions. *Trends Biotechnol* **20**: 79–84.

Sali, A., Glaeser, R., Earnest, T. and Baumeister, W. (2003) From words to literature in structural proteomics. *Nature* **422**: 216–225.

Stevens, R.C., Yokohoma, S. and Wilson, I.A. (2001) Global efforts in structural genomics. *Science* **294**: 89–92.

Terwilliger, T.C. (2000) Structural genomics in North America. *Nature Struct Biol* **7**: 935–939.

Yokoyama, S. *et al*. (2000) Structural genomics projects in Japan. *Prog Biophys Mol Biol* **73**: 363–376.

Zhang, C. and Kim. S.H. (2003) Overview of structural genomics: from structure to function. *Curr Opin Chem Biol* **7**: 28–32.

Internet resources

http://www.structuralgenomics.org/ NIGMS Protein Structure Initiative (PSI) homepage

http://www.spineurope.org/ Structural Proteomics in Europe (SPINE) homepage

http://www.rcsb.org/pdb/strucgen.html Protein Data Bank structural genomics page, with links to worldwide structural proteomics initiatives, meetings and funding sources

http://www.nature.com/nsb/structural_genomics/index.html Nature's structural genomics special supplementary issue, with free access

http://www.isgo.org/ International Structural Genomics Organization homepage

Interaction proteomics

7

7.1 Introduction

In the preceding chapter, we explored the link between protein structure and function, and showed that the tertiary structure of a protein determines the overall shape of the molecule, the distribution of surface charges and the juxtaposition of critical functional residues. Such residues might constitute the active site of an enzyme, the ligand-binding site of a receptor or the antigen-recognition domain of an antibody. The structure of a protein therefore influences its function by *determining the other molecules with which it can interact and the consequences of those interactions*. Protein interactions lie at the heart of most biological processes. Proteins may interact with small molecules, nucleic acids and/or other proteins. Indeed nearly all proteins are gregarious, functioning as part of larger complexes rather than working in isolation. Within such complexes the interactions between proteins may be static or transient, the latter often occurring in signaling and metabolic pathways. From the above it is clear that protein interactions and functions are intimately related, and it follows that the investigation of protein interactions can help in the functional annotation of uncharacterized, hypothetical proteins.

Interaction proteomics encompasses the investigation of protein interactions at multiple levels (*Figure 7.1*). The highest resolution methods are those we considered in the Chapter 6, i.e. X-ray crystallography and nuclear magnetic resonance spectroscopy. Such methods help to characterize interactions on the atomic scale, producing very detailed data that show the precise structural relationships between interacting atoms and residues. These methods can be used to study protein–protein interactions, but they are also useful for revealing interactions between proteins and small molecule ligands, substrates and cofactors. As discussed in the previous chapter, the presence of a bound ligand or cofactor may help to reveal the function of a hypothetical protein whose structure has been resolved (p. 127). Because of the detailed datasets produced by this type of analysis, however, atomic resolution methods are not yet applied to study protein interactions in a high-throughput manner. We do not discuss them further here.

The core of interaction proteomics is the study of direct interactions on the molecular scale. Methods for studying interactions between proteins can be divided into those that detect binary interactions (i.e. interactions between pairs of proteins) and those that detect complex interactions (i.e. interactions between multiple proteins that form complexes). These methods do not reveal the precise chemical nature of the interactions but simply report that such interactions take place. Many different techniques can be used to detect molecular interactions on a small scale but the major high-throughput technologies are the yeast two-hybrid system and its derivatives for binary interactions and systematic affinity purification followed by mass spectrometry for complex interactions (*Table 7.1*).

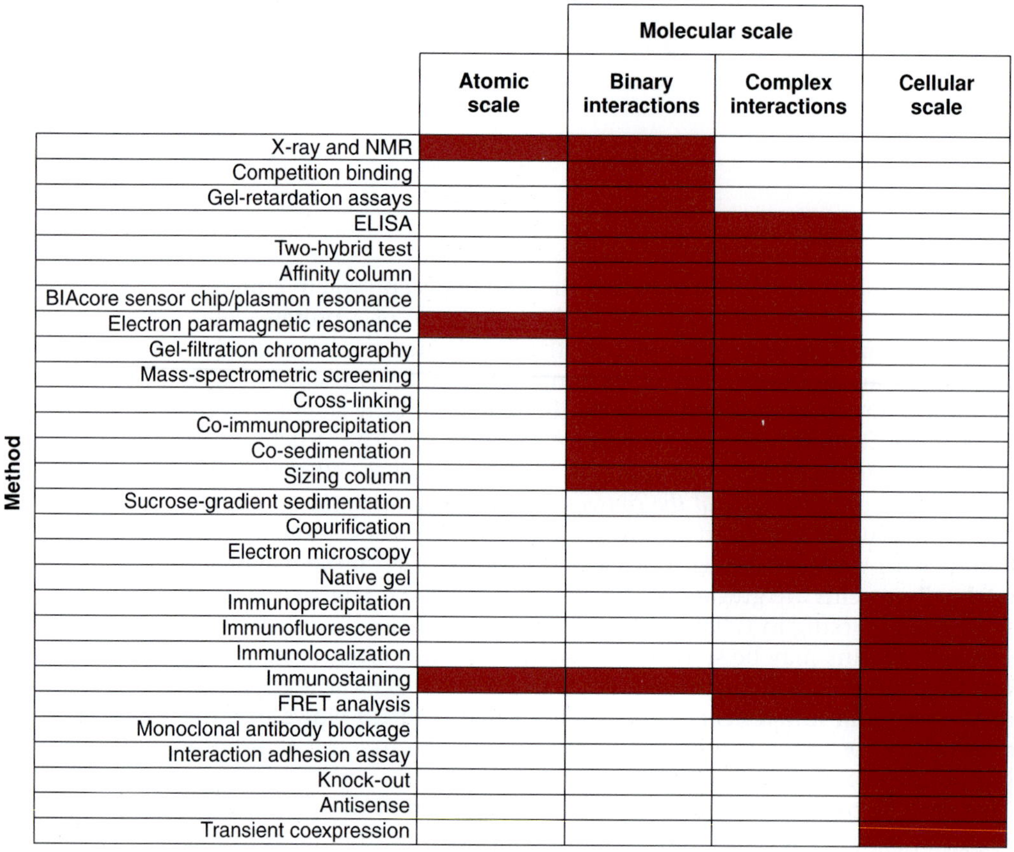

Figure 7.1

Methods to detect protein interactions have different resolutions from atomic, through molecular to cellular. The direct analysis of interactions on a molecular scale can focus on binary interactions (only two proteins) or complex interactions (more than two proteins). Reprinted from Current Opinion in Biotechnology, Vol. 12, Xenarios and Eisenberg, 'Protein interaction databases', pp 334–339, ©2001, with permission from Elsevier.

Protein chips are also emerging as useful tools for the characterization of protein interactions but we defer the discussion of these miniature devices until Chapter 9.

In reductionist terms, molecular interaction analysis is useful for the functional characterization of hypothetical proteins because proteins that interact are likely to be engaged in the same process (guilt by association). For example, if hypothetical Protein X interacts with Proteins Y and Z, both of which are required for mRNA splicing, then it is likely that Protein X is a splicing factor. Although this may not necessarily be the case, such associations at least provide useful leads that can be used to design further experiments. In global terms, molecular interaction analysis is useful because it can be applied on a massive scale, and can therefore be used for the construction of interaction maps of the entire proteome. These are graphs that show proteins or protein complexes as nodes and interactions as the links between them. As we shall see later, such graphs not only provide a holistic view of the functioning cell but they also show which

Table 7.1 Large-scale studies of binary and complex interactions. Reprinted from Current Opinion in Cell Biology, Vol 15, Drewes G. and Bouwmeester T., 'Global approaches to protein–protein interactions', pp 1–7, ©2003, with permission from Elsevier.

Organism (size of proteome)	Technology	Sample	Layout of screen	Number of interactions (number previously known)	Data availability
T7 bacteriophage (55)	Yeast two-hybrid	Proteome	Random library screened against random library	25 (4)	
Vaccinia virus (266)	Yeast two-hybrid	Proteome	266 ORFs screened against proteome array	37 (9)	
Hepatitis C virus (10)	Yeast two-hybrid	Proteome	Proteome and 22 ORF fragments screened against proteome	5 (2)	
Helicobacter pylori (1590)	Yeast two-hybrid	Subset of proteome	261 ORFs screened against genome-encoded library	1524	http://pim.hybigenica.com
S. cerevisiae (6131)	Yeast two-hybrid	Subset of proteome	a. 192 ORFs screened against arrayed proteome b. 5345 ORFs screened against pool (5341 ORFs)	a. 281 b. 691 (88)	http://portal.auragen.com
	Yeast two-hybrid	Proteome	62 × 62 matings of 96-ORF pads	2374 (233)	http://genome.c.kanazawa-u.sc.p/Y2H/
	TAP of protein complexes – peptide mass fingerprinting	Subset of proteome including human orthologs	1739 ORFs tagged 589 complexes purified	411 interactions (1440 individual proteins) in 589 purifications	http://yeast.cellzome.com
	Affinity purification of protein complexes – LC-MS/MS	Subset of proteome including kinases, phosphatases and DNA damage response proteins	725 ORFs tagged 493 complexes purified	3617 interactions (1578 individual proteins) in 493 purifications	http://www.mdsp.com./yeast
C. elegans (19 293)	Yeast two-hybrid	Proteins involved in vulval development	a. 27 × 27 matings in matrix b. 27 ORFs screened against random library	a. 8 (6) b. 148 (15)	http://vidal.cifci.harvard.edu/interactome.htm
	Yeast two-hybrid	Proteins involved in DNA-damage response	a. 75 × 75 matings in matrix b. 67 ORFs screened against random library	a. 26 (17) b. 165 (4)	http://vidal.cifci.harvard.edu/interactome.htm
	Yeast two-hybrid	Proteasome	a. 30 × 30 matings in matrix b. 30 ORFs screened against random library	a. 17 (4) b. 138	http://vidal.cifci.harvard.edu/interactome.htm
Crosophila (18 000)	Yeast two-hybrid Yeast two-hybrid	Proteome Proteome	ORF × library ORF × library	2135 4780	

proteins or complexes are vital hubs in the system and which are redundant. Ultimately, this can help in the selection of appropriate drug targets (Chapter 10).

Finally, interaction studies can be carried out at the cellular level by determining where proteins are localized. This important but often-overlooked component of interaction data can support molecular interaction studies by placing two proteins in the same place at the same time, and can provide evidence against spurious interactions. Also, it may be possible to determine the function of a protein directly from its localization, e.g. a protein localized at the spindle pole is likely to be required for the function of that organelle. Large-scale localization studies often utilize a technique called gene trapping (Chapter 1) to introduce reporter gene sequences or affinity tags into each gene, so that the fate of each protein can be followed in the cell by tracing the reporter tag.

This chapter begins by introducing the principles of interaction analysis and showing how these principles have been developed into high-throughput technologies. The accomplishments of proteome-scale interaction analysis are discussed and we conclude by considering the bioinformatic strategies for dealing with interaction data.

7.2   Principles of protein–protein interaction analysis

Protein–protein interactions are central to virtually every biological process and many different analytical methods have been developed over the years to investigate them. Most of these are suitable for studying interactions within a small group of proteins and cannot be employed on a proteomic scale. However, the small-scale methods employ similar principles to the large-scale technologies we discuss later so it is useful to understand them. The small-scale analysis methods are also useful in proteomics because the large-scale methods tend to produce a significant number of false positives. It is therefore necessary to have a selection of further methods available to confirm or reject such proposed interactions.

7.2.1   Genetic methods

Classical genetics can be used to investigate protein interactions by combining different mutations in the same cell or organism and observing the resulting phenotype. This sort of approach has been widely used in genetically amenable species such as the yeast *Saccharomyces cerevisiae*, the fruit fly *Drosophila melanogaster*, the nematode *Caenorhabditis elegans*, the mouse (*Mus musculis*) and the model plant *Arabidopsis thaliana*.

A straightforward example is a screen for suppressor mutants, i.e. secondary mutations that correct the phenotype of a primary mutation. As shown in *Figure 7.2*, the principle is that a mutation in the gene for Protein X that prevents its interaction with Protein Y will result in a loss of function that generates a mutant phenotype. However, a second mutation in the gene for Protein Y could introduce a compensatory change that restores the interaction. Suppressor mutants identified in the screen are then mapped and the corresponding genes and proteins identified.

The advantage of genetic screens is that they provide a shortcut to functionally significant interactions, sifting through the proteome for those interactions that have a recognizable effect on the overall phenotype.

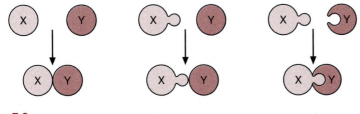

Figure 7.2

Suppressor mutations. Two proteins, X and Y, normally interact. A mutation in X prevents the interaction causing a loss of function phenotype, but this can be suppressed by a complementary mutation in Y which restores the interaction.

However, it is important to remember that genetic screens only provide indirect evidence for interactions and further direct evidence, at the biochemical level, must also be obtained. One potential problem is that the suppressor mutation may map to the same gene as the primary mutation, since second mutations in the same gene can suppress the primary mutant phenotype by introducing a compensatory conformational change within the same protein. Even if the suppressor maps to a different gene, the two gene products might not actually interact. For example, a mutation that abolishes the activity of an enzyme required for amino acid biosynthesis could be suppressed by a gain of function mutation in a transport protein that increases the uptake of that amino acid from the environment. Furthermore, the mutations do not necessarily have to change the structures of Proteins X and Y. An alternative explanation is that Protein X and Protein Y must be present at the correct ratio, which may mean they function in a stoichiometric complex or may simply indicate their activities must be balanced to maintain metabolic homeostasis. If the primary mutation changes the quantity of Protein X, e.g. by altering the promoter, it could be suppressed by a compensatory change in the amount of Protein Y caused by a similar mutation.

Another genetic approach is a screen for enhancer mutations, i.e. those that worsen the phenotype generated by a primary mutation. One example of this strategy is the synthetic lethal screen, where individual mutations in the genes for Proteins X and Y do not prevent interaction and are therefore viable, but simultaneous mutations in both genes prevent the interaction and result in a lethal phenotype (*Figure 7.3*). Tong

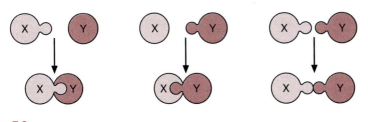

Figure 7.3

Synthetic lethal effect. The same two proteins can still interact if there is a mutation in either X or Y that does not drastically affect the interaction between them. However, if the mutations are combined, protein interaction is abolished and a loss of function phenotype is generated.

et al. (see Further Reading) have recently established the synthetic genetic array (SGA) system in which a mutation in one yeast gene can be crossed to a set of 5000 viable deletion mutants, allowing synthetic interactions to be mapped in a systematic fashion. This can be used to identify all the proteins involved in the same pathway or complex as a particular query protein. Mutations in different genes that generate similar phenotypes often indicate that the protein products are part of the same complex or the same biochemical or signaling pathway. For pathways, the order of protein function can often be established by epistasis. In this type of experiment, loss of function and gain of function mutations (with opposite phenotypes) are combined in the same cell or organism. If a loss of function mutation in Gene X overrides a gain of function mutation in Gene Y, it suggests that Protein X acts downstream of Protein Y in the pathway (*Figure 7.4*).

One final strategy worth mentioning is the dominant negative approach, where a loss of function mutation generates a dominantly interfering version of the protein that quashes the activity of any normally functioning version of the protein in the same cell. This generally suggests that the protein acts as a multimeric complex and that the nonfunctioning version of the protein interferes with the normal version when they are present in the same complex. Like suppressor mutants, however, these methods provide evidence that two gene products interact but they do not provide definitive proof. There are many other plausible explanations for such genetic effects and candidate protein interactions must be confirmed at the biochemical level.

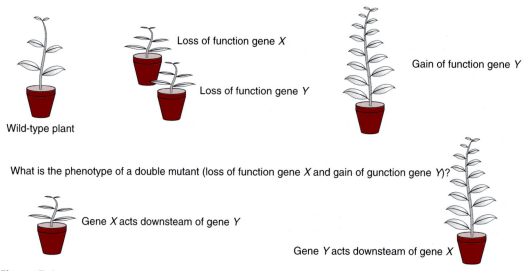

Figure 7.4

Establishing gene order in a pathway by epistasis. A loss of function mutation in either gene X or Y causes a plant to become stunted. A gain of function mutation in gene Y causes a growth burst. If the phenotype of the double mutant is stunted, then X acts downstream of Y, but if its phenotype is tall, then the converse is true.

7.2.2 Bioinformatic methods

The availability of complete genome sequences for many different organisms allows comparative genomics to be used for the functional annotation of proteins. Three methods have been developed to infer protein interactions directly from genomic data. These work best in bacteria because more bacterial genome sequences are available for comparison and because bacterial genomes are often organized into functional units called operons where the encoded proteins tend to have related functions.

The first is called the domain fusion or Rosetta stone method (*Figure 7.5*) and is based on the principle that protein domains are structurally and functionally independent units that can operate either as discrete polypeptides or as part of the same polypeptide chain. Therefore, multidomain proteins in one species may be represented by two or more interacting subunits in another. A well-known example is the *S. cerevisiae* topoisomerase II protein, which has two domains, and which is represented by the two separate subunits GyrA and GyrB in *Escherichia coli*. The domain fusion method can be summarized as follows:

- The sequence of Protein X, a single-domain protein from genome 1, is used as a similarity search query on genome 2. This identifies any single-domain proteins related to Protein X and also any multidomain proteins, which we can define as Protein X-Y.
- The sequence of Protein X-Y can then be used in turn to find the individual gene for Protein Y in genome 1. If the Protein Y gene in genome 1 was uncharacterized until this point, then the Rosetta stone method successfully provides the first functional annotation for Protein Y. It also provides indirect evidence that Protein Y interacts with Protein X.
- The sequence of Protein X-Y may also identify further domain fusions, such as protein Y-Z. This links three proteins into a functional group and possibly identifies an interacting complex.

As well as revealing previously unknown interactions between different protein families, iterative screening of multiple genomes can link many different proteins into an interaction map, based on gene fusion and gene fragmentation events that have occurred over an evolutionary timescale.

The second comparative genomic method is based on the knowledge that bacterial genes are often organized into operons and that such genes are often functionally related even if their sequences are diverse. Therefore, if two genes are neighbors in a series of bacterial genomes, it suggests they are functionally related and that their products may interact. Caution is required in expanding this conservation of gene position principle to all bacterial genomes, however, as it is becoming evident that genes whose functions are apparently unrelated may also be organized into operons. Furthermore, while there is some evidence for functionally related gene neighbors in eukaryotes, the value of conserved gene position as a predictive tool remains to be established.

The final method is based on phylogenetic profiling and exploits the evolutionary conservation of genes involved in the same function. For example, the conservation of three or four uncharacterized genes in 20 aerobic bacteria and their absence in 20 anaerobes might indicate that the products are required for aerobic metabolism. Since proteins usually function as complexes, the loss of one component would render the entire

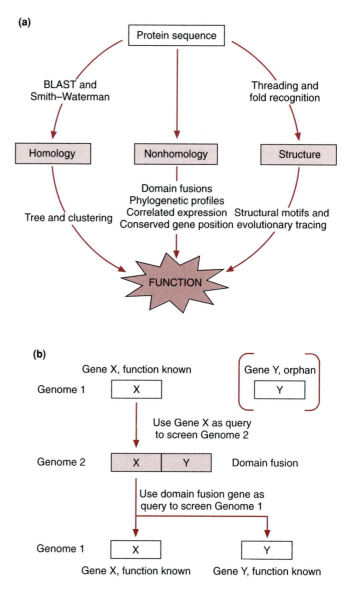

Figure 7.5

(a) As well as bioinformatic methods based on homology searching (Chapter 5) and structural analysis (Chapter 6), several additional nonhomology methods can be used to establish gene functions and predict interactions. Reprinted from Current Opinion in Structural Biology, Vol. 10, Marcotte, 'Computational genetics: finding protein function by nonhomology methods', pp 359 – 365, ©2000, with permission from Elsevier. (b) One of these approaches is the domain fusion method. The sequence of Gene X, of known function from Genome 1, is used as a search query to identify orthologs in Genome 2. The search may reveal single-domain orthologs of Gene X, but may also reveal domain fusion genes such as XY. As part of the same protein, domains X and Y are likely to be functionally related. The sequence of domain Y can then be used to identify single-domain orthologs in Genome 1. Thus, Gene Y, formerly an orphan with no known function, becomes annotated due to its association with Gene X. The two proteins are also likely to interact.

complex nonfunctional, and would tend to lead to the loss of the other components over evolutionary time since mutations in the corresponding genes would have no further detrimental effect. The use of phylogenetic profiling to assign a function to the yeast hypothetical protein YPL207W is shown as an example in *Figure 7.6*.

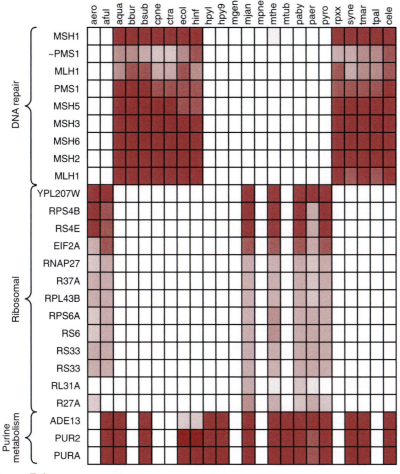

Figure 7.6

Phylogenetic profiles for three groups of yeast proteins (ribsomal proteins and proteins involved in DNA repair and purine metabolism) sharing similar coinheritance patterns. Each row is a graphical representation of a protein phylogenetic profile, with elements colored according to whether a homolog is absent (white box) or present (colored box) in each of 24 genomes (columns). When homology is present, the elements are shaded on a gradient from light red (low level of identity) to dark red (high level of identity). In this case, homologs are considered absent when no BLAST hits are found with expectation (E) values $< 1 \times 10^{-5}$. When homologs are present, the profile receives a score ($-1/\log E$) that describes the degree of sequence similarity with the best match in that genome. The uncharacterized protein (YPL207W) clusters with the ribsomal proteins and can be assigned a function in protein synthesis. Reprinted from Current Opinion in Structural Biology, Vol. 10, Marcotte, 'Computational genetics: finding protein function by nonhomology methods', pp 359–365, ©2000, with permission from Elsevier.

7.2.3 Affinity-based biochemical methods

Genetic and genomic methods infer protein interactions but biochemical methods are needed to prove them. This can be achieved by exploiting the affinity (selective binding ability) of a particular protein for its inter-action partners. If a particular protein, Protein X, can be expressed or purified, its interacting partners can be identified by affinity chromatog-raphy. In this method, Protein X is immobilized on a matrix such as a column packed with Sepharose beads, and a complex mixture of proteins (such as a cell lysate) is passed through the column under controlled conditions of temperature, pH and salt concentration (*Figure 7.7*). Immobilization of Protein X may be achieved by conjugating antibodies that are specific for Protein X to the affinity matrix, or by expressing Protein X as a fusion with glutathione-S-transferase (GST), which binds strongly to Sepharose beads coated with glutathione. Most of the proteins in the mixture will pass through the column but those that interact with Protein X will be retained (*Figure 7.7*). These can be eluted selectively by increasing the salt concentration or by adding SDS to the washing buffer, and then identified by mass spectrometry or immunoblotting (Chapter 3). Stepwise increments in salt or SDS concentration can be used to discriminate between proteins that bind with high or low affinity to Protein X. Controls are required to eliminate proteins that bind to irrele-vant components of the experiment, such as the antibody or the glutathione-S-transferase. The use of specific proteins as baits to trap interacting partners (prey) is widely exploited in the high-throughput

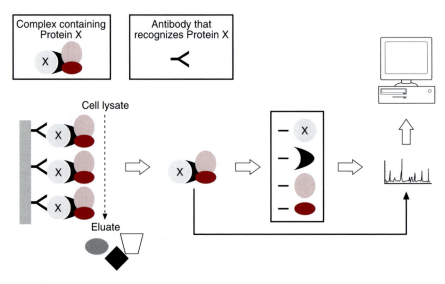

Figure 7.7

Affinity chromatography can be used to trap interacting proteins. If Protein X is immobilized on Sepharose beads (e.g. using specific antibodies), then proteins (and other molecules) interacting with Protein X can be captured from a cell lysate passed through the column. After washing away unbound proteins, the bound proteins can be eluted, separated by SDS-PAGE (optional) and analyzed by mass spectrometry.

interaction technologies discussed later in the chapter, and is one of the underpinning principles of large-scale interaction analysis.

Instead of immobilizing Protein X on a column, the affinity-based isolation of interacting proteins can be achieved in solution by techniques such as coimmunoprecipitation and GST pulldown (*Figure 7.8*). Coimmunoprecipitation (*Figure 7.8a*) is based on the principle that the addition of antibodies specific for Protein X to a cell lysate will result in the precipitation of the antibody–antigen complex. However, any proteins interacting with Protein X when the antibody is added will also precipitate. The technique is usually carried out with polyclonal antisera, although monoclonal antibodies can be used if a second antibody is added to facilitate cross-linking. The precipitated complexes are separated from the cell lysate by centrifugation, washed and then fractionated by SDS-PAGE, and the bound proteins can be identified by mass spectrometry. GST pulldown (*Figure 7.8b*) is an analogous technique in which the Protein X is expressed as a fusion to GST. After mixing the fusion protein with a

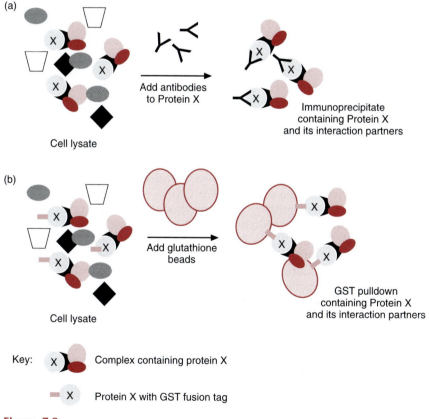

(a)

Cell lysate → Add antibodies to Protein X → Immunoprecipitate containing Protein X and its interaction partners

(b)

Cell lysate → Add glutathione beads → GST pulldown containing Protein X and its interaction partners

Key: X Complex containing protein X

       X Protein X with GST fusion tag

Figure 7.8

(a) Immunoprecipitation can be used to isolate proteins interacting with Protein X if a specific antibody is available. (b) Alternatively, Protein X can be expressed as a glutathione-S-transferase (GST) fusion protein and captured using glutathione beads. Only in the former case is the bait protein present at physiological levels.

cell lysate and allowing complexes to form, glutathione-coated beads are added to capture the GST part of the fusion. The beads are recovered by centrifugation, washed and the recovered proteins fractionated and identified by mass spectrometry as above. As is the case for chromatography-based methods, appropriate controls must be used to eliminate irrelevant interactions. Note that coimmunoprecipitation has the advantage of characterizing protein interactions in the context of a normal physiological concentration of the bait protein. Because GST pulldown requires the addition of a fusion bait protein to the cell lysate, it is likely that there will be much more of the bait than is normally found in the cell, and this may have unanticipated effects such as altering the normal stoichiometry of certain protein interactions.

In the descriptions above, the affinity methods have been used to characterize binary interactions (i.e. interactions between a bait protein and one or more individual partners). However, all affinity methods have the potential to purify not only proteins that interact directly with the bait but also those that interact indirectly. Indeed, careful application allows the isolation of entire protein complexes with >50 components, a strategy that can be combined with mass spectrometry to facilitate systematic protein complex analysis (p. 155). Direct interactions within a complex can be characterized by cross-linking, where interacting proteins are covalently joined together. A useful strategy is shown in *Figure 7.9a*. This involves the use of a photoactivated cross-linking reagent, which contains a radioactive label. If this reagent is covalently joined to purified Protein X *in vitro* then the conjugate can be added to a cell lysate and cross-linking can be induced by exposure to light. However, because the label is on the photoactivated moiety of the cross-linking reagent, it is transferred to the interacting partner of Protein X allowing it to be purified and characterized. Cross-linking followed by two-dimensional gel electrophoresis has been widely used to study the architecture of protein complexes (*Figure 7.9b*). Note that cross-linking is also a useful method to study protein interactions with nucleic acids (see *Box 7.1*).

A final note about affinity trapping methods is that they are not limited to single bait proteins. By switching from homogeneous (in solution) assay formats to solid phase assays (where the bait is immobilized on a solid surface such as a nitrocellulose membrane, or in the wells of microtiter dishes) the interactions of many proteins can be studied in parallel. Traditional techniques for protein analysis and quantitation, such as western blotting and the enzyme-linked immunosorbent assay (ELISA) (see *Box 4.1*) are optimized for the use of a single probe. That is, thousands of protein targets may be immobilized on the surface, but the idea is to detect interactions between a single probe and target – usually an antibody probe and a complementary antigen. Although not yet very suitable for high-throughput interaction assays, solid-phase affinity-based methods can be regarded as the forerunners of some of the higher-throughout techniques discussed later, such as phage interaction display (p. 146) and functional protein chips (p. 202).

7.2.4 Physical methods

A number of methods for studying protein interactions exploit the principles of physics rather than biochemistry. X-ray crystallography and

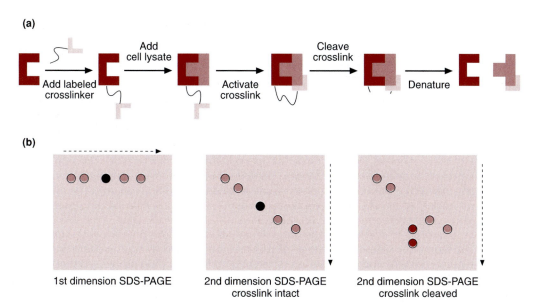

Figure 7.9

(a) Interacting proteins can be identified by crosslinking. A labeled crosslinker is added to Protein X *in vitro* and the cell lysate is added so that interactions can occur. If the crosslink is activated at this stage, interacting proteins become covalently attached to the bait. After purification, the crosslink can be cleaved and the interacting proteins separated. The label remains on the interaction partner. (b) Mapping complex architecture by 2D-PAGE. Interacting proteins are crosslinked and separated by SDS-PAGE in two dimensions. If the crosslink remains intact, proteins will form a diagonal pattern because the smallest proteins move farthest in both dimensions. However, if the crosslink is cleaved between the two gel runs, formerly crosslinked proteins can be identified because they move off the diagonal.

nuclear magnetic resonance spectroscopy are examples. They employ the principles of X-ray diffraction and nuclear magnetic resonance, respectively, to yield data about the relative spacing of atoms (see Chapter 6). These techniques provide high-resolution models of proteins, protein complexes, and proteins interacting with various ligands and cofactors.

BOX 7.1

Protein–nucleic acid interactions

Protein–nucleic acid interactions underlie some of the most fundamental biochemical processes, including DNA replication, DNA repair, recombination, transcription, mRNA processing and translation. They are also important for packaging nucleic acids (e.g. histones in chromatin) and transporting them around the cell (e.g. chromosome segregation, RNA export from the nucleus and RNA localization). All nucleic acids associate with proteins at some stage and often exist as permanent or semipermanent nucleoprotein complexes. Some proteins interact nonspecifically with DNA and/or RNA whereas others only bind to particular sequences. The latter are the most interesting because they often have a regulatory function. The first reports of global studies of transcription factor binding are beginning to appear (see Lee *et al.* and Horrack *et al.*, Further Reading). The functions of proteins can also be predicted by promoter analysis (see Wener, Further Reading).

Biochemical techniques for the investigation of protein–nucleic acid interactions can be divided into two major categories.

Affinity-dependent purification and screening methods
Nucleic acid-binding proteins can be purified by exploiting their affinity for DNA or RNA. A successful early method for the isolation of RNA-binding proteins was simply to filter cell lysates through nitrocellulose. The RNA, and any associated proteins, would bind to the nitrocellulose while other proteins would be washed through. Slightly more sophisticated methods are required to isolate sequence-specific binding proteins. First the cell lysate must be mixed with an excess of total genomic DNA or tRNA (as appropriate) in order to block the nonspecific binding proteins. Sequence-specific binding proteins can then be isolated by affinity chromatography in which a particular oligonucleotide is used as the affinity matrix. The affinity of proteins for nucleic acids can also be exploited to identify DNA- and RNA-binding proteins on membranes or in expression libraries. After blocking with nonspecific DNA, a labeled DNA or RNA probe is applied to the membrane and will only bind to those proteins with affinity for that specific sequence. One disadvantage of this method, known as southwestern screening for DNA-binding proteins and northwestern screening for RNA-binding proteins, is that nucleic acid-binding proteins made up of several different subunits will not be detected because the components will be present as separate clones. A variant of the yeast two-hybrid system, known as the yeast one-hybrid system, is useful for the identification of transcription factors. Essentially, this involves the transformation of yeast with a construct comprising a minimal promoter and reporter gene, with several tandem copies of a candidate transcription factor-binding motif placed upstream. A cDNA expression library is then prepared in which all proteins are expressed as transactivation domain hybrids. These will activate the target gene only if they contain a DNA-binding domain that interacts with the chosen promoter sequence. This system can only identify proteins that bind to DNA autonomously. The one-and-a-half hybrid system is similar, but can detect proteins that bind DNA as heterodimers with a second, accessory protein. The one–two hybrid system can search for both autonomous binders and proteins that bind only as heterodimers. Another variant of the two-hybrid system, known as bait and hook or three-hybrid is useful for the identification of RNA-binding proteins or protein interactions with small ligands. In this system, one of the components (the hook) comprises the DNA-binding domain of a transcription factor and a sequence-specific RNA-binding protein that attaches to one end of a synthetic RNA molecule. The other end of the RNA molecule contains the sequence for which candidate interactors are sought. A prey library is constructed as normal, with each protein expressed as a fusion to a transactivation domain. Only in cells where the prey interacts with the RNA sequence attached to the hook will the transcription factor be assembled and the reporter gene activated.

Methods for the precise characterization of protein–nucleic acid interactions
These methods are diverse and are usually designed to identify the sequence to which a particular protein binds. The gel retardation assay is used to demonstrate protein–DNA interactions but it can also identify the approximate location of protein-binding sites in DNA or RNA when DNA fragments with a putative binding site are used. It is based on the fact that nucleic acid–protein complexes move through electrophoretic gels more slowly than naked DNA or RNA. DNase footprinting can identify the exact nucleotides covered by a protein because these will be protected from nuclease digestion. Methylation interference and methylation protection are techniques that identify the specific bases that make contact with a binding protein because these are either protected from methylation when the protein is bound or because they interfere with the normal interaction if they are already modified. RNA–protein interactions in complexes are often studied by chemical cross-linking or treatment with nucleases. A very useful technique is the hybridization of short DNA oligonucleotides to RNA molecules in an RNA–protein complex followed by digestion with RNaseH, which is specific for DNA/RNA hybrids. This allows the systematic functional testing of parts of the RNA component.

Other techniques, which have a lower resolution, can provide some details about the structure of a protein complex. These include electron crystallography and electron tomography, the latter of which can be used to study protein complexes *in situ*. Several manufacturers of protein chips have developed systems that exploit surface plasmon resonance to detect protein interactions. This is an optical effect that occurs when monochromatic polarized light is reflected off thin metal films. The amount of resonance that occurs is determined by the material adsorbed to the metal film, and surface plasmon resonance spectroscopy is therefore being developed as a method to detect and characterize protein interactions occurring on the surface of gold-coated glass chips. We do not discus this technology any further at this point but the interested reader can refer to Chapter 9, which considers protein chip technology in more detail.

Another major area of research involves the use of fluorescence resonance energy transfer (FRET) to detect protein interactions. FRET is the energy transfer that occurs when two fluorophores are close together, and one of the fluorophores (the donor) has an emission spectrum that overlaps the excitation spectrum of the other fluorophore (the acceptor). When a lone donor fluorophore is excited, light is produced with a characteristic emission spectrum. However, when the donor fluorophore is excited in close proximity to the acceptor fluorophore, energy is transferred to the acceptor fluorophore with the result that the intensity of emission from the donor is reduced (quenched) while that of the acceptor is increased (enhanced). To investigate the interaction between two known proteins *in vitro*, each can be conjugated to a different fluorophore, such as Cy3 and Cy5. If the detector is calibrated to read the enhanced emission of the acceptor fluorophore then a signal will be obtained only when the two proteins interact. The advantage of this method is that transient as well as stable interactions are detected. More recently, derivatives of green fluorescent protein have been used to generate bioluminescent protein fusions, which can be expressed in living cells and used to detect protein interaction *in vivo*. For example, protein–protein interactions in living plant cells have been studied using bait proteins fused to cyan fluorescent protein and candidate prey fused to yellow fluorescent protein. The technique of immunoelectron microscopy can also be used to confirm that two proteins interact, and can also reveal their approximate relative locations within a complex.

7.3 Library-based methods for the global analysis of binary interactions

The genetic, biochemical and physical techniques discussed above each have limitations in terms of the number of interactions that can be studied simultaneously and this makes them rather unsuitable for interaction analysis on a global scale. The reasons for this become clear if we think about the number of potential interactions that could take place in even a simple cell. The yeast *Saccharomyces cerevisiae* is a useful example because there is a relatively small number of genes in the genome (~ 6000) and processes such as alternative splicing are the exception rather than the rule, which means that the basic proteome is likely to be very similar in size to the gene catalog (at least if we ignore diversity generated by post-translational modifications). Even so, this provides scope for 36 000 000 possible binary interactions and even larger numbers of higher-order interactions. The actual number of interactions will be much lower than this because most proteins will have a small number of very specific interacting partners. In part, this will reflect spatial and temporal separation either through gene regulation or protein compartmentalization within the cell. Mostly, however, the number of interactions is limited by the affinities of different proteins for each other. The total number of interactions in this particular organism is probably only an order of magnitude higher than the size of the proteome. But all 36 000 000 possible interactions need to be tested in order to establish the few tens of thousands that are functionally significant.

At the current time, the testing of binary protein interactions on such a grand scale can only be carried out using library-based methods. As well as the benefit of high-throughput screening, such methods are advantageous because the protein is always associated in some way with the gene that encodes it, allowing the direct annotation of interacting proteins by database homology searching. Three library-based methods have been used to study protein interactions as described below.

7.3.1 Standard expression libraries

Standard cDNA expression libraries, such as those constructed using the λgt11 vector, can be used to investigate protein–protein interactions if a labeled bait protein is used as the probe. This is really an extension of the protein detection and quantitation techniques discussed in *Box 4.1*, with the important difference that the proteins are released from phage particles that also contain the corresponding cDNA, allowing them to be identified by DNA sequencing. Expression libraries are usually screened with labeled antibodies, and since antibodies are proteins this process of immunoscreening can be thought of as a rather specialized form of interaction analysis. In place of antibodies, other proteins can be used as probes. For example, labeled calmodulin has been used to screen for calmodulin-binding proteins and a probe corresponding to the phosphorylated internal domain of the EGF receptor has been used to identify signaling proteins containing the SH2 domain. DNA and RNA probes have also been used on protein expression libraries to identify transcription factors and RNA-binding proteins (see *Box 7.1*).

While expression libraries have been useful for protein interaction screening there are numerous disadvantages, perhaps the most important of which in the context of proteomics is the relatively low throughput of the technique. For example, in order to study the 36 000 000 possible interactions of the yeast proteome, 6000 separate screenings would have to be performed unless some sort of pooling strategy were used. Added to this, the *in vitro* assay format does not provide the native conditions for the folding of all proteins, so a significant number of interactions would not be detected.

7.3.2 Phage interaction display

Phage display is an expression cloning strategy in which proteins are expressed on the surface of phage particles. This is achieved by inserting

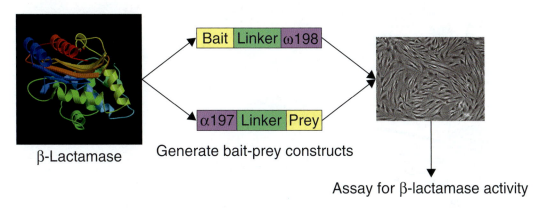

β-Lactamase

Bait | Linker | ω198

α197 | Linker | Prey

Generate bait-prey constructs

Assay for β-lactamase activity

Plate 8

Mapping mammalian protein interactions using a β-lactamase assay. In this approach, a construct is made to create a fusion protein of a protein-bait and the ω198 fragment of β-lactamase. A second construct is also designed to create a fusion protein between a protein-prey and the α197 fragment of β-lactamase. Stable cell lines that express both fusion proteins are generated. If the bait protein binds to the prey proteins β-lactamase activity is observed. Image courtesy of Protein DataBank.

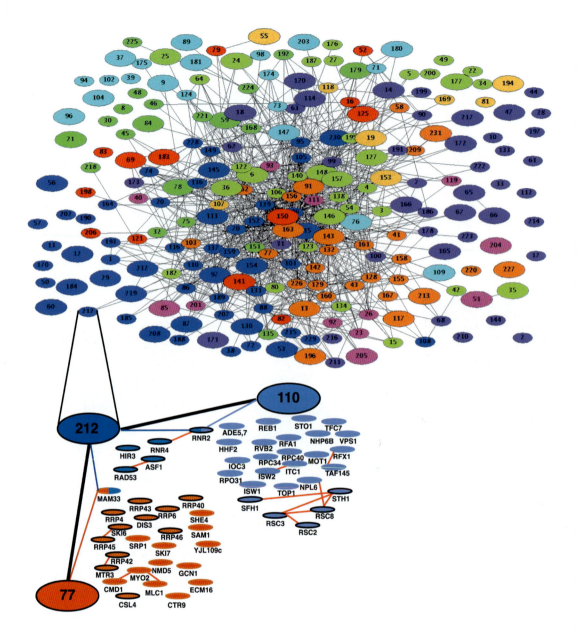

Plate 9

The protein complex network, and grouping of connected complexes. Links were established between complexes sharing at least one protein. For clarity, proteins found in more than nine complexes were omitted. The graphs were generated automatically by a relaxation algorithm that finds a local minimum in the distribution of nodes by minimizing the distance of connected nodes and maximizing distance of unconnected nodes. In the upper panel, cellular roles of the individual complexes are color coded: red, cell cycle; dark green, signaling; dark blue, transcription, DNA maintenance, chromatin structure; pink, protein and RNA transport; orange, RNA metabolism; light green, protein synthesis and turnover; brown, cell polarity and structure; violet, intermediate and energy metabolism; light blue, membrane biogenesis and traffic. The lower panel is an example of a complex (TAP-C212) linked to two other complexes (TAP-C77 and TAP-C110) by shared components. It illustrates the connection between the protein and complex levels of organization. Red lines indicate physical interactions as listed in the Yeast Proteome Database. ©Nature Publishing Group, Nature, Vol. 415, 114–117, 'Functional organization of the yeast proteome by systematic analysis of protein complexes' by Gavin A.-C., *et al.*

the relevant cDNA sequence into the phage coat protein gene and either transfecting bacterial cells with the recombinant phage DNA or transducing them with phage particles that have been packaged with the recombinant DNA *in vitro*. A purified fusion phage will bind to any protein that interacts with the component expressed on its surface.

The phage display technique has a number of applications in proteomics in addition to interaction screening, mostly involving the production of antibodies. Such applications include the rapid and high-throughput production of recombinant antibodies for protein chips (see Chapter 9) and the creation of antibodies against peptides translated from ESTs for rapid expression profiling at the protein level.

For interaction screening, a phage display library is created in which each protein in the proteome is displayed on the phage surface (*Figure 7.10*). The wells of microtiter plates are then coated with particular bait proteins of interest, and the phage display library is pipetted into each well. Phage with interacting proteins on their surface will remain bound to the surface of the well while those with noninteracting proteins will be washed away. A particular advantage of the technique is that the retained phage, displaying interacting proteins, can be eluted from the wells and used to infect *E. coli*, resulting in massive amplification of the corresponding cDNA sequence. This can be used to identify the interacting proteins by database searching.

Phage display is suitable for proteome-scale interaction analysis because highly parallel screenings can be carried out and the technique is amenable to automation. In theory, 6000 bait proteins in microtiter dishes could be screened with a single phage display library and phage from each well could be eluted individually and amplified in *E. coli* in preparation for DNA sequencing. As with standard library screening, however, the *in vitro* assay format would not allow all proteins to adopt their native structures. Furthermore, only short peptides can be displayed on the phage surface because larger proteins disrupt replication. It is likely that some interactions, requiring more extensive contacts between the interacting partners, would not be detected for this reason.

Although phage display has not been used for the systematic large-scale analysis of interactions in any proteome, it has been used in a combined approach with the yeast two-hybrid system (see below) to define protein interaction networks for peptide recognition modules, which mediate many protein–protein interactions. Tong *et al.* (see Further Reading) combined the computational prediction of interactions from phage-display ligand consensus sequences with large-scale two-hybrid physical interaction tests to study interactions involving yeast SH3 domains. This revealed 394 interactions among 206 proteins and a two-hybrid network containing 233 interactions among 145 proteins. Many of these interactions were confirmed *in vivo* by coimmunoprecipitation experiments.

7.3.3 The yeast two-hybrid system

The yeast two-hybrid system addresses the problems of the *in vitro* assay format by testing for protein interactions within the yeast cell. The principle of the system is the assembly of an active transcription factor from two fusion proteins and the detection of this assembly by the activation of a marker gene. The general scheme is shown in *Figure 7.11*. The bait

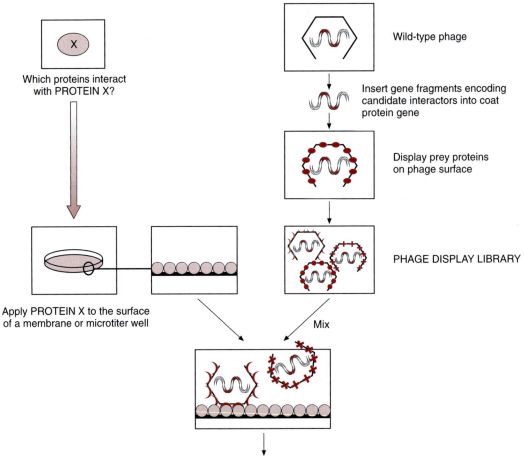

Which proteins interact
with PROTEIN X?

Wild-type phage

Insert gene fragments encoding
candidate interactors into coat
protein gene

Display prey proteins
on phage surface

PHAGE DISPLAY LIBRARY

Apply PROTEIN X to the surface
of a membrane or microtiter well

Mix

Recover bound phage, sequence and characterize the foreign gene insert

Figure 7.10

The principle of phage display as applied to high-throughout interaction screening. Protein X, for which interactors are sought, can be immobilized on the surface of microtiter wells or membranes. All other proteins in the proteome are then expressed on the surface of bacteriophage, by cloning within a phage coat protein gene, to create a phage display library. The wells or membranes are then flooded with the phage library. Phage-carrying interacting proteins will be retained while those displaying noninteracting proteins will be washed away. The bound phage can be eluted in a high-salt buffer and used to infect *E. coli*, producing a large amount of phage particles containing the DNA sequence of the interacting protein.

protein, for which interactors are sought, is expressed as a fusion with a DNA-binding domain from a transcription factor such as GAL4 that on its own is unable to activate the marker gene. This bait fusion is expressed in one haploid yeast strain. Another haploid yeast strain is used to create a cDNA expression library in which all the proteins in the proteome are expressed as fusions with a transactivation domain of GAL4, which is also unable to activate the marker gene on its own. The two strains of yeast are then mated to yield a diploid strain expressing both the hybrid bait protein and one candidate hybrid prey protein. In those cells where the bait and prey do not interact, the transcription factor remains unassembled

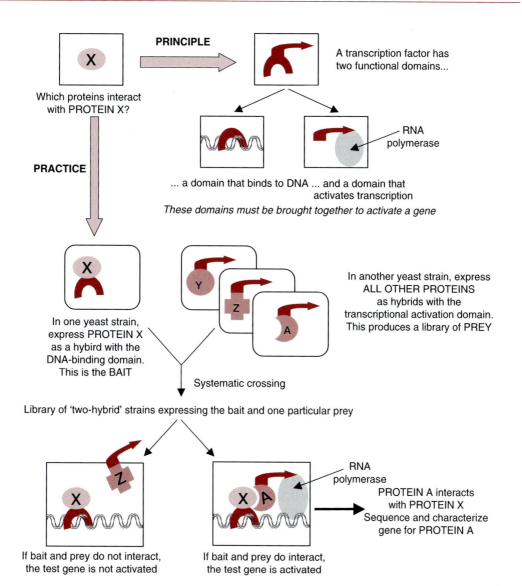

Figure 7.11

The principle of the yeast two-hybrid system. Transcription factors generally comprise two functionally independent domains, one for DNA binding and one for transcriptional activation. These do not have to be covalently joined together, but can be assembled to form a dimeric protein. This principle is exploited to identify protein interactions. Bait proteins are expressed in one yeast strain as a fusion with a DNA-binding domain and candidate prey are expressed in another strain as fusions with a transactivation domain. When the two strains are mated, functional transcription factors are assembled only if the bait and prey interact. This can be detected by including a reporter gene activated by the hybrid transcription factor.

and the marker gene remains silent. However, in those cells where there is an interaction between the bait and the prey, the transcription factor is assembled and the marker gene is activated. Cells with interacting proteins can therefore be identified and the corresponding cDNAs characterized.

7.4 Interaction proteomics using the yeast two-hybrid system

The yeast two-hybrid system was the first technology to facilitate global protein interaction analysis. By arraying panels of haploid yeast strains in microtiter dishes and carrying out pairwise matings in a systematic fashion, tens of thousands of interactions can be screened in a single experiment. Several very comprehensive large-scale studies have been published (*Table 7.1*), including some in bacteria and yeast that have encompassed the entire interactome (the sum of all binary interactions between proteins). Several variations of the standard two-hybrid method have been used in these studies, the advantages and disadvantages of which are discussed below. Several derivative techniques have been developed to address the limitations of the standard yeast two-hybrid system, and these are described in *Box 7.2* (see *Plate 8*).

7.4.1 Matrix screening

The matrix screening method is a systematic approach in which panels of defined bait and prey strains are mated in an array format (this can be expressed as ORF × ORF meaning that specific and defined open reading frames are used in each construct). Each bait and prey construct is made individually by PCR and introduced into yeast cells that are maintained in isolation. The different transformed cell lines are then arranged in microtiter dishes and crossed in all possible pair-wise combinations (*Figure 7.12a*). Since individual constructs are required for every protein, whole interactome analysis is possible only in those species with fully sequenced genomes and completed gene catalogs. The advantage of the matrix approach is that it is comprehensive and can provide exhaustive interactome coverage. However, the preparation stage is laborious, and the amount of work required increases in proportion to the size of the proteome being investigated.

The first complete and systematic interactome analysis using the matrix screening method was reported by McCraith and colleagues in 2000 (see Further Reading). They tested all 266 proteins of the vaccinia virus proteome against each other, representing a total of nearly 71 000 possible interactions. The actual number of interactions detected was 37, nine of which were already known. The same approach was adopted by Uetz and colleagues to screen the yeast proteome (see Further Reading). A panel of nearly 200 baits was assembled and screened against >5000 preys. In this study, 87 of the baits were shown to be involved in a total of 281 interactions. These numbers of interactions are perhaps lower than might be expected and some possible reasons for this are considered later.

7.4.2 Pooled matrix screening

In order to increase the throughput and scale of the matrix approach, Uetz *et al.* also described a modified strategy, which they called the pooled matrix screening method (*Figure 7.12b*). Like the standard matrix screening method, defined strains were produced for each bait construct in this case representing >5000 individual proteins in the proteome. The preys, however, were screened in pools rather than as individual strains. Yeast

BOX 7.2

Derivatives of the yeast two-hybrid system

The original yeast two-hybrid system was developed to test or screen for interactions between pairs of proteins. Once established, however, investigators turned their attention towards improvements and enhancements that allowed the detection of different types of interactions. One of the earliest adaptations made it possible to detect interactions between proteins and small peptides, which can be useful to define minimal sets of conserved sequences in inter-action partners. Other derivatives allowed higher-order complexes to be studied, by expressing the bait with a known interaction partner in the hope of attracting further complex compo-nents. A major disadvantage of yeast for the analysis of higher eukaryotic protein interactions is the limited amount of post-translational protein modification that occurs (Chapter 8). This was addressed by carrying out two-hybrid screens in a strain of yeast expressing a mammalian kinase, therefore enabling the usual phosphorylation target sites to be occupied. The one-hybrid system and its derivatives for the detection of DNA-binding proteins, and the bait and hook/three-hybrid systems for the detection of RNA-binding proteins and protein–ligand inter-actions are described in *Box 7.1*. Another interesting variant is the reverse two-hybrid system, which uses counterselectable markers to screen for the loss of protein interactions. This is used to identify mutations that disrupt specific interaction events, and could conceivably be used to find drugs that disrupt interactions between disease-causing proteins. Various systems using dual baits have also been described, and these can be used to find mutations that block specific interactions between a given prey protein and one of two distinct baits.

As well as derivative systems based on transcriptional activation as described above, a number of related technologies have been developed that do not rely on transcription, and therefore circumvent problems of autoactivation. The split ubiquitin system (ubiquitin-based split protein sensor, USPS) involves fusing a bait protein to the amino-terminal portion of ubiquitin and prey proteins to the separated carboxy-terminal. Interactions reassemble an active ubiquitin molecule, which then causes protein degradation, a process that can be monitored by western blot. The SOS recruitment system (SRS) or CytoTrap involves the fusion of bait proteins to a myristoylation signal, thus targeting them to the plasma mem-brane, while prey are expressed as fusions to the mammalian signal transduction protein SOS. In yeast strains deficient for CDC25 (the yeast ortholog of SOS) survival is possible only if SOS is recruited to the membrane, and this can only occur if the bait and prey proteins interact and form a membrane-targeted complex. The RAS recruitment system (RRS) is based on similar principles (i.e. the prey proteins are expressed as RAS fusions) in a yeast strain deficient for RAS.

Further systems have been devised which do not depend on yeast at all. Several bacterial two-hybrid systems have been developed in *E. coli*, one of which is based on the reconstruc-tion of a split adenylyl cyclase enzyme and its activation of the *lac* or *mal* operons. A mammalian two-hybrid system has been developed in which interactions between bait and prey assemble the enzyme β-lactamase, so that the enzyme activity can be monitored in real time (*Plate 8*). Similarly, the protein complementation assay (PCA) involves the reassembly of the enzyme dihydrofolate reductase (DHFR) from two inactive components. This is used to monitor protein interactions in plant cells. Interaction between bait and prey reassembles the enzyme and allows it to bind a fluorescein-conjugated derivative of its normal substrate methotrexate. Free methotrexate is exported from plant cells but the enzyme–substrate complex is retained allowing fluorescence to be monitored.

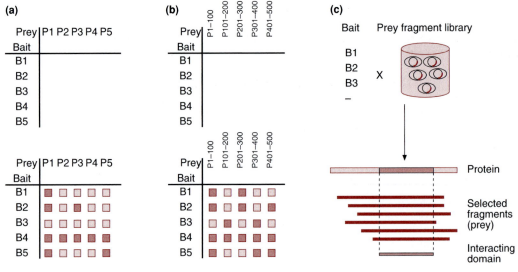

Figure 7.12

The matrix and library screening approaches to build large-scale protein interaction maps. (a) The matrix approach is systematic and uses the same collection of proteins (1–5) as bait (B1–B5) and prey (P1–P5). The results can be drawn in a matrix. Autoactivators (for example, B4) and 'sticky' prey proteins (for example, P1 interacts with many baits) are identified and discarded. The final result is summarized as a list of interactions that can be heterodimers (e.g. B2–P3) or homodimers (e.g. B5–P5). (b) The pooled matrix approach is a variation on the above in which prey are pooled to allow higher-throughout screening. For example, no interactions occur between B1 and P301–500, so 200 individual screens can be omitted. Prey pool P201–300 can be deconvoluted to identify specific interactors. (c) The library screening approach is random and identifies the domain of interaction for each prey protein interacting with a given bait. Sticky prey proteins are identified as fragments of proteins that are often selected regardless of the bait protein. Reprinted from Trends in Genetics', Vol. 17, Legrain *et al.*, 'Protein-protein interaction maps: a lead towards cellular functions', pp 346 – 352, ©2001, with permission from Elsevier.

cells were transformed with mixtures of prey constructs and screened *en masse*. In this way, many more potential interactions could be screened in each mating (ORF × pooled ORF). Where interactions were detected, the mixed strains could be deconvoluted in order to identify individual interactors. Uetz and colleagues identified nearly 700 interactions in this experiment, about 90 of which were already known. The pooled matrix approach was also used by Ito *et al.* (see Further Reading) in another comprehensive study of the yeast interactome. In this case, all 36 000 000 potential interactions were screened by pooling both the bait and the prey constructs (pooled ORF × pooled ORF). Initially, pools of 96 baits and 96 prey were tested against each other in 430 combinations to investigate about 4 000 000 interactions. A total of 175 interacting pairs of proteins was identified, 12 of which were already known. The experiment was then scaled up ten-fold to embrace the entire interactome. Almost 1000 highly reliable interactions were detected in this second screen.

7.4.3 Random library screening

The labor-intensive task of producing individual bait and prey constructs for every protein in the proteome can be side-stepped by the use of random libraries of fusion constructs. Apart from savings in time and materials, each protein is represented not by a single defined ORF but by a collection of overlapping clones. This has an added advantage in that interactions can often be narrowed down to a specific protein domain, common to all the clones representing a single bait or prey.

The random library method has been used predominantly for moderate-scale analyses of protein complexes or pathways, and the general approach has been to use defined bait constructs to screen a random library of prey (ORF × library). The first studies of this nature focused on the yeast spliceosome and RNA polymerase III complex. A highly complex prey library containing over one million clones was produced for this purpose. In the initial investigation, the library was screened with 15 yeast splicing proteins leading to the identification of 170 interactions involving 145 prey. Three interaction screens have also been carried out in *C. elegans*, one to study proteins involved in vulval development, one to study proteins involved in the DNA damage response and one to study the 26S proteosome. In each case, a pilot matrix study (ORF × ORF) has preceded the larger-scale analysis in which a panel of approximately 30–70 ORFs was used to screen the random library. In each of these systems, roughly 150 interactions were detected.

Thus far only two interactome-wide studies have been carried out using random libraries. The first was an investigation of bacteriophage T7, whose proteome contains 55 proteins. In this case a random library of baits was screened against a random library of prey (library × library) and 25 interactions were identified, four being previously known. The other study was a large-scale analysis of the bacterium *Helicobacter pylori*, using a panel of 261 baits to screen a random library of prey (ORF × library). The genome of this bacterium encodes approximately 1600 proteins and 1524 interactions were identified. Because few protein interactions had been identified previously in this relatively uncharacterized bacterium, the results of the screen were compared to data available for *E. coli*. Surprisingly, only about half of the interactions known to occur in *E. coli* were detected in *H. pylori*.

7.4.4   Limitations of the yeast two-hybrid system

The yeast two-hybrid system is the only available *in vivo* technology for the high-throughput systematic analysis of binary interactions on a proteomic scale, but the wide coverage has a trade off in that the data are of lower quality than other, more laborious approaches. The problems can be divided into three groups as described below.

First, where independent groups have carried out similar, large-scale studies, the degree of overlap in the reported interactions is very low (10–15%). This suggests either that the screens were not comprehensive or that even minor differences in experimental conditions could influence the types of interactions that are detected. The large-scale studies of the yeast interactome carried out by Uetz *et al.* and Ito *et al.* employed similar pooled matrix strategies but quite different culture conditions and selection strategies. Among the >2000 interactions detected by Ito and colleagues only 141 were in common with the 700 or so interactions reported by Uetz *et al.*

Second, a significant number of well-characterized interactions are not detected in the large-scale screens, suggesting there is a high level of false negatives. This problem appears to arise for different reasons in matrix-type assays and random library screens. In matrix assays, many interactions are missed because full-length proteins are used (these often do not work in two-hybrid assays). In the case of random library screens, the screens may not be saturated due to incomplete representation of genes in the library or because the numbers of sequenced positives are too small.

Third, a significant number of interactions that are detected in large-scale screens appear spurious when investigated in more detail, suggesting there is also a high level of false positives.

In addition to a lack of comprehensive coverage, there are probably many factors that affect the reliability of data obtained from yeast two-hybrid screens. One likely contributor to the high false-negative rate in matrix-type assays is the occurrence of PCR errors during the preparation of bait and prey constructs. Another is the possible inability of some proteins to fold properly when expressed as fusions. This would be a more serious limitation in matrix assays because only one version of each construct is prepared. In the random library method, several variants of each construct are present and thus there is a greater chance that such a folding problem could be overcome. False negatives could also arise due to intrinsic limitations of the assay system. The detection of interactions relies on the formation of a transcription factor in the yeast nucleus. Entry into the nucleus would be problematical for certain classes of proteins, such as integral membrane proteins, while other proteins normally resident in compartments with different ionic and pH conditions might become denatured and unable to bind to their normal interaction partners when forced into the nucleus. Again, this problem might be more pronounced in matrix-type assays because each ORF is present in full, whereas in random libraries it would be possible to find partial ORFs encoding the globular intracellular domains of integral membrane proteins but not the hydrophobic membrane-spanning domains. An extreme example of the difference between matrix and random library methods was reported by Flajolet and colleagues (see Further Reading) who investigated interactions between the ten mature polypeptides of hepatitis C virus. A 10×10 matrix analysis in which each polypeptide was expressed as an independent ORF showed no interactions at all, whereas a library approach revealed both interactions that were already known and three novel ones.

False positives can reflect nonspecific interactions, where the prey interacts with many different bait proteins (sticky prey). This might be expected for proteins whose normal function requires diverse interactions, such as molecular chaperones or components of the protein degradation machinery. In other cases, the bait and/or prey may be capable of auto-activation (spontaneous activation of the marker gene in the absence of any interaction). This is especially problematical if either the bait or the prey encodes a transcriptional activator, which might account for up to 10% of the proteome. A further source of false positives is irrelevant interactions between proteins that would never encounter each other under normal circumstances, such as those normally found in different tissues, those expressed at different times of development or those resident in different intracellular compartments. This may be a common source of error if several members of the same protein family are differentially expressed or localized, but pairwise interactions occur if they are deliberately expressed in the same compartment.

The only way to verify that an interaction detected in a two-hybrid screen is genuine is to seek conformation in the form of supportive evidence from other experiments, i.e. benchmarking against datasets of reliable interactions and looking at overlaps between independent datasets. However, many false positives can be eliminated by using statistical analysis to attach a confidence score to each interaction. In matrix assays, confidence is proportional to reproducibility and most interactions are accepted only if they are detected in several independent screens. In the analysis of the vaccinia virus interactome, each mating assay was carried out four times and only those interactions occurring in three or all four of the assays were accepted. Confidence in random library screens is increased by independent hits from overlapping clones, and is also related to the size of the interacting fragments and the total number of hits. When interaction data are assembled into a topological map, then dense nodes (i.e. groups of 5–10 proteins showing interactions with each other) are likely to represent complexes within which the interactions are true.

7.5 Systematic complex analysis by mass spectrometry

The limitations of the yeast two-hybrid method are predominantly related to the nonphysiological nature of the assay system. As discussed above, protein interactions are not studied in their natural context, but are reconstituted artificially in the yeast nucleus. This does not accurately reflect the conditions under which most interactions occur (leading to false negatives) and brings together proteins that would not usually encounter each other in the cell (leading to false positives). Overall, only about half of the interactions predicted from yeast two-hybrid screens are expected to be true.

Affinity-based methods allow interactions to be studied in their natural context, reducing the appearance of irrelevant interaction data. Unlike the yeast two-hybrid system, they also allow the investigation of higher-order interactions, including the purification and categorization of entire complexes. The major bottleneck to large-scale affinity-based interaction analysis, that of identifying the proteins in each complex, has been removed by advances in mass spectrometry that allow the characterization of very low-abundance protein samples (in the low femtomole range). These developments have culminated in the use of affinity purification and mass spectrometry for the systematic analysis of protein complexes, providing a global view of protein interactions known as the complexome.

The first reports of complex analysis by mass spectrometry, such as the analysis of the yeast U1 snRNP complex by Neubauer and colleagues (see Further Reading), involved the antibody-based affinity purification of specific, known components, and thus relied on the availability of suitable antibodies. For whole complexome analysis, a less-selective approach is required for bait preparation and affinity tags have been used instead. These can be attached to any protein of interest and used to capture that protein on a suitable affinity matrix. Two large-scale studies of the yeast complexome were carried out in 2002. In one of these studies (see Ho *et al.* 2002, Further Reading), 725 bait proteins selected to represent multiple functional classes were transiently expressed as fusions with the FLAG epitope, a short peptide that can be recognized by a specific antibody. Cell lysates were prepared from each yeast strain and complexes isolated by affinity capture of an anti-FLAG antibody. Over 1500 captured complexes were separated by SDS-PAGE and characterized by MS/MS analysis (Chapter 3). When redundant and nonspecific interactions were eliminated, this revealed a total of 3617 interactions among 1578 proteins. In the second study (see Gavin *et al*. 2002, Further Reading) the tandem affinity purification (TAP) procedure was used. This involves the expression of each bait protein as a fusion to a calmodulin-binding peptide and staphylococcal protein A, with the two elements separated by a protease recognition site (*Figure 7.13*). Instead of expressing these constructs transiently, the investigators used gene targeting to replace nearly 2000 yeast genes with a TAP fusion cassette. Yeast cells expressing each bait–TAP fusion cassette were lysed and the cell lysate was passed through an immunoglobulin affinity column to capture the protein A component of the bait fusion. After washing to remove nonspecific binding, the bound

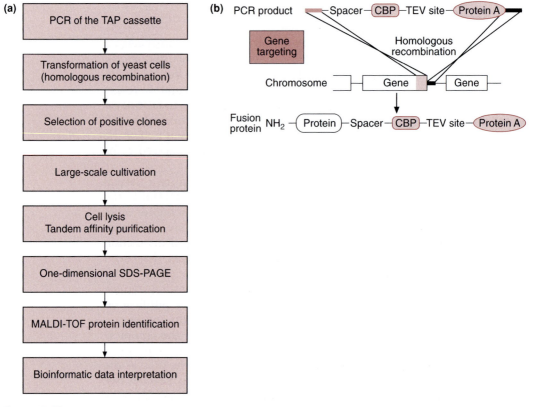

Figure 7.13

(a) Strategy for systematic protein complex analysis in yeast. (b) The tandem affinity purification (TAP) cassette, consisting of a PCR-derived gene-specific homology region for targeting each yeast gene, and a generic region comprising of a spacer, a calmodulin-binding peptide, a protease cleavage site recognized by tobacco etch virus protease and staphylococcal protein A. The TAP procedure itself is described in the text. © Nature Publishing Group, Nature **415**:141–147, 'Functional organization of the yeast proteome by systematic analysis of protein complexes', by Gavin A-C. *et al*. (TEV, tobacco etch virus; CBP, calmodulin-binding protein.)

complexes were selectively eluted by the addition of the protease. Highly selective binding was then carried out in a second round of affinity chromatography using calmodulin as the affinity matrix in the presence of calcium ions. The proteins retained in this step were eluted by adding the calcium-chelating agent EGTA, and were examined by mass spectrometry. Gavin and colleagues found 4111 interactions involving 1440 proteins. Only 10% of the identified complexes had been completely characterized beforehand. In about 30% of the complexes, new components were identified while nearly 60% were entirely novel. Half of the complexes had five or fewer components, and most had fewer than 20. About 10% of complexes had over 30 components and the largest complex contained 83 proteins.

The mass spectrometry approaches were more sensitive than the large-scale yeast two-hybrid experiments when compared to literature benchmarks but still failed to detect about 60% of known interactions, suggesting a high false-negative rate. In part, this may reflect the fact that affinity-based methods favor the recovery of stable complexes rather than transient ones. In contrast, the yeast two-hybrid system can detect transient interactions because even short-lived interactions will cause some activation of the reporter gene. The two mass spectrometry studies of the yeast complexome also showed a low degree of overlap, perhaps because of the different experimental approaches. As described on p. 142, the recovery of interacting proteins depends to a large degree on the amount of bait. Gavin *et al.* used a gene-targeting strategy such that each bait was expressed at roughly physiological levels, whereas Ho *et al.* overexpressed their baits, which may have had a significant effect on complex architecture. Overall, it appears there is no ideal method for the large-scale collection of interaction data and that interaction maps should be built from a variety of complementary sources.

7.6   Protein localization in proteomics

Knowledge of protein localization can provide important evidence either to support or challenge the data from interaction screens. At the very least, showing that two proteins exist in the same cell and in the same subcellular compartment at the same time, indicates that such interactions *could* happen. If this is backed up by FRET analysis or cross-linking studies (pp. 143–145), then the interactions are almost certainly genuine. However, care must be taken to ensure that such experiments are conducted on intact cells with normal levels of gene expression, since both cellular damage and protein overexpression can result in proteins escaping from their normal compartments and contaminating others.

As well as helping to confirm or dismiss claimed interactions, protein localization data can be useful in their own right. As discussed earlier, it is in some cases possible to propose a protein's function based solely on its location, e.g. proteins located in the thykaloid membrane of a chloroplast are probably involved in photosynthesis. For these reasons, many investigators have carried out studies of subcellular or organellar proteomes (organelle proteomics) and several attempts have been made to catalog protein localization data on an even larger scale.

In one such study, thousands of yeast strains have been generated in which a particular gene was replaced with a substitute bearing an epitope sequence. Each strain therefore produced one protein labeled with an epitope tag, allowing the protein to be localized using antibodies and fluorescence microscopy. High-throughput imaging was used to determine the localization of nearly 3000 proteins. The results suggested that about half of the yeast proteome is cytosolic, about 25% is nuclear, 10–15% is mitochondrial and 10–15% is found in the secretory pathway. Within the above classifications, about 20% of the proteome was represented by transmembrane proteins. About 1000 proteins of unknown function were included in the analysis and knowledge of their locations may help in the design of further experiments to determine more precise functions. More recently, Huh and colleagues (see Further Reading) have carried out a similar study in which proteins were labeled with green fluorescent protein, allowing real time analysis and the localization of 70% of the yeast proteome into 22 compartment categories.

A pilot experiment has also been performed using mammalian cells, where the cells were grown on a DNA chip containing arrays of expression constructs. The array was first coated with a transfection reagent, a chemical that promotes DNA uptake, and then immersed in a dish of rapidly growing cells. The cells covered the array, took up the DNA in each area of the array and expressed the corresponding proteins. After a few days, the array was recovered, the cells were fixed *in situ*, and cells in each area were examined by indirect immunofluorescence to determine where the proteins were located. A number of well-characterized proteins were correctly localized, validating the accuracy of the method (e.g. the transcription factor MEFC2 was observed in the nucleus). The major advantage of this method is that the number of proteins investigated simultaneously is limited only by the number of expression constructs that can be fitted on an array. It may therefore be possible to study 5000–10 000 different proteins in parallel.

Several companies are developing imaging technology that is compatible with high-throughput localization studies, with the ultimate aim of building up a three-dimensional map of the cell containing localization and interaction data.

7.7 Protein interaction maps

The presentation of interaction data represents an interesting challenge because of its overall complexity. Each interaction must be annotated to show how it was identified, binary interactions need to be distinguished from interactions within complexes, transient interactions need to be distinguished from permanent associations, there needs to be some representation of interaction stoichiometry, and there should also be a system to assign confidence to interactions identified in different ways. All this must be integrated with existing sequence, structure, metabolic pathway and ontology databases and must be presented in such a way that the interested researcher can switch between simplified views encompassing the entire cell or subcellular compartment and detailed views of particular interaction networks. Other cellular components, such as DNA, RNA and small molecules, will also have to be built in.

With these issues in mind, a number of interaction databases have been established, most of which can be accessed over the Internet (*Table 7.2*). Most of them originated from the large-scale interaction screens described in *Table 7.1*, and are largely focused on the yeast proteome (e.g. the Biomolecular Interaction Network Database, the Database of Interacting Proteins, the Comprehensive Yeast Genome Database and the Saccharomyces Genome Database). Several tens of thousands of interactions are listed, many of which await further functional validation. These databases have been augmented with additional data from other sources. Importantly, a potentially very large amount of data concerning individual protein interactions is 'hidden' in the scientific literature going back many years. It will be a challenge to extract this information and integrate it with that obtained from recent high-throughput experiments. Several bioinformatics tools have been developed to trawl through the literature databases and identify keywords that indicate protein interactions so that such references can be scrutinized by the human curators of interaction databases.

The complexity of interaction networks is shown in *Figure 7.14*. The top panel shows a binary interaction network representing 1548 yeast proteins (25% of the proteome) and a total of 2358 interactions that had been identified at the time of publication (2000). As might be expected, proteins

Table 7.2 Protein interaction databases and resources available free on the Internet. Many companies also make interaction datasets available free to academic institutions

Database	Acronym	URL	Content
Database of Interacting Proteins	DIP	http://dip.doe-mbi.ucla.edu	Experimentally determined protein–protein interactions
Database of ligand receptor partners	DLRP	http://dip.doe-mbi.ucla.edu/dip/DLRP.cgi	Ligand–receptor complexes involved in signal transduction
Biomolecular Interaction Network Database	BIND	http://www.blueprint.org/bind/bind.php	Molecular interactions, complexes and pathways
Protein-Protein-Interaction and Complex Viewer	MIPS-CYDB	http://mips.gsf.de/proj/yeast/CYGD/interaction/	Protein–protein interactions from large scale screens
Hybrigenics	PIM	http://www.hybrigenics.fr	Protein interactions in *Helicobacter pylori*
General Repository for Interaction Datasets	GRID	http://biodata.mshri.on.ca/grid	Central repository for yeast protein interactions
Molecular Interactions Database	MINT	http://cbm.bio.uniroma2.it/mint/	Protein interactions with proteins, nucleic acids and small molecules
Curagen Drosophila interactions database		http://portal.curagen.com/cgi-bin/interaction/flyHome.pl	Protein interactions in *Drosophila*
Curagen yeast interactions database		http://portal.curagen.com/cgi-bin/interaction/yeastHome.pl	Protein interactions in yeast
Saccharomyces Genome Database	SGD	http://www.yeastgenome.org/	Comprehensive structural and functional information, including interactions

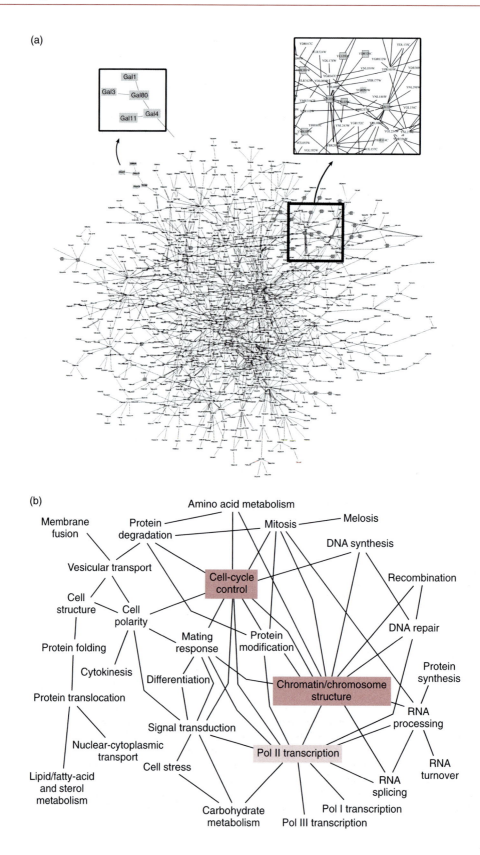

with a similar general function (e.g. membrane transport) tend to interact with each other rather more than with functionally unrelated proteins, such as those involved in the maintenance of chromatin structure. The lower panel shows a simplified version in which proteins have been clustered according to their function. This provides a good overview of the whole interaction map, which can be probed for more detail if required. Although the map is not topological, i.e. it does not reflect the architecture of the cell, proteins that are colocalized also tend to interact more often than those that are located primarily in different compartments, and tracing interaction routes from protein to protein does allow signaling, regulatory and metabolic pathways to be identified. *Plate 9* shows the complex interaction map resulting from the yeast protein complex screen published in 2002. This has been simplified by omitting proteins found in more than nine complexes. As shown in the insert, each complex can be inspected for individual proteins, again providing the researcher with multiple levels of detail. As with the binary map, complexes with similar functions tend to share components and interactions, while there are fewer interactions between functionally unrelated complexes.

The databases described in this section, and the maps derived from them, are useful not only to collate interaction data and allow cross-referencing to other databases, but they also provide a benchmark against which further interaction data can be judged. For example, if several studies have shown that Protein X is located in the nucleus, interacts with four other proteins that are all involved in transcriptional regulation and binds to DNA, while Protein Y is associated with the plasma membrane, binds external signaling molecules and forms a transient signaling complex with seven other proteins, then an unexpected interaction between them revealed in a yeast two-hybrid screen is likely to be a false positive. Conversely, an interaction identified between proteins that are already known to exist in separate complexes both of which are involved in RNA processing would suggest that the interaction was genuine.

Figure 7.14 facing page

(a) Binary interaction map including 1200 interacting proteins based on published interactions (taken from Tucker *et al.*, 2001; see Further Reading). Inset shows close-up of region highlighted in box. Highlighted as dark gray boxes are cell structure proteins (a single functional class). Proteins in this category can be observed to cluster primarily in one region. Although interacting proteins are not depicted in a way that is consistent with their known cellular location (i.e. those proteins known to be present in the nucleus in the center of the interaction map and those present in plasma membranes in the periphery), signal-transduction pathways (or at least protein contact paths) can be inferred from this diagram. (b) Functional group interaction map derived from the detailed map. Each line indicates that there are 15 or more interactions between proteins of the connected groups. Connections with fewer than 15 interactions are not shown because one or a few interactions occur between almost all groups and often tend to be spurious – that is, based on false positives in two-hybrid screens or other assays. Note that only proteins with known function are included and that about one-third of all yeast proteins belong to several classes. Reprinted from Trends in Cell Biology, Vol. 11, Tucker *et al.* 'Towards an understanding of complex protein networks', pp 102–106, ©2001, with permission from Elsevier.

7.8 Proteins and small molecules

We touch briefly on the subject of protein interactions with small molecules to finish this chapter but return to the subject in more detail in Chapter 10 which looks at some of the applications of proteomics, particularly in drug development. Small molecules can act as cofactors, enzyme substrates, ligands for receptors or allosteric modulators, and the function of many proteins is to transport or store particular molecules. On a proteomic scale, screening methods can be employed to isolate proteins that interact with particular small molecules, e.g. through the use of labeled substrates as probes or the immobilization of those substrates on chips. Protein interactions with small molecules can be studied at atomic resolution using X-ray crystallography, and occasionally a protein is accidentally purified along with its ligand, providing valuable information about its biochemical function.

Large-scale screens for protein interactions with small molecules are often carried out to identify lead compounds that can be developed into drugs (Chapter 10). This process can be simplified considerably by choosing compounds based on a known ligand or screening for potential interacting compounds *in silico* using a chemical library. If the structure of the target protein is available at high resolution, docking algorithms can be used in an attempt to fit small molecules into binding sites using information on steric constraints and bond energies. Some of this software is available for free on the Internet, and is listed in *Table 7.3*. One of the most established docking algorithms is Autodoc, which determines ligand coordinates, bonds that have axes of free rotation and interaction energies before carrying out the docking simulation. Another widely used program is DOCK, in which the arrangement of atoms at the binding site is converted into a set of spheres called site points. The distances between the spheres are then used to calculate the exact dimensions of the binding site, and this is compared to a database of chemical compounds. Matches between the binding site and a potential ligand are given a confidence score, and ligands are then ranked according to their total scores. This modeling approach has the disadvantage that the binding site and every potential ligand are considered to be stiff and inflexible. Other algorithms can incorporate flexibility into the structures. A more recent development called CombiDOCK considers each potential ligand as a scaffold decorated with functional groups. Only spheres on the scaffold are initially used in the docking prediction and then individual functional groups are tested using a variety of bond torsions. Finally, the structure is bumped (checked to make sure none of the positions predicted for individual functional groups overlap) before a final score is presented.

Chemical databases can be screened not only with a binding site (searching for complementary molecular interactions) but also with another ligand (searching for identical molecular interactions). Several available algorithms can compare two-dimensional or three-dimensional structures and build a profile of similar molecules. This approach is important, for example, if a ligand has been shown to interact with a protein but has negative side effects, or if a structurally distinct ligand is required in a drug-development project to avoid intellectual property issues. In each case a molecule of similar shape with similar chemical properties is required, but with a different structure.

Table 7.3 Chemical docking software available over the Internet

URL	R/F	Description	Availability
http://www.scripps.edu/pub/olson-web/doc/autodock/index.html	F	Autodock, discussed in main text	Download for UNIX/LINUX
http://swift.embl-heidelberg.de/ligin/	R	LIGIN, a robust ligand–protein interaction predictor limited to small ligands	Download for UNIX or as a part of the WHATIF package
http://www.bmm.icnet.uk/docking/	R	FTDock and associated programs RPScore and MultiDock. Can deal with protein-protein interactions. Relies on a Fourier transform library.	Download for UNIX/LINUX
http://reco3.musc.edu/gramm/	R	GRAMM (Global Range Molecular Matching), an empirical method based on tables of inter-bond angles.GRAMM has the merit of coping with low-quality structures.	Download for UNIX or Windows.
http://cartan.gmd.de/flex-bin/FlexX	F	FlexX, which calculates energetically favorable molecular complexes consisting of the ligand bound to the active site of the protein, and ranks the output.	Apply on-line for FlexX workspace on the server.

R/F means rigid or flexible, and indicates whether the program regards the ligand as a rigid or flexible molecule.

Further reading

Boulton, S.J., Vincent, S. and Vidal, M. (2001) Use of protein-interaction maps to formulate biological questions. *Curr Opin Chem Biol* **5**: 57–62.

Davis, T.N. (2004) Protein localization in proteomics. *Curr Opin Chem Biol* **8**: 49–53.

Drewes, G. and Bouwmeester, T. (2003) Global approaches to protein–protein interactions. *Curr Opin Cell Biol* **15**: 1–7.

Figeys, D. (2003) Novel approaches to map protein–protein interactions. *Curr Opin Biotechnol* **14**: 1–7.

Flajolet, M., Rotondo, G., Daviet, L., et al. (2000) A genomic approach of the hepatitis C virus generates a protein interaction map. *Gene* **241**: 369–379.

Gavin, A.C., Bosche, M., Krause, R., et al. (2002) Functional organization of the yeast proteome by systematic analysis of protein complexes. *Nature* **415**: 141–147.

Giot, L., Bader, J.S., Brouwer, C., et al. (2004) A protein interaction map of Drosophila melanogaster. *Science* **302**: 1727–1736.

Ho, Y., Gruhler, A., Heilbut, A., et al. (2002) Systematic identification of protein complexes in *Saccharomyces cerevisiae* by mass spectrometry. *Nature* **415**: 180–183.

Horak, C.E., Luscombe, N.M., Quain, J.A., et al. (2002) Complex transcriptional circuitry at the G1/S transition in *Saccharomyces cerevisiae*. *Genes Dev* **16**: 3017–3033.

Huh, W.K., Falvo, J.V., Gerke, L.C., Carroll, A.S., Howson, R.W., Weissman, J.S. and O'Shea, E.K. (2003) Global analysis of protein localization in budding yeast. *Nature* **425**: 686–691.

Ito, T., Chiba, T., Ozawa, R., Yoshida, M., Hattori, M. and Sakaki, Y. (2001) A comprehensive two-hybrid analysis to explore the yeast protein interactome. *Proc Natl Acad Sci USA* **98**: 4569–4574.

Ito, T., Tashiro, K., Muta, S., *et al.* (2000) Toward a protein–protein interaction map of the budding yeast: a comprehensive system to examine two-hybrid interactions in all possible combinations between the yeast proteins. *Proc Natl Acad Sci USA* **97**: 1143–1147.

Lee, T.I., Rinaldi, N.J., Robert, F., *et al.* (2002) Transcriptional regulatory networks in *Saccharomyces cerevisiae*. *Science* **298**: 799–804.

Li, S., Armstrong, C.M., Bertin, N., *et al.* (2004) A map of the interactome network of the metazoan C. elegans. *Science* **303:** 540–543.

McCraith, S., Hotzam, T., Moss, B. and Fields, S. (2000) Genome-wide analysis of vaccinia virus protein–protein interactions. *Proc Natl Acad Sci USA* **97**: 4879–4884.

Neubauer, G., Gottschalk, A., Fabrizio, P., Séraphin, B., Lührmann, R. and Mann, M. (1997) Identification of the proteins of the yeast U1 small nuclear ribonucleoprotein complex by mass spectrometry. *Proc Natl Acad Sci USA* **94**: 385–390.

Pelletier, J. and Sidhu, S. (2001) Mapping protein–protein interactions with combinatorial biology methods. *Curr Opin Biotechnol* **12**: 340–347.

Phizicky, E.M. and Fields, S. (1995) Protein–protein interactions: methods for detection and analysis. *Microbiol Rev* **59**: 94–123.

Phizicky, E., Bastiaens, P.I.H., Zhu, H., Snyder, M. and Fields, S. (2003) Protein analysis on a proteomic scale. *Nature* **422**: 208–215.

Schwikowski, B., Uetz, P. and Fields, S. (2000) A network of protein–protein interactions in yeast. *Nature Biotechnol* **18**: 1257–1261.

Titz, B., Schlesner, M. and Uetz, P. (2004) What do we learn from high-throughput protein interaction data? *Expert Rev. Proteomics* **1**: 111–121.

Tong, A.H., Evangelista, M., Parsons, A.B., *et al.* (2001) Systematic genetic analysis with arrays of yeast deletion mutants. *Science* **294**: 2364–2368.

Tong, A.H.Y., Lesage, G., Bader, G.D., et al. (2004) Global mapping of the yeast genetic interaction network. *Science* **303**: 808–813.

Uetz, P. (2001) Two-hybrid arrays. *Curr Opin Chem Biol* **6**: 57–62.

Uetz, P., Giot, L., Cagney, G., *et al.* (2000) A comprehensive analysis of protein–protein interactions in *Saccharomyces cerevisiae*. *Nature* **403**: 623–627.

Vorm, O., King, A., Bennett, K.L., Leber, T. and Mann, M. (2000) Protein-interaction mapping for functional proteomics. *Proteomics: A Trends Guide* **1**: 43–47.

Walhout, A.J.M. and Vidal, M. (2001) Protein interaction maps for model organisms. *Nature Rev Mol Cell Biol* **2**: 55–62.

Werner, T. (2003) Promoters can contribute to the elucidation of protein function. *Trends Biotechnol* **21**: 9–13.

Xenarios, I. and Eisenberg, D. (2001) Protein interaction databases. *Curr Opin Biotechnol* **12**: 334–339.

Internet resources

Useful Internet resources for protein interactions are listed in *Tables 7.1* and *7.2*.

Protein modification in proteomics

8.1   Introduction

Almost all proteins are modified in some way during or after synthesis, either by cleavage of the polypeptide backbone or chemical modification of specific amino acid side chains. This phenomenon, which is known as post-translational modification (PTM), provides a direct mechanism for the regulation of protein activity and greatly enhances the structural diversity and functionality of proteins by providing a larger repertoire of chemical properties than is possible using the 20 standard amino acids specified by the genetic code. Several hundred different forms of chemical modification have been documented, some of which influence protein structure, some of which are required for proteins to interact with ligands or each other, some of which have a direct impact on biochemical activity and some that help sort proteins into different subcellular compartments (*Table 8.1*). Modifications are often permanent, but some, such as phosphorylation, are reversible and can be used to switch protein activity on and off in response to intracellular and extracellular signals. Post-translational modification is therefore a dynamic phenomenon with a central role in many biological processes. Importantly, inappropriate post-translational modification is often associated with disease, and particular post-translational variants can be used as disease biomarkers or therapeutic targets (Chapter 10). While the above types of modification are typical of normal physiological processes, others are associated with damage, aging or occur as artifacts when proteins are extracted in particular buffers.

The complexity of the proteome is increased significantly by post-translational modification, particularly in eukaryotes where many proteins exist as a heterogeneous mixture of alternative modified forms. Ideally, it would be possible to catalog the proteome systematically and quantitatively in terms of the types of post-translational modifications that are present, and specify the modified sites in each case. However, such attempts are frustrated by the sheer diversity involved. Every protein could potentially be modified in hundreds of different ways, and might contain multiple modification target sites allowing different forms of modification to take place either singly or in combination. Thus, it remains the case that most post-translational modifications are discovered accidentally when individual proteins, complexes or pathways are studied. Modifications cannot be predicted accurately from the genome sequence, since even where a definitive modification motif is present, it is not necessarily the case that such a modification will take place.

Until recently, the analysis of post-translational modifications at the proteomic level has received little attention because of the lack of suitable methods. However, many of the techniques discussed in this book can now be adapted for this type of experiment. For example, the protein separation

Table 8.1 A summary of programmed enzymatic protein modifications with roles in protein structure and function, protein targeting or processing and the flow of genetic information

Covalent modification	Examples
Substitutions (minor side chain modifications)	
Minor side chain modification – permanent and associated with protein function	Hydroxylation of proline residues in collagen stabilizes triple helical coiled coil tertiary structure Sulfation of tyrosine residues in certain hormones Iodination of thryroglobulin γ-carboxylation of glutamine residues in prothrombin
Formation of intra- and intermolecular bonds	Formation of disulfide bonds in many extracellular proteins, e.g. insulin, immunoglobulins
Minor side chain modification – reversible and associated with regulation of activity	Phosphorylation of tyrosine, serine and threonine residues regulates enzyme activity, e.g. receptor tyrosine kinases, cyclin-dependent kinases Many side chains are also methylated although the function of this modification is unknown Acetylation of lysyl residues of histones regulates their ability to form higher-order chromatin structure and plays an important role in the establishment of chromatin domains
Augmentations (major side or main chain modifications)	
Addition of chemical groups to side chains – associated with protein function	Addition of nucleotides required for enzyme activity (e.g. adenyl groups added to glutamine synthase in *E. coli*) Addition of *N*-acetylglucosamine to serine or threonine residues of some eukaryotic cytoplasmic proteins Addition of cholesterol to Hedgehog family signaling proteins controls their diffusion Addition of prosthetic groups to conjugated proteins, e.g. heme group to cytochrome C or globins
Addition of chemical groups to side chains – associated with protein targeting or trafficking	Acylation of cysteine residue targets protein to cell membrane Addition of GPI membrane anchor targets protein to cell membrane *N*-glycosylation of asparagine residues in the sequence Asn-Xaa-Ser/Thr is a common modification in proteins entering the secretory pathway *O*-glycosylation of Ser/Thr occurs in Golgi Ubiquitinylation of proteins targeted for degradation
End group modification	Acetylation of N-terminal amino acid of many cytoplasmic proteins appears to relate to rate of protein turnover Acylation of N-terminal residue targets proteins to cell membrane, e.g. myristoylation of Ras
Cleavage (removal of residues)	
Cleavage of peptide bonds	Co- or post-translational cleavage of initiator methionine occurs in most cytoplasmic proteins Cotranslational cleavage of signal peptide occurs during translocation across endoplasmic reticulum membrane for secreted proteins Maturation of immature proteins (proproteins) by cleavage: e.g. activation of zymogens (inactive enzyme precursors) by proteolysis, removal of internal C-peptide of proinsulin, cleavage of Hedgehog proteins into N-terminal and C-terminal fragments Processing of genetic information: e.g. cleavage of polyproteins synthesized from poliovirus genome and mammalian tachykinin genes, splicing out of inteins

techniques discussed in Chapter 2 can generally resolve different post-translational variants, and gels can be stained with reagents that recognize particular types of modified proteins. If the modified group can be removed by chemical or enzymatic treatment, then 'before and after' 2D gels can identify the positions of modified proteins. Edman sequencing is the method used most frequently to characterize proteolytic modifications, but mass spectrometry is preferred for the characterization of chemical additions and substitutions. Once a modified protein has been isolated, it is typically digested with a protease and the peptides are separated by HPLC. Mass spectrometry or Edman sequencing can then be used to identify peptides carrying specific chemical adducts and can pinpoint their positions in the protein sequence. Having said this, it should not be assumed that the detection of modifications is an easy task – only abundant protein variants can be detected using the above methods, and one must be careful to avoid introducing artefactual modifications.

The sensitivity of detection is a key issue. Reversible modifications such as phosphorylation are often used to control the activities of signaling proteins and regulatory molecules, which are the least abundant proteins in the cell. Since the stoichiometry of phosphorylation is usually low, i.e. only a small proportion of the total intracellular pool of a given protein is likely to be modified at a particular time, the modified target protein may be present in limiting amounts and may be difficult to detect and quantify. Even when the 'parent' protein is abundant, the heterogeneity of modification can mean that the amount of protein with a defined, single-modification state is very low. This is often the case with glycoproteins. Finally, even if adequate amounts of a particular variant are available, much more of the sample is required for the full characterization of modifications compared to the relatively simple matter of protein identification. At the current time, researchers rely on affinity-based enrichment techniques to improve the chances of detecting their targets by isolating subproteomes with particular types of modification. This chapter considers the three types of modification that have been subject to the most extensive analysis in proteomics research: phosphorylation, glycosylation and ubiquitinylation. These are also the three most widespread forms of modification in the eukaryotic cell and together probably affect over 90% of all proteins.

8.2 Phosphoproteomics

8.2.1 Overview of protein phosphorylation

Phosphorylation is a ubiquitous form of post-translational modification, and is certainly the most important form of regulatory modification in both prokaryotic and eukaryotic cells. Phosphorylation lies at the heart of many biological processes, including signal transduction, gene expression and the regulation of cell division. In humans, the aberrant phosphorylation of proteins is often associated with cancer.

The esterification of an amino acid side chain through the addition of a phosphate group introduces a strong negative charge, which can change the conformation of the protein and alter its stability, activity and potential for interaction with other molecules. The enzymes that phosphorylate proteins are termed protein kinases and those that remove phosphate groups are termed protein phosphatases (*Figure 8.1*). The substrates for

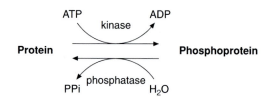

Figure 8.1

Protein phosphorylation is a reversible modification catalyzed by kinases and phosphatases.

these enzymes, i.e. the proteins that are subject to phosphorylation and dephosphorylation, are termed phosphoproteins. In bacteria, proteins are phosphorylated predominantly on aspartic acid, glutamic acid and histidine residues, but this is rare in eukaryotes, where serine, threonine and tyrosine are the major targets. Some proteins in both prokaryotes and eukaryotes are also phosphorylated on arginine, lysine or cysteine residues (*Figure 8.2*). Genes encoding protein kinases and phosphatases account for 2–4% of the eukaryotic genome (there are about 120 kinase and 40 phosphatase genes in the yeast genome and about 500 kinase and 100 phosphatase genes in the human genome). It is thought that up to one third of all the proteins in a eukaryotic cell are phosphorylated at any one time and that there may be as many as 100 000 potential phosphorylation sites in the human proteome, the majority of which are presently unknown. Most phosphoproteins have more than one phosphorylation site and exist as a mixture of alternative phosphoforms.

Since phosphorylation plays such an important role in the regulation of cellular activities, our understanding of the functioning cell would be incomplete without a comprehensive inventory of the phosphoproteome, i.e. a catalog of all the phosphoproteins in the cell, showing the distribution of phosphorylation sites and the abundance of alternative phosphoforms under different conditions. The quantitative aspect of this inventory is important because the phosphoproteome is not only complex but also extremely dynamic. However, only recently has such analysis become possible, with the development of phosphoprotein enrichment methods and improved techniques for the analysis of phosphopeptides by mass spectrometry. The methods for studying phosphoproteins are described in the following sections. However, it should be noted that similar methods could potentially be applied to any form of modification that involved the addition of a small chemical group, e.g. sulfation, methylation and hydroxylation.

8.2.2 Sample preparation for phosphoprotein analysis

Phosphoprotein analysis begins with a mixture of phosphorylated and nonphosphorylated proteins, e.g. a cell lysate or serum sample. The overall aim is to recognize the phosphoproteins, identify them, determine the phosphorylated sites and, if possible, carry out a quantitative analysis of phosphorylation under different conditions. There are various different experimental methods that can be used to achieve these aims, and these

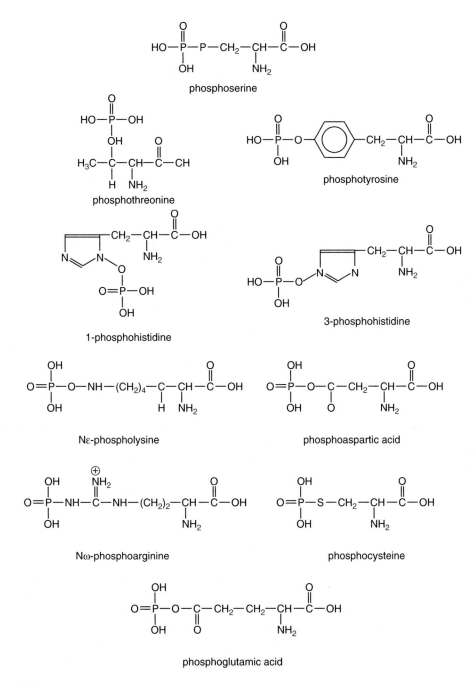

Figure 8.2

Ten different amino acids are known to be phosphorylated in a natural biological context, but only pSer, pThr and pTyr are common in eukaryotes, and only pHis, pAsp and pGlu are common in prokaryotes.

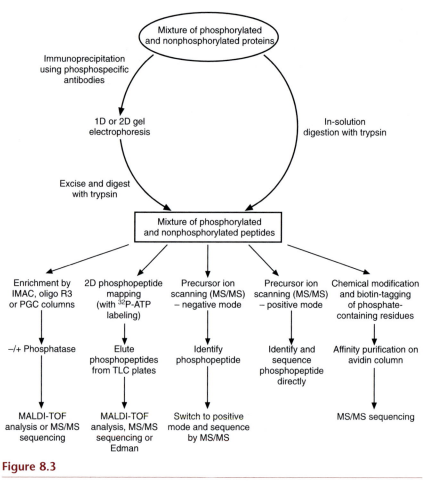

Figure 8.3

Techniques for the enrichment and analysis of phosphoproteins. Reprinted from Trends in Biotechnology, Vol. 20, Mann *et al.*, 'Analysis of protein phosphorylation using mass spectrometry: deciphering the phosphoproteome', pp 261–268, ©2002, with permission from Elsevier.

are summarized in *Figure 8.3*. However, because of the low abundance of many phosphoproteins, enrichment of the sample prior to analysis is usually necessary. As discussed below, enrichment is also necessary to overcome some of the limitations of phosphoprotein analysis by mass spectrometry. Enrichment can be achieved by affinity purification either with or without chemical modification of the phosphate groups.

Affinity purification without chemical modification is advantageous because only small amounts of starting material are required. The simplest method involves antibodies that bind specifically to phosphorylated proteins. If one particular phosphoprotein is sought, it may be possible to use an antibody that binds specifically to that protein. However, for large-scale analysis a more general approach is required. A number of companies market antiphosphotyrosine antibodies, and these can be used as generic reagents to isolate phosphotyrosine-containing proteins by immunoprecipitation. Antibodies that bind other phosphorylated residues, e.g. serine and threonine, have also been produced, but they are less satisfactory for immunoprecipitation and are not widely used. This means that antibody enrichment is generally confined to the analysis of proteins phosphorylated on tyrosine residues (*Box 8.1*). Another disadvantage is that the antibodies do not bind phosphopeptides very strongly. Although it is possible to isolate phosphopeptides from proteolytic digests and analyze them by MALDI-TOF MS while still bound to the antibodies, the antibodies are usually employed prior to digestion, enriching for phosphoproteins that are subsequently fractionated, digested and analyzed by other means.

An alternative affinity-based enrichment strategy, which is widely used to isolate phosphopeptides from pre-digested samples, is immobilized metal-affinity chromatography (IMAC). This exploits the attraction between negatively charged phosphate groups and positively charged metal ions, particularly Fe^{3+} and Ga^{3+}. The method is advantageous because it is relatively easy to combine with downstream analysis by mass spectrometry. Thus, several research groups have carried out off-line analysis of phosphopeptides isolated by IMAC, while others have coupled IMAC to on-line ESI-MS either with or without an intervening fractionation step. It has even been possible to analyze phosphopeptides by MALDI-MS while

BOX 8.1

Probing signaling pathways with antiphosphotyrosine antibodies

Protein phosphorylation plays an important role in the regulation of signaling pathways in both prokaryotes and eukaryotes. Two studies published in 2000 neatly demonstrated the power of phosphotyrosine-specific antibodies for the analysis of the epidermal growth factor (EGF) pathway, which is regulated by tyrosine phosphorylation. The EGF receptor oligomerizes in response to EGF, inducing a latent kinase activity and resulting in the phosphorylation of each subunit of the oliomeric receptor by the tyrosine kinase activity of another subunit (autotransphosphorylation). Cytosolic proteins are then recruited to the receptor if they contain a SRC homology 2 domain (SH2) or phosphotyrosine interaction domain (PID), which bind specifically to phosphotyrosine residues. These cytosolic proteins may also be phosphorylated.

To analyze the entire EGF signaling pathway in a single step, a combination of two antiphosphotyrosine antibodies was used to immunoprecipitate phosphotyrosine-containing proteins from HeLa cells that had or had not been stimulated with EGF. Side-by-side comparison of the recovered proteins identified nine proteins that were tyrosine-phosphorylated specifically in response to EGF. Seven of these proteins were known components of the EGF pathway while the eighth, a ubiquitous protein called VAV2, was not previously known to be a substrate of EGFR. A ninth protein, named STAM2, was novel, but was found to be related to a signaling protein induced by interleukin-2.

In 2002, a novel mass spectrometry technique known as phosphotyrosine-specific immonium ion scanning (or PSI scanning, see main text) was also used to look at the EGF pathway. This identified ten pathway components, two of which were novel, but more importantly it found five novel phosphorylation sites on the proteins SHIP-2, Hrs, Cbl, STAM and STAM2.

still bound to the IMAC column. One drawback of this method is that IMAC columns also bind other negatively charged amino acid residues, such as aspartic acid and glutamic acid. This problem can be circumvented by methyl esterification of all carboxylate groups in the protein sample prior to chromatography. Other chromatography methods that can be used for phosphoprotein or phosphopeptide enrichment include elution from reversed-phase or porous graphitic carbon (PGC) beads.

Affinity purification with prior chemical modification of phosphates is limited by the requirement for larger amounts of starting material, but two methods have been described which may be useful for the isolation of more abundant phosphoproteins and phosphopeptides. In the first method, ethanedithiol is used to replace the phosphate group of phosphoserine and phosphothreonine residues by β-elimination under strongly alkaline conditions, leaving a thiol group that can be used to attach a biotin affinity tag (*Figure 8.4*). The phosphoproteins or phospho-peptides can then be isolated from complex mixtures using streptavidin-coated beads. Cysteine and methionine residues are also derivatized by this method, so they must be oxidized with performic acid prior to the reaction. The major disadvantage of ethanedithiol treatment is that it does not work with phosphotyrosine residues. Furthermore, serine and threonine residues that are O-glycosylated (see later in the chapter) are also derivatized, so further experiments are necessary to confirm that the protein is indeed phosphorylated. In contrast, all three phosphorylated residues are modified in the second method, in which cystamine is added to phosphate groups via a carbodiimide condensation reaction (*Figure 8.4*). This allows affinity-based isolation using iodoacety-lated beads.

8.2.3 Detection of phosphoproteins after protein separation

A general picture of the phosphoproteome can be gained by selectively staining or labeling phosphoproteins, allowing them to be identified in gels or on membranes, or in fractions eluting from a chromatography column. Gel/membrane staining is not a particularly sensitive technique and only allows the most abundant phosphoproteins to be detected, but it helps to identify groups of phosphoforms (these tend to migrate in gels at slightly different rates, forming chains of spots) and can show on/off differences and overt quantitative differences between samples.

The classical technique, which is applicable to all downstream separation methods, is to radiolabel phosphoproteins selectively with ^{32}P, either *in vitro* using [γ-^{32}P]-ATP and a purified kinase or *in vivo* by equilibrating the cellular ATP pool with [γ-^{32}P]-ATP or ^{32}PO$_4$ (orthophosphate). The proteins are then separated by SDS-PAGE, 2DGE or thin-layer chromatography, and the labeled proteins are detected by autoradiography or phosphorimaging. Individual proteins can then be excised from the gel or membrane for fur-ther analysis. Alternatively, radiolabeled fractions can be collected as they elute from a chromatography column. Before a phosphorylation event detected *in vitro* can be accepted as biologically significant, it must also be shown to occur *in vivo*. This is because kinases *in vitro* may act on many pro-teins with which they never come into contact under physiological conditions, perhaps because they are expressed in different cells or located in different subcellular compartments. Unfortunately, *in vivo*

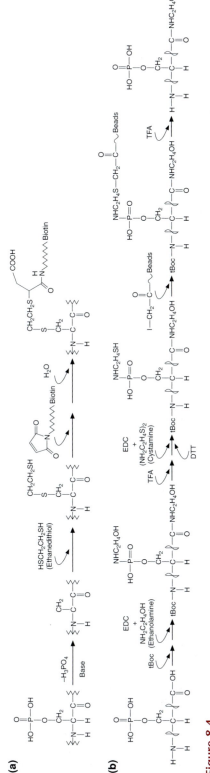

Figure 8.4

Chemical derivatization for the isolation of phosphoproteins and phosphopeptides. (a) Chemical modification based on β-elimination: samples containing phosphoproteins are first treated with a strong base, leading to β-elimination reactions in the case of phosphoserine (pictured here) and phosphothreonine residues. A reactive species containing an α,β unsaturated bond is formed. This serves as a Michael acceptor for the nucleophile (in this case, ethanedithiol or an isotopic variant may be substituted for quantitation purposes). The biotinylated reagent reacts with sulfhydryl (-SH) groups at acidic to neutral pH. Biotinylated phosphoprotein is now tagged for enrichment on avidin columns in later steps. (b) Chemical modification based on carbodiimide condensation reaction. The amino termini of peptides are first protected with tert-butyl oxycarbonyl (tBoc) chemistry. A condensation reaction then occurs between the carboxyl groups as well as the phosphate moiety in the presence of excess amine (ethanolamine) in a reaction catalyzed by N,N' dimethylaminopropyl ethyl cabodiimide HCl (EDC). The condensation reaction results in the formation of an amide bond and a phosphoamidate bond from carboxyl and phosphate bonds, respectively. The phosphate group is regenerated by rapid hydrolysis with acid and the sample is desalted on reverse phase material (this intermediate step is not shown here). A second condensation reaction (also catalyzed by EDC) is performed next with excess cystamine. The sample is reduced with dithiothreitol (DTT), converting the disulfide bond of cystamine to a sulfhydryl group and thereby tagging the phosphate moiety. The sample is again desalted using reverse phase material. The tagged peptides are captured on glass beads containing bound iodoacetyl groups that will react with sulfhydryl groups. The recovery of phosphopeptides is performed by strong acid hydrolysis that cleaves both the phosphoamidate bond and the tBoc protective group, thus regenerating the phosphate moiety and the N-terminus, respectively. Reprinted from Trends in Biotechnology, Vol. 20, Mann et al., 'Analysis of protein phosphorylation using mass spectrometry: deciphering the phosphoproteome', pp 261–268, ©2002, with permission from Elsevier.

incorporation also depends on the metabolic phosphorylation rate and the equilibrium between phosphorylated and nonphosphorylated forms of the target protein. If the pool of a given protein is already saturated with phosphate groups, then no further incorporation will occur regardless of the activity of the kinase, and the phosphoprotein will not be detected.

To avoid such problems, a number of staining methods have been developed which will stain all phosphoproteins in 1D and 2D gels, on membranes or in chromatography fractions. One example is the Pro-Q Diamond stain, available from Molecular Probes Inc., which can detect as little as 1 ng of phosphoprotein and can be used in combination with the general SYPRO staining agents (Chapter 3). Western blotting with antiphosphotyrosine antibodies, or the chemical modification of phosphate residues with fluorescent labels, are examples of such methods based on the enrichment procedures discussed above. Although antiphosphoserine and antiphosphothreonine antibodies have insufficient affinity to be used for immunoprecipitation, they are adequate for immunoblot analysis and can be used to identify the corresponding phosphorylated proteins immobilized on membranes.

8.2.4   Identification of phosphorylated residues

If a relatively pure protein sample can be obtained, e.g. a spot excised from a 2D-gel or membrane, partial hydrolysis under alkaline conditions or via enzyme cleavage can release individual phosphoamino acids, which can be used to confirm the presence of a phosphoprotein and identify the phosphorylated residue. If related samples are available, e.g. healthy and diseased tissue, this method also allows the abundance of phosphoamino acids in each sample to be compared.

The method used for separation of the phosphoamino acids depends on the type of sample and how it has been treated. Proteins taken directly from an *in vitro* kinase reaction, in which [γ-^{32}P]-ATP has been used to incorporate a radiolabel, are generally separated by gel electrophoresis or thin-layer chromatography after digestion, since phosphoserine, phosphothreonine and phosphotyrosine are readily identified by this method. For proteins labeled *in vivo* with ^{32}PO$_4$, there may be contaminating labeled compounds and 2D-separation is required to give better resolution. If proteins or released phosphoamino acids can be derivatized with a fluorogenic reagent, then HPLC can be used in combination with UV detection to identify and quantify the phosphorylated residues. Mass spectrometry can also be used to identify phosphoamino acids, although improved techniques for the analysis of phosphopeptides (see below) make this approach obsolete.

8.2.5   Identification of phosphoproteins and prediction of phosphorylated sites

Edman degradation and mass spectrometry

Until the late 1990s, the standard approach to phosphorylation site analysis was to label the isolated phosphoprotein with ^{32}P, digest it into peptides and separate the peptides by first-dimension thin-layer electrophoresis and second-dimension thin-layer chromatography (an approach known as 2D-peptide mapping). Phosphopeptides could then be identified by autoradiography, and these were excised and sequenced using Edman chemistry. The phosphorylated site was determined by the release of a radiolabeled amino acid in the corresponding sequencing cycle. Variations on this theme included the use of chemically derivatized phosphopeptides, which released amino acids that could be recognized by their particular retention times or because they carried a fluorescent label. Although 2D peptide mapping and Edman sequencing continues to be used today for phosphorylation site analysis, it is very laborious to apply on a large scale.

As in other areas of proteomics, the analysis of phosphoproteins has been revolutionized by mass spectrometry. Two main principles are exploited, namely that peptides containing a single phosphate modification will show a mass shift of 79.983 compared to the nonphosphorylated peptide, and that phosphopeptides will yield diagnostic fragment ions that are not found on unmodified peptides. In practice, MS analysis is more challenging because phosphopeptides are often far less abundant than their unmodified counterparts. Furthermore, due to factors that are not completely understood, an equimolar mixture of peptides will generate signals of varying intensity and some will be lost altogether, resulting in incomplete coverage of the protein. This phenomenon affects phosphopeptides more strongly than unmodified peptides because they are more difficult to ionize; the signal from the unmodified peptide is said to suppress that of the modified peptide. These problems can be addressed by enriching the phosphopeptide pool using one of the methods discussed earlier in the chapter, and fractionating the peptides by HPLC prior to mass spectrometry. Another difficulty is that phosphate groups tend to inhibit proteolytic cleavage by trypsin at nearby peptide bonds, making full coverage of the protein even more unlikely. Therefore, Edman degradation remains useful as a complementary approach where MS fails to provide adequate data.

Analysis of intact phosphopeptide ions by MALDI-TOF MS

As discussed in Chapter 3, MALDI-TOF MS is most often used to analyze intact peptides, and correlative database searching (peptide mass fingerprinting) allows the derived masses to be matched against the theoretical peptides of known proteins. Therefore, if the identity of the protein is known or can be deduced from the peptide masses, phosphopeptides can be identified simply by examining the mass spectrum for mass shifts of 79.983 compared to predicted masses. Parallel analysis in which the sample has been treated with alkaline phosphatase can also be helpful, since peaks corresponding to phosphopeptides in the untreated sample should be absent from the treated sample (*Figure 8.5*). This method does not identify phosphorylated residues directly, but if the peptide sequence contains only one possible phosphorylation site, if a consensus kinase target site is present (*Table 8.2*) or if the phosphorylated residue has been chemically identified using one of the methods described in Section 8.2.3, then it is most likely that the site can be identified accurately.

Analysis of fragment ions

The analysis of fragment ions (see Chapter 3 for a general overview) serves two purposes in phosphoproteomics. First, phosphopeptides preferentially

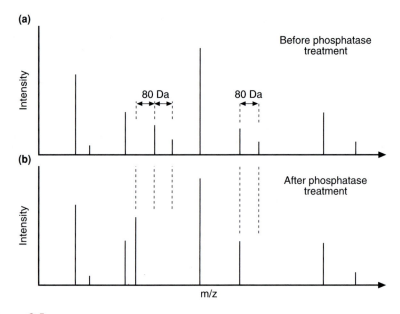

Figure 8.5

Phosphopeptide identification by MALDI-TOFMS mapping combined with alkaline phosphatase treatment. (a) The MALDI-TOF MS spectrum of a proteolytic digest. Phosphopeptides are indicated by peaks shifted by multiples of 80 Da (HPO_3 = 80 Da) relative to predicted unphosphorylated peptide masses. (b) The disappearance of such peaks upon treatment with a phosphatase confirms their identity as phosphopeptides. Reprinted from Current Opinion in Chemical Biology, Vol. 5, McLachlin and Chait, 'Analysis of phosphorylated proteins and peptides by mass spectrometry', pp 591–602, ©2001, with permission from Elsevier.

yield diagnostic, phosphate-specific fragment ions such as $H_2PO_4^-$, PO_3^- and PO_2^-, which have masses of approximately 97, 79 and 63 respectively. Phosphoserine and phosphothreonine are more labile in this respect than phosphotyrosine. The presence of such ions in a mass spectrum therefore indicates the presence of a phosphopeptide in the sample. Secondly, fragmentation along the polypeptide backbone can yield peptide fragments that allow a sequence to be built up *de novo* (p. 65). This sequence will include the phosphoamino acid, providing a definitive location for the phosphorylated residue.

Since the phosphate group provides a negative charge, phosphate-specific fragment ions are usually obtained by MS/MS using an ESI ion source in negative ion mode. Collision-induced dissociation (CID) is used to generate the fragments and analysis is usually carried out using a triple quadrupole or more sensitive hybrid quadrupole-quadrupole-TOF machine (an ion trap can also be used, although this is less common because the instrumentation is not widely available). Three general strategies are used. The first is called in-source CID and requires excess energy during ionization to induce multiple collisions and produce the phosphate reporter ions in the emerging ion stream (*Figure 8.6*). This method also

Table 8.2 Summary of phosphorylation sequence motifs recognized by various kinases. Reprinted from J. Chromatog. A., Vol 808, Yan *et al.*, 'Protein phosphorylation: technologies for the identification of phosphoamino acids.' pp 23–41, ©1998, with permission from Elsevier.

Sequence motif	Enzyme	Protein (substrate)
Ser/Thr phosphorylation		
Ser–Ser–Xaa–Ser(P)	Bone morphogenetic proteins receptor kinase	TGF-beta family mediator Smad 1
Arg–Xaa–Arg–Yaa–Zaa–Ser(P)/Thr(P)–Hyd	Protein kinase B	Synthetic peptide
Ser(P)–Xaa–His	Protein kinase C	Alpha 1 Na,K-ATPase
Ser(P)–Leu–Gln–Xaa–Ala	cGMP-dependent kinase	Lentivirus Vif proteins
Glu–Val–Glu–Ser(P)	c-Myb kinase	Vertebrate c-Myb proteins
Arg–Xaa–Xaa–Ser(P)	Phosphotransferase	Serum response factor, c-Fos, Nur77 and the 40S ribosomal protein S6
Ser(P)/Thr(P)–Pro–Xaa (basic), Pro–Xaa–Thr(P)–Pro–Xaa (basic)	Cyclin-dependent kinase 2	Cyclin A or E
Thr(P)–Leu–Pro	Ceramide-activated protein kinase	Raf protein
Arg–Xaa–Ser(P)	cAMP-dependent protein serine kinase	PII protein (glnB gene product)
Ser–Xaa–Xaa–Xaa–Ser(P)	Glycogen synthase kinase 3	cAMP responsive element binding protein
Arg–Xaa–(Xaa)–Ser(P)/ Thr(P)–Xaa–Ser/Thr	Autophosphorylation-dependent protein kinase	Myelin basic protein
Hyd–Xaa–Arg–Xaa–Xaa–Ser(P)/ Thr(P)–Xaa–Xaa–Xaa–Hyd	Ca²⁺/calmodulin-dependent protein kinase Ia	Peptide analogs
Ser–Xaa–Glu–Ser(P)	Casein kinase	Bovine osteopontin, vitamin K-dependent matrix Gla protein from shark, lamb, rat, cow and human
Ser–Xaa–Xaa–Glu–Ser(P)	Casein kinase II	Bovine osteopontin
Xaa–Ser(P)/Thr(P)–Pro–Xaa	Proline-directed protein kinase	Tau protein
Ser–Pro–Arg–Lys–Ser(P)–Pro–Arg–Lys Ser(P)–Pro–Lys/Arg–Lys/Arg	Histone H1 kinase	Sea-urchin, sperm-specific histones H1 and H2B
Lys–Ser(P)–Pro	Serine kinase	Murine neurofilament protein
Tyr phosphorylation		
Tyr(P)–Met–Asn–Met, Tyr(P)–Xaa–Xaa–Met, Tyr(P)–Met–Xaa–Met	Phosphatidylinositol 3-kinase, in cytoplasmic tail	CD28 T cell costimulatory receptor
Asn–Pro–Xaa–Tyr(P)	Focal adhesion kinase, in cytoplasmic domain	Integrin beta-3
Tyr(P)–Xaa–Xaa–Leu	Protein Tyr kinase, in cytoplasmic tail	Mast cell function-associated antigen
Glu–Asp–Ala–Ile–Tyr(P)	Protein Tyr kinase	Synthetic peptides
Dual Thr and Tyr phosphorylation		
Thr(P)–Xaa–Tyr(P)	Mitogen-activated protein kinase	p38 mitogen-activated protein
Thr(P)–Glu–Tyr(P)	Mitogen-activated protein kinase kinase	Mitogen-activated protein kinase

Xaa is any amino acid, Yaa and Zaa are small residues other than Gly, Hyd is hydrophobic amino acid residue Phe or Leu.

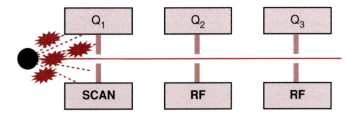

Figure 8.6

Detection of phosphopeptides using in-source CID in a triple quadrupole mass spectrometer. Excess energy used during ionization causes fragmentation to occur at the ion source. The ion stream is scanned in Q_1 for phosphate reporter ions such as PO_3^- (m/z = 79$^-$). These pass through the other quadrupoles (running in RF mode) to the detector.

fragments the peptide backbone to a lesser extent and can therefore provide some peptide sequence information (see below). Normal ionization energy levels are used in precursor ion scanning. In this mode, the first quadrupole (Q_1) is used to scan the ion stream, CID occurs in Q_2 (running in RF mode) and the third analyzer (Q_3 or TOF) is set to detect phosphate reporter ions, such as PO_3^-, induced by collision. Phosphopeptides are thus identified when a precursor ion scanned in Q_1 yields a phosphate fragment that is detected in Q_3 (*Figure 8.7*). In neutral loss scan mode, both Q_1 and Q_3 are set to scan the ion stream. Q_1 scans the full mass range, Q_2 is used as the collision cell and Q_3 scans a parallel range to Q_1 but at an m/z ratio that is 98/z lower, with the intention of detecting the neutral loss of H_3PO_4 (*Figure 8.8*).

All these methods can be combined with in-line HPLC, either using reversed-phase material alone or in combination with a second-dimension separation matrix, such as a strong cation exchange resin. This is currently the only way in which protein modifications can be analyzed in a high-throughout manner and is advantageous also because it can be coupled

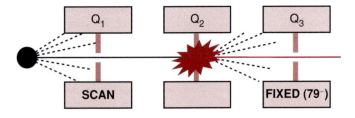

Figure 8.7

Detection of phosphopeptides using precursor ion scan mode in a triple quadrupole mass spectrometer. The entire ion stream is scanned in Q_1, allowing selected ions through to the collision chamber in Q_2. The fragmented ions then pass through Q_3, which is fixed to detect phosphate reporter ions such as PO_3^- (m/z = 79$^-$). Only if intact phosphopeptide ions pass through Q_1 will reporter ions pass through Q_3 to the detector.

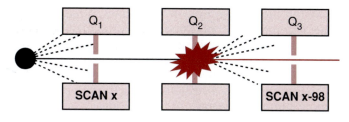

Figure 8.8

Detection of phosphopeptides using neutral loss scan mode in a triple quadrupole mass spectrometer. The entire ion stream is scanned in Q_1, allowing selected ions (x) through to the collision chamber in Q_2. Q_3 is set to scan the fragmented ions in parallel to Q_1, but at a lower mass range (e.g. x-98, where 98 is the mass of H_3PO_4). Only phosphopeptide ions which lose H_3PO_4 during CID will pass through Q_3 to the detector.

to an IMAC phosphopeptide enrichment step therefore helping to simplify the analyte and reduce the ion suppression effects discussed earlier. A good example of this approach was published in 2002 by Ficarro and colleagues (see Further Reading). They digested yeast protein lysates with trypsin converted the peptides into methyl esters and enriched the phosphopeptide pool using IMAC. This was coupled to a nanoflow HPLC column that fed fractions directly into an ESI-mass spectrometer. Over 1000 phosphopeptides were identified in this procedure, and the sequences of 216 peptides were obtained allowing 383 phosphorylation sites to be determined.

Fragment ions for protein sequencing are obtained in positive ion mode, so samples analyzed in negative ion mode as above need to be split or rebuffered prior to sequence analysis. More recently, instruments have been developed that can easily detect the immonium ion (mass 216.043) generated by double fragmentation of the polypeptide backbone on either side of a phosphotyrosine residue (phosphotyrosine-specific immonium ion scanning, PSI scanning). This method is not applicable to other phosphorylated residues but can be carried out in positive ion mode, which means it can be used in combination with strategies to identify the phosphorylation site. PSI scanning has been used to identify components of the EGF signaling pathway, as discussed in *Box 8.1*.

Generally, sequencing and the determination of phosphorylation sites are carried out by MS/MS using the full product scan mode, where specific precursor ions are gated at Q_1, fragmented in Q_2 and scanned for product ions in Q_3 (Chapter 3). The uninterpreted CID spectra can be used to search for matching proteins in the databases as long as mass shifts caused by the phosphate group are taken into account, or the mass spectra can be interpreted to produce an amino acid series. As discussed in Chapter 3, the interpretation of CID spectra is a complex process which involves the identification of fragment ions corresponding to a nested set of peptides that can be built into a complete series. The series is produced by calculating the mass differences between consecutive ions and correlating those mass differences to a standard table of amino acids. The only adjustment necessary in this application is that the mass of the phosphate group must also be allowed in the calculations. In some cases, it has been possible to facilitate the recognition of phosphorylated residues in ion series by chemical derivation. For example, β-elimination can be used to convert phosphoserine into S-ethylcysteine and phosphothreonine into β-methyl-S-ethylcysteine. This also removes these labile phosphate groups so that fragmentation is more evenly distributed along the polypeptide backbone, providing more complete coverage of the peptide.

Although ESI-MS/MS is the most widely used method for phosphoprotein analysis, some researchers have used post-source decay in MALDI-TOF instruments to obtain both phosphate reporter ions and fragments of the phosphopeptide itself. A relatively new development is electron capture dissociation, which is carried out in a Fourier transform ion cyclotron resonance mass spectrometer (FT-ICR MS) by bombarding the ion stream with subthermal electrons. This method is not widely used because FT-ICR MS instruments are expensive and require specialized operators. However, it does offer increased sensitivity and coverage, resulting in extended ion series that are much easier to interpret than CID spectra. Phosphorylation sites can also be identified in small proteins without proteolytic digestion.

8.2.6 Quantitative phosphoproteomics

Chapter 4 deals with quantitative proteomics in detail, and many of the techniques and principles discussed in that chapter for the analysis of proteins in general are equally applicable to the analysis of protein modifications. Rough estimates of the stoichiometry phosphorylation in a single sample, or differences in phosphorylation levels between two samples, can be made by separating the phosphorylated and corresponding unmodified peptides by HPLC, carrying out quantitative amino acid analysis and comparing the peaks. Rough quantitative data can also be obtained by comparing the intensity of signals on 2D gels. As discussed above, however, it is not possible simply to compare the intensity of signals obtained from the phosphorylated and unmodified peptides in a mass spectrometer, because of the differences in overall detection and the occurrence of suppression. Instead, quantitation is based on the incorporation of stable isotopes or mass tags, which produce two very similar chemicals that can be detected with equal efficiency, but which can be distinguished due to a mass shift when the samples are combined and analyzed together.

For the analysis of phosphoproteins, the general labeling methods discussed in Chapter 4 are not always suitable because they are not selective for phosphopeptides. For example, the standard ICAT method (p. 79) labels cysteine-containing peptides, and its use in phosphoprotein analysis would depend on whether the phosphorylated residue resided on the same peptide as the labeled cysteine. Metabolic labeling *in vivo* with ^{15}N or using heavy amino acids and the SILAC procedure (p. 82) would be more useful, since this is nonselective and all peptides would be labeled in the same way. When comparing two related samples, each phosphopeptide should be represented by four peaks, one phosphorylated and labeled, one unmodified and labeled, one phosphorylated and unlabeled and one unmodified and unlabeled. The labeled/unlabeled pairs should occur as doublets separated by the mass value of the chosen label, while the mass difference between each unmodified peptide and its phosphorylated counterpart should be about 80 (*Figure 8.9*). A variation of the ICAT method, which results in the specific labeling of phosphoserine and phosphothreonine residues, has been described. In this case, only phosphopeptides would be labeled and each would be represented by just two peaks, one labeled and one unlabeled, allowing direct comparison between samples.

As an alternative to labeling, quantitative differences in the phosphorylation of a given peptide between samples can be determined by including a chemically synthesized heavy derivative of a peptide in each sample as an internal standard. This approach cannot be applied on a proteomic scale but it is useful for the analysis of known phosphoproteins.

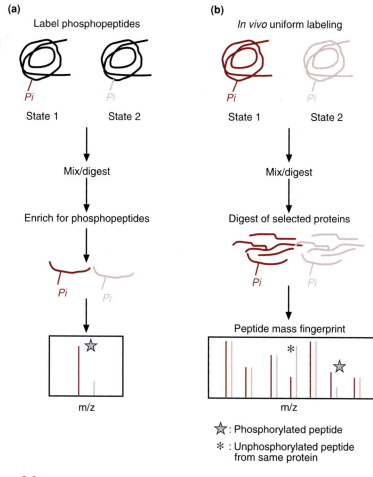

Figure 8.9

Quantitation of phosphoproteins by mass spectrometry. (a) If phosphoproteins can be labeled with mass tags and isolated by affinity capture, direct quantitative comparison across samples is possible by comparing peak intensities. (b) If peptides are labeled uniformly, peaks corresponding to the phosphorylated and unmodified versions of the same peptide will appear about 80 mass units apart. If protein abundance is the same in each sample, only phosphopeptides should show any quantitative variation. Reprinted from Current Opinion in Chemical Biology, Vol. 7, Sechi and Oda, 'Quantitative Proteomics using mass spectrometry', pp 70–77, ©2003, with permission from Elsevier.

8.3   Glycoproteomics

8.3.1   Glycoproteins

Glycosylation involves the addition of short-chain carbohydrate residues (oligosaccharides or glycans) to proteins during or after synthesis. This type of modification is very common in eukaryotes (>50% of all proteins are glycosylated), but it also occurs to a lesser extent in prokaryotes. In eukaryotes, the vast majority of glycosylated proteins, or glycoproteins, pass through the secretory pathway. However, not all of them are actually secreted. Some are retained within the endoplasmic reticulum (ER) or Golgi apparatus, some are targeted to lysosomes, and many are inserted into the plasma membrane. The three major types of glycosylation that occur in the secretory pathway of mammalian cells are N-linked glycosylation, O-linked glycosylation and the addition of glycosylphosphatidylinositol (GPI) anchors. N-linked glycans are attached to asparagine residues in the context Asn-Xaa-Ser/Thr, where Xaa can be any amino acid except proline. O-linked glycans are linked to the hydroxyl group of serine or threonine residues. GPI anchors are attached to the C-terminus of the protein following the removal of a C-terminal signal sequence. More rarely, proteins in the cytosol or those targeted to the nuclear pore complex may be modified by the addition of a single O-linked GlcNAc residue.

N-linked glycosylation occurs only in eukaryotes. It begins with the attachment of a branched, 14-residue oligosaccharide – the core glycan $GlcNAc_2Man_9Glc_3$. This modification occurs only in the ER because the enzyme responsible for the reaction is localized in the ER membrane. The core glycan is then trimmed by glycosidases to remove some of the residues, and the partially glycosylated protein moves to the Golgi apparatus. In this compartment, further modifications take place, involving the substitution of certain core glycan residues and the elaboration of the glycan chains. More than 30 different types of sugar molecule can be added, and the structure and architecture of chains can vary significantly. This process of elaboration produces three major types of glycan structure, known as high mannose, hybrid and complex types (*Figure 8.10*). The modifications that take place are different in plants, mammals, yeast and insects, resulting in glycan structures that are distinct to each species in terms of complexity, composition, branching structure and the linkages between residues. Since N-linked glycosylation does not take place in bacteria, recombinant mammalian proteins produced in bacteria lack the glycan chains. For some proteins, this appears to have no effect on biological activity (e.g. growth hormone) whereas in others the aglycosylated version is less active or completely nonfunctional (e.g. interleukin-2, thyroperoxidase).

There is generally a degree of heterogeneity in N-glycan modification, so that each protein is produced not as a single, defined molecule but a collection of glycoforms. Proteins may have more than one acceptor site for N-linked glycosylation, so there may be different glycan chains at the same site on different molecules (microheterogeneity) and different site occupancy (macroheterogeneity). This provides immense scope for structural diversity, although it is apparent that glycoproteins do not necessarily exist as all possible glycoforms and not all potential acceptor sites are modified.

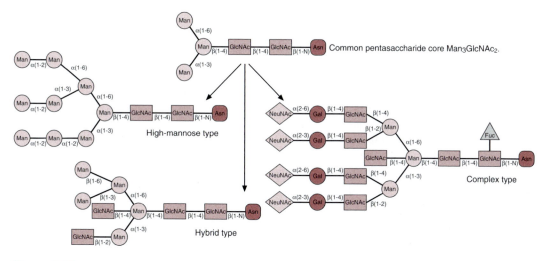

Figure 8.10

The three major types of N-linked glycans – high-mannose, hybrid and complex – are all built from a common pentasaccharide core.

Many proteins with N-linked glycans also undergo O-linked glycosylation in the Golgi apparatus, which involves the addition of sugars to exposed hydroxyl groups on serine and threonine side chains (and occasionally hydroxylysine and hydroxyproline). There does not appear to be a consensus sequence for the addition of mucin-type glycans, the most common form of O-linked glycosylation, indicating that modification may depend on secondary and tertiary structure. However, it is not uncommon to find O-linked glycosylation in proline-rich domains. Mucin-type glycans are structurally very heterogeneous and are usually classified according to their core structure (*Figure 8.11*). Other O-linked glycans include single glucosamine, fucose, galactose, manose or xylose residues, and these require specific consensus sequences.

A third major form of glycosylation that occurs in the secretory pathway is the addition of GPI moieties to proteins that need to be anchored in the plasma membrane. GPI-anchored proteins are attached at the C-terminus to a trimannosyl-nonacetylated glucosamine (Man$_3$-GlcN) core through a phosphodiester linkage involving phosphoethanolamine. This may be further modified in some cell types. The reducing end of the GlcN residue is linked through another phosphodiester bond to phosphatidylinositol (PI), which is anchored in the membrane (*Figure 8.12*).

8.3.2 The role of glycoproteins in the cell

Although most secreted proteins in eukaryotes are glycosylated, the purpose of the glycan chains remains unclear in many cases. It is apparent that glycans are required for some proteins to fold properly, and in other cases the carbohydrate residues act as address labels that facilitate protein sorting to the appropriate subcellular compartments. This is the case for proteins targeted to the lysosome, which have exposed mannose-6-phosphate residues, and membrane proteins containing GPI anchors.

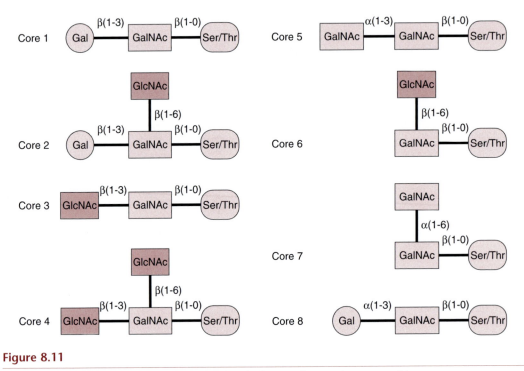

Figure 8.11

O-linked glycans are very diverse and are classified according to the core residues.

The stability of some proteins appears to be improved by the presence of glycan chains, possibly because they prevent proteases gaining access to the protein surface. One of the most important functions, however, is the control of protein interactions with each other and with other ligands. In this context, glycan chains are important for cell signaling, cell recognition during fertilization, in development and in the modulation of the immune response. Deficiencies or alterations to the glycan component of several proteins have been linked to disease, and a number of examples are shown in *Table 8.3*.

8.3.3 Glycoanalysis

Conventional glycoanalysis techniques are laborious and time-consuming because multiple steps are required, and they do not provide exhaustive data (*Figure 8.13*). Initially, the glycan or glycans must be removed from the isolated parent protein. With N-glycans, this can be achieved in a single step using the enzyme peptide-N-glycosidase F (PNGase F). Despite its name, PNHGase F is a deamidase rather than an endoglycosidase, which means that the Asn residue to which the glycan chain is attached is deamidated to Asp. This modification provides a useful signature when mass spectrometry is used to identify potential glycopeptides, since a database error of +1 is obtained compared to the predicted mass of the unmodified protein. However, this enzyme does not work on glycans containing α(1-3)-fucose (a residue which is found in plants and some worms, but not in mammals) and the alternative PNGase A must be used. There is no

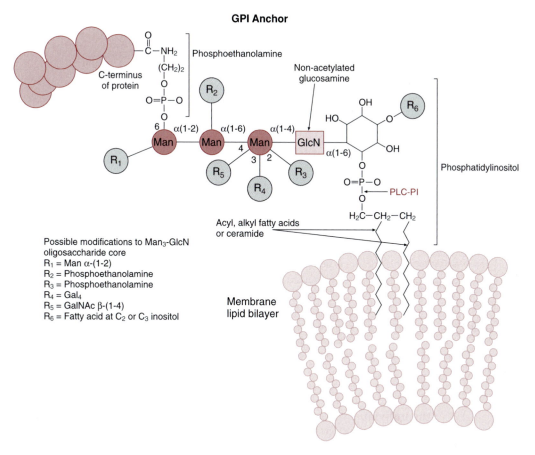

Figure 8.12

The GPI anchor is a carbohydrate-rich structure which tethers proteins to the plasma membrane.

equivalent enzyme for O-linked glycans, although mild alkaline treatment resulting in β-elimination is a useful and successful approach.

If the protein has multiple glycosylation sites or is present as multiple glycoforms, the collection of glycan chains must be fractionated and individual glycan species must be isolated. Several different types of analysis can then be carried out to determine the glycan structure. Each glycan can be broken up into its constituent monosaccharides by acid hydrolysis and

Table 8.3 Some diseases associated with altered glycan chains on glycoproteins

Disease	Glycoprotein	Alteration
Hepatic cancer	α-fetoprotein	Different N-glycan structures
Immune disorders	CD43	Different O-glycan structures
Rheumatoid arthritis	IgG	N-glycans, reduction in terminal galactosylation
Choriocarcinoma	hCG	N- and O-linked glycans, hyperbranching
Alcohol abuse	Transferrin	N-glycans, desialylation

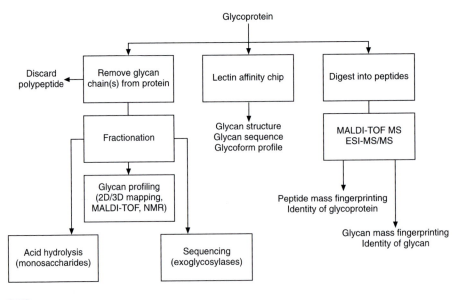

Figure 8.13

The full analysis of glycoproteins must involve characterization of both the polypeptide and glycan components. At the current time, this is usually achieved by parallel analysis of unglycosylated peptides and released glycans. Lectin chips, a new innovation, now allow the characterization of intact glycoproteins.

the individual sugars can be identified. This provides the monosaccharide composition of each glycan, but does not reveal any sequence or structural information. Nevertheless, monosaccharide composition is still a useful approach since all hexoses have the same mass (as do GlcNAc and GalNAc) and cannot therefore be distinguished by mass spectrometry. One traditional way to obtain sequences and structures is to carry out 2D/3D mapping, where glycans are resolved into their sugars by multiple rounds of chromatography, and the structures are worked out by comparing the elution positions to those of standards. Further structural information can be derived from mass spectrometry and NMR spectroscopy experiments. Each glycan can also be labeled and digested with specific exoglycosylases to determine the sequence. By combining these techniques, the sequence and branching pattern of each glycan, and its relative abundance in the original protein sample can be deduced. This sort of approach has been optimized for the analysis of individual glycoproteins produced in recombinant expression systems and is the method of choice for monitoring batch-to-batch differences in recombinant protein drugs.

What this type of analysis does not reveal is the distribution of glycan chains within a protein sample. For example, if a protein has two glycosylation sites (A and B) and there are two types of glycan chain (1 and 2), what does it mean if conventional glycoanalysis shows that each glycan is equally abundant? It could mean that all the proteins in the sample have glycan 1 at site A and glycan 2 at site B, or the reverse could be true, or 50% of the proteins might have two glycan 1 chains while the other 50% have two glycan 2 chains (*Figure 8.14*). Novel lectin chip technologies have been developed to address such problems (Section 8.3.6).

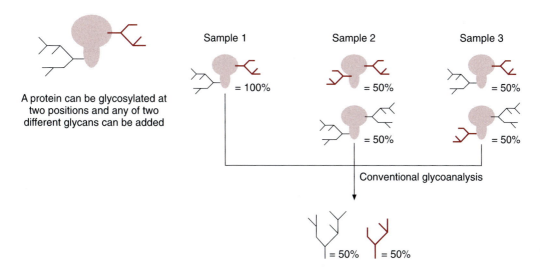

A protein can be glycosylated at
two positions and any of two
different glycans can be added

Sample 1 = 100%

Sample 2 = 50% = 50%

Sample 3 = 50% = 50%

Conventional glycoanalysis

= 50% = 50%

Figure 8.14

Conventional glycoanalysis, which involves removal of the glycan chains, can reveal glycan sequence and structure, and the relative proportions of each type of glycan in a mixture, but cannot resolve a mixture of different glycoforms. The three samples shown in the figure are not the same but they cannot be distinguished by conventional methods.

For glycoanalysis at the whole proteome level, higher-throughput and more information-rich analysis techniques are required. As discussed above for phosphoproteins, glycoproteomic analysis requires methods for the selective detection and isolation of glycoproteins and the identification of the glycosylated sites. In this case, however, structural and compositional analysis of the glycan chains has to be included in the investigation making comprehensive glycoprotein analysis an order of magnitude more complex than the analysis of phosphoproteins.

8.3.4 Separation and detection of glycoproteins

All of the separation techniques discussed in Chapter 2 are applicable to glycoproteins, and 2DGE is the method of choice for visualizing the glycoproteome. Standard techniques for in-gel or on-membrane protein staining appear to work poorly with glycoproteins and special methods are required. One of the earliest to be described was the periodic acid/Schiff (PAS) method, which relies on the oxidation of sugar moieties for the detection of glycoproteins in gels or on membranes. This can be combined with a more sensitive detection assay if the glycans are modified, e.g. with biotin-hydrazide (detected with streptavidin-peroxidase and appropriate colorimetric or chemiluminescent substrates) or with fluorescein semi-carbazide hydrazide (for sensitive fluorometric detection). More recently, several companies have developed universal stains that work well with glycoproteins, such as the SYPRO series of stains marketed by Molecular Probes Inc. (see p. 72). The same company has also produced a glycoprotein-specific staining reagent called Pro-Q Emerald, which is 50 times more sensitive than the PAS method and can be combined with SYPRO staining.

A problem with 2DGE is that glycan heterogeneity causes each glycoprotein to appear as a series of discrete spots, representing glycoforms with different molecular masses or different pI values (*Figure 8.15*). The same protein can therefore appear in several or many different spots, often in a chain, and the concentration of that protein in each individual spot is reduced. The analysis of individual spots by MS (see below) has revealed, perhaps surprisingly, that each spot is not homogeneous for a particular glycoform. In some cases, this may be because the same protein contains identical glycan chains at different acceptor positions, but generally there also appears to be heterogeneity in glycan size and charge (e.g. sialic acid content) suggesting that the relationship between glycoprotein structure and the migration on 2D gels is complex. Higher-resolution glycoform separation is possible by combining methods such as reversed phase HPLC, strong anion exchange chromatography and capillary electrophoresis.

More recently, robust methods have been described that allow the analysis of N- and O-linked oligosaccharides released from glycoproteins separated by 2D-PAGE and then electroblotted onto PVDF membranes. Nicole Packer and colleagues (see Wilson *et al.*, Further Reading) have described a technique in which N-linked oligosaccharides are released by treatment with PNGase F followed by the chemical release of O-linked oligosaccharides using β-elimination. The released species are then separated and characterized by LC-ESI-MS. N-linked site-specific information was obtained by trypic digestion of the remaining proteins and analysis by MALDI-MS.

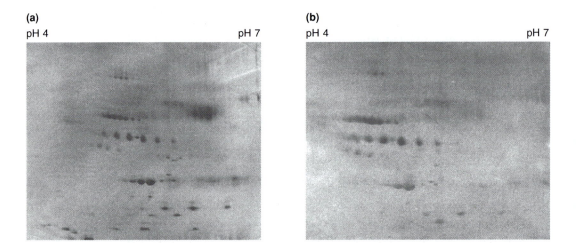

(a)
pH 4   pH 7

(b)
pH 4   pH 7

Figure 8.15

Fluorescent staining of glycoproteins on a PVDF membrane: (a) Coomassie Brilliant Blue stain; (b) fluorescein carbohydrate stain. One micoliter of serum was loaded by rehydration, separated by 2DGE and electroblotted to a PVDF membrane. The fluorescent stain used periodate oxidation of the sugars as contained in the Bio-Rad glycoprotein detection kit, but used a solution of 0.05 mg/ml fluroescein semicarbazide hydrazide (Molecular Probes) in 50% (v/v) methanol in 1 mM sodium acetate pH 5.5, instead of sandwich antibody color development. Fluorescence was vizualized with a Fluor S imager (Bio-Rad). Courtesy of Nicolle Packer.

8.3.5   Enrichment of glycoproteins

Glycoprotein enrichment is generally carried out by lectin-affinity chromatography. Lectins are proteins that bind carbohydrates. Many lectins are available that have very specific ligands, including concanavalin A (Con A) which binds specifically to mannosyl and glucosyl residues, wheat germ lectin which binds specifically to di-N-acetylglucosamine and N-acetylneuraminic acid residues, and m-aminophenylboronic acid, which binds to 1,2-cis-diol groups. Other lectins, such as *Riccinus communis* lectin, have broader specificities. Several lectin-affinity procedures may be used one after the other to select different classes of glycan chains progressively. Alternatively, fractionation within a class of glycoforms can be achieved by gradient elution (using stepped increases in a competitive binding agent). Lectin-affinity chromatography is also useful for the purification of glycopeptides following proteolytic digestion, and the purification of glycan chains derived from glycoproteins in preparation for enzymatic or mass spectrometry-based sequencing.

Recently, Mann and Jensen (see Further Reading) have reported a novel method for the selective enrichment of proteins modified with GPI anchors. The technique involves treating cell membrane preparations with an enzyme that specifically cleaves the GPI anchor. This releases the GPI-modified proteins into the buffer and allows them to be extracted and characterized by LC MS/MS.

8.3.6   High-throughput identification and characterization of glycoproteins

Glycoproteomics is a relatively new subdiscipline of proteomics and the technology for high-throughout glycoprotein characterization is still in the early stages of development. At the current time, direct and simultaneous analysis of both the protein and carbohydrate components is difficult unless the glycan chain is relatively simple. For example, peptides with mass shifts of +162 or multiples thereof are indicative of proteins modified with hexose sugars, but large N-glycan-substituted peptides are difficult to study by MALDI-MS because of their mass, and their tendency to be heterogeneous (which results in broad peaks). The analysis of individual glycoforms resolved by capillary electrophoresis or HPLC is more straightforward, but the complexity of the glycan chain still makes it difficult to resolve the structure without data from additional glycan sequencing experiments (see above).

The few glycoproteomics strategies that have been developed to date therefore involve separate analysis of the protein and glycan components. An example is the 'glyco-catch' procedure of Hirabayashi and Kim (see Further Reading) (*Figure 8.16*). This involves the isolation of glycoproteins from cell lysates using lectin-affinity chromatography. Subsequent rounds of affinity separation using different lectins can be used to simplify the glycoprotein pool. Selected glycoproteins are then digested with protease and the glycopeptides selected using the same affinity procedure. The peptides are then fractionated by HPLC and sequenced using Edman chemistry or mass spectrometry. Meanwhile, the glycans are removed with PNGase F, derivatized with pyridylamine and subjected to 2D/3D

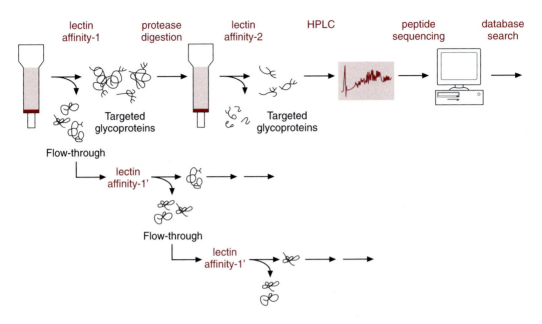

Figure 8.16

The GLYCOCATCH procedure for high-throughput analysis of glycoproteins. Reprinted from Medline, Vol. 771, Hirabayashi and Kasai, 'Separation technologies for glycomics', pp 67–87, ©2002, with permission from Elsevier.

mapping, mass spectrometry and frontal affinity chromatography with lectins to determine binding constants.

Another recent development in glycoproteomics is the use of lectin chips to generate glycan profiles. These chips, which are manufactured and marketed by Procognia Inc., are arrayed with specific lectins and can be used to screen protein samples for particular glycans. When intact glycoproteins are bound via their glycan moieties to the lectin array, their presence can be detected with labeled probes bound to some other site on the glycoproteins. An intensity scan from the chip, when normalized and interpreted by proprietary algorithms, produces a fingerprint of the glycoprotein sample. Database analysis then allows the fingerprint to be converted into the sequences of all the glycans in a sample and the proportion of each glycan present to create a glycan profile. Because the technique is nondestructive, the algorithms and software can further identify the different glycoforms, as well as the proportion of each in a mixture to produce a glycoform profile. Information derived from the glycan structures and their relationships on different glycoforms helps to guide the rational design of protocols for the affinity separation of individual glycoforms from the mixture. Although designed primarily as a diagnostic tool to test the quality of recombinant proteins, such technology could become very useful for the characterization of glycoproteins on a wider scale.

8.4 Ubiquitinomics

A final class of protein modification that has been dealt with at the proteomic level is ubiquitinylation. It is fitting that we discuss this form of modification last because this is almost certainly the last form of modification any protein will undergo. The function of ubiquitin, an 8.5-kDa protein found in all eukaryotic cells, is to tag old, damaged or defective proteins for degradation. Proteins differ widely in their half-lives, some existing for only a few minutes and others lasting for days or weeks. Some proteins have different half-lives under different circumstances, showing that the destruction of proteins is regulated. It has been estimated that up to 30% of newly synthesized protein may be degraded immediately because they contain defects, while other proteins are destroyed because they have suffered oxidation or other forms of chemical damage.

Proteins targeted for destruction are covalently attached to ubiquitin through an isopeptide bond which joins the C-terminal lysine of ubiquitin to the ε-amino group of an internal lysine residue of the substrate protein (*Figure 8.14*). Several lysine residues in the same protein may be modified, and further ubiquitin molecules may attach to the ubiquitins that are already attached. The ubiquitinylated protein is then digested by a multisubunit complex known as the 26S proteosome, and the ubiquitin is recycled.

In 2003, Gygi and colleagues (see Further Reading) set out to investigate protein ubiquitinylation in the yeast *Saccharomyces cerevisiae* on a global scale. The first step was to replace the endogenous yeast ubiquitin gene with a cassette in which six codons for histidine had been added to the 5′ end of the gene. This resulted in the expression of a recombinant ubiquitin with an N-terminal polyhistidine tag. Proteins thus labeled can be isolated from cell lysates using specific antibodies or, more frequently, IMAC. The recombinant yeast strain was cultured under normal growth conditions, and then the cells were harvested and lysates were obtained. Ubiquitin-tagged proteins were recovered from the lysates by affinity chromatography, digested with trypsin, fractionated by multidimensional liquid chromatography and analyzed by MS/MS. Over 1000 ubiquitinylated proteins were identified in this experiment, and 110 precise ubiquitin-acceptor sites were mapped in 72 ubiquitin-protein conjugates. The method is generally applicable to the large-scale analysis and characterization of protein ubiquitinylation and will be useful for examining changes in the regulation of protein degradation in response to different stimuli.

Further reading

Conrads, T.P., Issaq, H.J. and Veenstra, T.D. (2002) New tools for quantitative phosphoproteome analysis. *Biochem Biophys Res Commun* **290**: 885–890.

Ficarro, S.B., McCleland, M.L., Stukenberg, P.T., et al. (2002) Phosphoproteome analysis by mass spectrometry and its application to *Saccharomyces cerevisiae*. *Nature Biotechnol* **20**: 301–305.

Hirabayashi, J. and Kasai, K. (2002) Separation technologies for glycomics. *J Chromatog B* **771**: 67–87.

Jensen, O.N. (2000) Modification-specific proteomics: strategies for systematic studies of post-translationally modified proteins. *Proteomics: A Trends Guide,* **(1)**: 36–42.

Jensen, O.N. (2004) Modification-specific proteomics: characterization of post-translational modifications by mass spectrometry. *Curr Opin Chem Biol* **8**: 33–41.

Kalume, D.E., Molina, H. and Pandey, A. (2003) Tackling the phospho-proteome: tools and strategies. *Curr Opin Chem Biol* **7**: 64–69.

Mann, M. and Jensen, O.N. (2003) Proteomic analysis of post-translational modifications. *Nature Biotechnol* **21**: 255–261.

Mann, M., Ong, S.E., Grønborg, M., Steen, H., Jensen, O.N. and Pandey, A. (2002) Analysis of protein phosphorylation using mass spectrometry: deciphering the phosphoproteome. *Trends Biotechnol* **20**: 261–268.

McLachlin, D.T. and Chait, B.T. (2001) Analysis of phosphorylated protein and peptides by mass spectrometry. *Curr Opin Chem Biol* **5:** 591–602.

Opiteck, G.J. and Scheffler, J.E. (2004) Target class strategies in mass spectrometry-based proteomics. *Expert Rev. Proteomics* **1**: 57–66.

Packer, N.H. and Keatinge, L. (2001) Glycobiology and proteomics. In: Pennington, S.R. and Dunn, M.J. (eds) *Proteomics: From Protein Sequence to Function*, 257–275. Bios Scientific Publishers, Oxford, UK.

Peng, J.M., Schwartz, D., Elias, J.E., *et al.* (2003) A proteomics approach to understanding protein ubiquitination. *Nature Biotechnol* **21**: 921–926.

Wilson, N.L., Schulz, B.L., Karlsson, N.G. and Packer, N.H. (2002) Sequential analysis of N- and O-linked glycosylation of 2D-PAGE separated glycoproteins. *J Proteome Res* **1**: 521–529.

Yan, J.X., Packer, N.H., Gooley, A.A. and Williams, K.L. (1998) Protein phosphorylation: technologies for the identification of phosphoamino acids. *J Chromatog A* **808**: 23–41.

Internet resources

http://www.indstate.edu/thcme/mwking/protein-modifications.html A nice introduction to the subject of post-translational modification on the Indiana University School of Medicine medical biochemistry page.

http://www-lecb.ncifcrf.gov/phosphoDB/ The Phosphoprotein Database.

http://www.abrf.org/index.cfm/dm.home?AvgMass=all Delta Mass, a database of protein post-translational modifications and the mass differences that need to be used in mass spectrometry experiments.

http://pir.georgetown.edu/cgi-bin/resid RESID, database of post-translational modifications and associated information.

http://us.expasy.org/tools/ A list of tools that can be used to predict modification sites on proteins.

http://www.netconferences.net/tgn/inf_res.htm A list of sites and resources that deal with the analysis of glycans and glycoproteins.

Protein chips and functional proteomics

9.1 Introduction

All of the proteomics technologies described in this book share one common feature, i.e. that they can be used for the parallel analysis of large numbers of proteins in a single experiment. As in other areas of biological research, the trend towards higher throughput has been matched by a trend towards miniaturization and automation. One only has to look at the success of DNA chips and the impact they have had on sequence analysis and expression profiling to see how crucial such devices have become in large-scale biology (Chapter 1). DNA chips are miniature appliances upon which many cDNA sequences, genomic DNA fragments or oligonucleotides can be arrayed in the form of a grid. The resulting DNA microarray covers an area no bigger than a postage stamp, but it allows thousands of genes to be analyzed in parallel using only a few tens of microliters of analyte. Because only small sample volumes are required, high signal intensities can be achieved with a low background. DNA microarray experiments are therefore very sensitive. Microarray assays are also easy to automate, making them suitable for today's high-throughput, genome-scale experiments. With the creation of in-house microarray printing services in many academic and industrial settings, global expression profiling has become economical and practical, and the experiments yield immense amounts of useful data. Not surprisingly, there has been a strong drive towards the development of similar devices for the analysis of proteins, i.e. protein chips and protein microarrays.

The concept of the protein array is not new. Miniaturized, multiplexed, solid-phase immunoassays were developed in the 1980s using protein microdots spotted manually onto nitrocellulose sheets and other solid supports. It was shown quite clearly that this multianalyte immunoassay format was far more sensitive than standard immunoassays carried out in microtiter plates because the sample volumes were so much smaller. At about the same time, the first gridded cDNA expression libraries were developed, allowing the functions and binding capacities of large numbers of arrayed, immobilized proteins to be tested in parallel. The arrays were printed on big sheets of nitrocellulose or nylon, which by today's standards would be regarded as quite cumbersome. At the time, however, these were much more convenient to use than standard libraries taken from plate imprints (where the clones were distributed randomly) and also allowed data to be shared more efficiently between laboratories. More recently, protein arrays have evolved into microarrays as the materials, apparatus, surface chemistries and printing technologies developed for the manufacture of DNA microarrays have been modified and exploited to develop analogous devices for protein analysis. However, protein chip technology does not stop at the microarray. Almost any conceivable proteomics method can be miniaturized and developed in a chip format, including protein separation by chromatography or electrophoresis, the processing of samples for mass spectrometry and the large-scale analysis of fluids, cells or tissue samples for protein abundance and localization.

This chapter begins with an overview of protein chip technology and the different types of chip that have been developed. We then discuss how microarrays are made, how they are printed, how different types of array are used and how signals can be detected. To maintain clarity in this very diverse area of proteomics, the main text sticks to technical and practical issues while case studies are discussed in boxes. Despite the technological hurdles that remain to be overcome, protein chips represent the fastest growing sector of the proteomics market, with particular interest in the area of functional proteomics – the direct analysis of protein biochemical and cellular functions on a large scale. Thus far, there have been very few attempts to study biochemical functions systematically on a large scale. The most significant study was that of Martzen and colleagues (see Further Reading) in which 6144 yeast strains were produced, in each of which a particular gene was expressed as a GST-fusion. Strains were grown in defined pools, assayed for a number of biochemical activities and then the pools were deconvoluted to identify strains with particular functions. This study revealed the biochemical activities of three erstwhile uncharacterized proteins. An increasing number of functional affinity reagents are being used to identify protein in gels and on chips, e.g. peptidyl chloromethyl ketone affinity probes for the detection of serine proteases, and labeled penicillin probes to detect penicillin-binding proteins (*Table 9.1*). Protein chips provide a novel platform for the high-throughput screening of protein functions.

9.2   Different types of protein chips

The term 'protein chip' encompasses a bewildering number of quite different devices linked only by their overall function, which is the large-scale analysis of proteins. First we can distinguish between *bona fide* arrays, i.e. chips with arrayed molecules on their surfaces, and other devices based on microfluidics technology. The latter are not arrays, but miniature bioanalytical devices that can separate molecules such as proteins by controlling the movement of small volumes of liquids and gases. These chips are generally prototypical in nature, they exploit very new innovations in microfluidics and nanotechnology, and their full impact on proteomics and other areas of biology is currently difficult to judge. The ultimate aim is to provide a one-stop device for complete proteomics analysis – e.g. separation, protease digestion and analysis by mass spectrometry – in a parallel chip-based format. Many companies founded in the last few years are developing such lab-on-a-chip contrivances and some examples are provided in *Box 9.1*. We do not discuss this type of protein chip any further in the rest of the chapter.

Protein arrays can be further classified in a number of different ways, according to how they are made, their surface chemistry, their specificity, the density of features, the target molecules in the analyte, what they measure and how the signal is generated and detected. Perhaps the most important distinction is between analytical arrays, which are used predominantly for expression profiling (quantitative analysis), and

Table 9.1   A selection of function specific affinity reagent that can be used to identify functional classes of proteins in gels, on membranes and on chips. Modified from Current Opinion in Chemical Biology, Vol 7, Campbell, D.A. and Szardenings, A.K., 'Functional profiling with affinity labels', pp 296–303, ©2003 with permission from Elsevier.

Affinity probe	Protein family
	Serine protease
	Serine hydrolase
	Cysteine protease
	Cysteine protease
	Tyrosine phosphatases
	Aldehyde dehydrogenase
	Thiolase NAD/NADP-dependent oxidoreductase Enoyl CoA hydratase Epoxide hydrolase Glutathione S-transferase
	Penicillin-binding proteins
	Kinases (IKKβ)
	NF-κB and unknown target

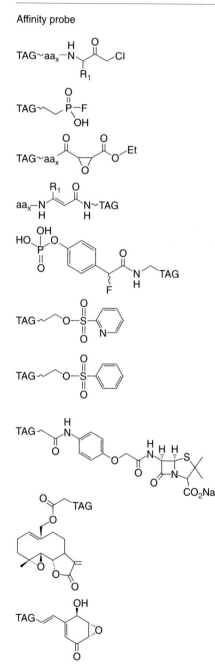

BOX 9.1

The lab-on-a-chip

Several companies have developed miniature devices that allow proteomics separation technology to be applied to very small volumes of liquid. This increases sensitivity and throughput, reduces the experimental timescale and allows almost total automation. For example, consider the widely used conventional separation method of 2DGE (Chapter 2). This requires relatively large sample volumes, separations can take more than 24 hours to complete and the maximum sensitivity is somewhere in the low-nanogram range. The gels are large and cumbersome, and they are difficult to integrate with downstream analysis procedures such as mass spectrometry. In contrast, on-chip separations can be carried out on tiny analyte volumes in less than 30 minutes, and ten or more separations can be carried out simultaneously. Recent innovations allow on-chip protease digestion, peptide separation and mass spectrometry using trypsin-membranes and microscale capillary zone electrophoresis. Chips have been developed than can perform electrophoretic and/or chromatographic separations in two dimensions in a matter of minutes, and the elimination of hands-on sample processing means that there is no loss of analyte, providing picomole sensitivities.

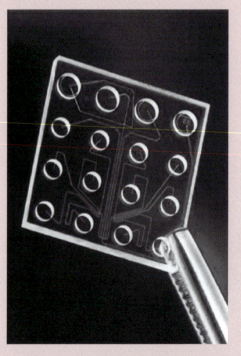

Figure 9.1 shows the prototype microfluidic channel system developed by Agilent Technologies, which allows ten electrophoretic separations to be completed in less than an hour in combination with real-time viewing of separations. ©(2004) Agilent Technologies, Inc. Reproduced with permission.

functional arrays, which can be used to investigate biochemical activities and interactions (*Figure 9.2*). The difference between these devices is as follows. In the case of functional arrays, the proteins under investigation are immobilized on the chip surface and are either tested for their biochemical functions or used to probe the analyte for interacting

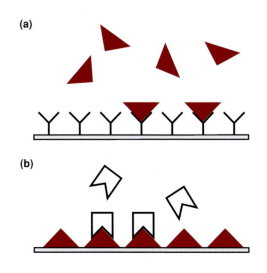

Figure 9.2

Analytical and functional protein arrays. (a) Analytical arrays contain immobilized capture agents (which may or may not be proteins) and the proteins under investigation are in the analyte. (b) Functional arrays operate on the reverse principle, where the proteins under investigation are immobilized and used as probes to capture interacting molecules in the analyte. The proteins under investigation are shown in red.

molecules. In contrast, in the case of analytical arrays the proteins under investigation are in the solution applied to the chip, and the device itself contains immobilized capture agents which act as probes. The capture agents can be proteins (usually antibodies) but other types of molecules can be used instead, including nucleic acids, peptides, small organic molecules, carbohydrates and synthetic polymers. Their designation as protein arrays therefore refers to what they capture and analyze rather than their own make-up. The terms protein chip, microchip, biochip, array and microarray appear to be used interchangeably to describe a whole host of different devices and the choice is mostly a matter of personal preference. Several functionally specific types of analytical and functional protein arrays are discussed below.

9.2.1 Antibody arrays

The most common type of analytical protein chip is the antibody array, which is a coated glass slide or silicon wafer containing a high-density array of specific antibodies. The antibodies may be conventional full-size immunoglobulins produced in hybridoma cells, or recombinant derivatives such as single-chain Fv (scFv) or Fab fragments expressed in bacteria. The chip is flooded with the analyte, allowing the antibodies to capture any antigens that are present, and then washed to remove unbound proteins. The proteins in the analyte may be labeled, allowing direct detection by fluorescence scanning or autoradiography, they may be detected using a label-free procedure such as surface plasmon resonance spectroscopy, or the bound, unlabeled antigen may be detected using a second, labeled antibody in a sandwich assay (*Figure 9.3*). The pros and cons of different probe detection methods are discussed in Section 9.4.

The two major technological problems limiting the development of antibody arrays are the difficulty in obtaining and expressing sufficient numbers of antibodies for large-scale studies and the difficulty in obtaining antibodies of adequate specificity. At the time of writing, commercial chips have been manufactured containing up to 500 different antibody probes (Antibody Microarray 500, BD Biosciences Clontech, Palo Alto, California) but most experimental and commercial chips contain fewer than 150 probes because not enough suitable antibodies are available. While small numbers of probes are suitable for moderate-scale experiments, e.g. monitoring the expression profiles of key proteins, proteome-scale analysis would require at least a ten-fold increase in complexity, and even this would only allow the analysis of relatively simple proteomes, such as those of bacteria and yeast.

Conventional hybridoma technology is too labor-intensive and time-consuming to achieve the scale of antibody production needed for the manufacture of whole-proteome analytical chips, so alternative methods are required. The best option at the current time is phage antibody display technology, which allows the production of very complex libraries of scFv

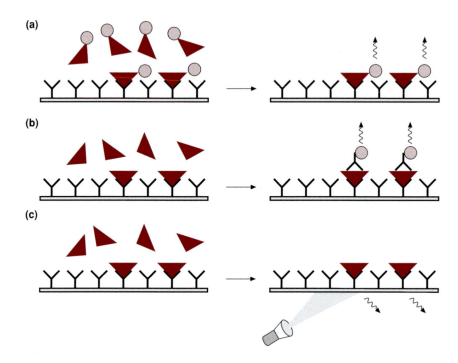

Figure 9.3

Signal detection strategies used with antibody arrays and similar analytical devices. (a) The proteins in the analyte may be labeled universally, e.g. with a fluorescent conjugate. (b) The proteins in the analyte may be unlabeled and detected using a labeled antibody. (c) The proteins in the analyte may be unlabeled and detected using a label-free method, such as surface plasmon resonance spectroscopy.

or Fab antibodies displayed on the surface of phage particles (see Chapter 7). In a recent demonstration of the power of this technology for proteomic applications, a phage display library was used to probe human proteins that had been separated by 2DGE and blotted onto PVDF membranes (see Liu *et al.*, Further Reading). Automation of this process would allow panels of specific antibodies to be generated, and since phage display antibodies are linked to phage particles containing the DNA sequences that encode them, it would be relatively simple to move from affinity-based identification to cloning in recombinant bacteria and large-scale expression. De Wildt and colleagues have developed scFv arrays containing over 18 000 probes (see Further Reading).

Phage display not only allows the rapid generation of antibodies, but also facilitates the selection of high-affinity binders through several rounds of maturation and affinity panning. This may help to address the second limitation of current antibody arrays, that of insufficient antibody specificity. The specificity problem reflects the fact that most antibody arrays are currently used to detect particular, restricted classes of proteins, often cytokines or other secreted factors that are released into the serum or culture medium. Such antibodies have been developed especially for serum profiling and in many cases have not been checked for broader cross-reactivity, e.g. in cell lysates. In the few studies that have addressed this issue, the data suggest that up to 50% of antibodies used on chips cross-react with nontarget antigens (see *Box 9.2*). The proteins in a typical analyte cover a broad dynamic range, so antibodies with high affinity for a scarce target antigen and low cross-affinity for an abundant nontarget antigen might bind both antigens equally well. This would provide a completely false indication of the relative abundances of the two antigens in the analyte. It is therefore likely that many of the antibodies currently used for specific analytical applications will be unsuitable for proteome-wide applications. The problem of cross-reactivity is eliminated in the sandwich assay approach, because two noncompeting antibodies (i.e. antibodies recognizing different epitopes of the antigen) would be required for each target protein. However, this in itself generates another volume problem because twice as many antibodies would need to be produced. Several companies, e.g. Cambridge Antibody Technologies, Cambridge, UK, are using phage display or ribosome display to develop large panels of highly specific antibodies for array manufacture, and are cooperating with chip producers for the development of commercial arrays.

9.2.2 Alternative capture agents

Antibodies are not the only specific capture molecules that can be immobilized on chips for the detection of proteins. Indeed, certain antibodies, such as scFvs, may be nonideal in any case due to their poor stability. A variety of alternative reagents have been developed which might offer a longer shelf life. Among these, perhaps the most promising are oligonucleotide and peptide aptamers, which can be obtained from highly complex libraries and can be optimized for specific binding activity using *in vitro* evolution methods. There is great interest in peptide arrays not only because they are more stable than antibody arrays but also because they can be printed directly onto the chip surface using photolithographic techniques developed by Affymetrix Inc. for the manufacture of DNA chips (Chapter 1). An alternative strategy is to use completely synthetic antibody mimics or protein scaffolds, such as affibodies (Affibody, Stockholm) and Trinectin reagents, which are recombinant fibronectin structures (Phylos, Lexington, Massachusetts). Other nonprotein molecules that can be used as affinity reagents include synthetic ligands identified by combinatorial chemistry, enzyme substrates and ribozymes (Ribo-Reporters, developed by Archemix, Cambridge, Massachusetts). A novel class of capture reagents known as molecular imprinted polymers (MIPs) could potentially be used to mimic any specific binding event. In this platform technology, a polymerization reaction is induced on the surface of a chip that has been flooded with a particular target molecule. The polymer forms around the target and becomes embossed with its shape. When the target molecule is removed, the imprint remains and can be used to capture similar molecules from solution. It is not known if these imprints will ever attain the sensitivity or specificity of antibodies, or if they can be developed on a scale suitable for proteomic applications. Other capture agents may be used to detect specific functional classes of proteins. Carbohydrate arrays, for example, can be used to capture lectins and other carbohydrate-binding proteins. In contrast, lectin chips can be used to capture glycoproteins and analyze their glycan structures (see Chapter 8).

BOX 9.2

Analytical protein chips: Case studies with dual color antibody arrays

Dual labeling is widely used with DNA microarrays to compare gene expression levels across multiple samples. Typically, two samples are obtained, the mRNA or derived cDNA is universally labeled with one of two fluorescent molecules, and both samples are applied to the array. The array is scanned at the excitation wavelength of each fluorophore in turn, and the signals are read at the corresponding emission wavelengths. The images from each fluorophore are then rendered in false color and combined, providing a global snapshot of differential gene expression (Chapter 1).

Dual labeling technology has been applied less frequently in proteomics because uniform labeling is more difficult to achieve (see Section 9.4). The technique of difference gel electrophoresis, which incorporates dual labeling, is discussed on p. 76. There have also been several reports in which dual labeling has been used with protein microarrays. An early and extensive study into the feasibility of dual fluorescence microarray analysis was published Brian Haab and colleagues in 2001 (see Further Reading). These investigators obtained 115 well-characterized antibody–antigen pairs from three commercial sources, and transferred the antibodies onto glass slides that had been coated with poly-L-lysine. They then made various different preparations of the antigens, wherein each protein varied in concentration from 1.6 µg ml^{-1} to 1.6 ng ml^{-1}. Six different preparations were made, and each was labeled with the fluorescent molecule Cy5. The antigen preparations were then mixed with a reference preparation that had been labeled with Cy3, wherein each antigen was present at a concentration of 1.7 µg ml^{-1}. The different combined samples were applied to the arrays and the levels of Cy3 and Cy5 fluorescence at each address were determined by laser scanning. The results showed that only about 18% of the antibodies were specific and accurate over the range of concentrations used in the experiment, but that these antibodies could detect target antigens at levels down to 100 pg ml^{-1}, which is suitable for clinical evaluation applications.

Sreekumar and colleagues (see Further Reading) applied the same dual labeling technology to protein profiling in colon cancer. They produced a microarray with 146 antibodies (1920 features in total) recognizing proteins involved in cell cycle regulation, stress response and apoptosis. VoLo carcinoma cells were irradiated with a cobalt-60 source and cultured for 4 hours before protein extracts were obtained and labeled with Cy3. Protein extracts from parallel cultures of nontreated cells were labeled with Cy5 (*Figure 9.4*). The two samples were mixed and applied to the array. These experiments identified 11 proteins that were up-regulated in colon cancer, six of which were previously not known to be involved. Most of these proteins had roles in apoptosis, and increased apoptosis of the cells was observed after radiation treatment. Another protein, the carcinoembryonic antigen, was shown to be down-regulated.

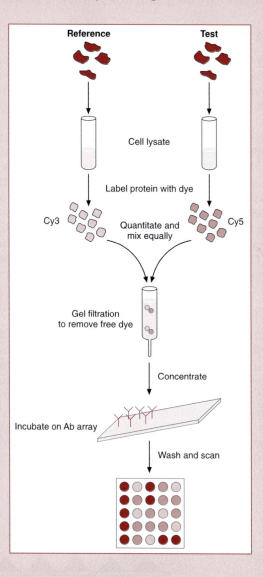

Figure 9.4

Dual labeling technology for differential protein profiling using antibody microarrays. Reprinted from Drug Discovery Today, Vol. 7, Lal *et al.* 'Antibody arrays: an embryonic but rapidly growing technology', pp S143–S149, ©2002, with permission from Elsevier.

9.2.3 Antigen arrays

Antigen arrays are the converse of antibody arrays. They are spotted with antigens and are used to capture antibodies from solution, e.g. for antibody profiling in serum (*Figure 9.5*). The antigens may be proteins or other molecules such as peptides or carbohydrates. Several reports have been published in which arrays of allergens have been used to screen serum samples for IgE reactivity in allergic responses and autoimmune diseases. In some cases it has proven possible not only to confirm the presence of such antibodies but also to carry out quantitative analysis. More recently, antigen arrays have been used to serodiagnose patients with viral infections.

9.2.4 Broad-specificity capture chips

Some protein chips do not contain arrays of specific capture agents, but instead possess various surface chemistries to capture broad classes of chemically similar proteins. For example, Ciphergen Biosystems Inc., Fremont, California, produce a range of protein chips, marketed under the name *ProteinChips*, which retain different classes of proteins on a number of alternative chromatographic surfaces. Although relatively nonspecific compared to antibodies, complex mixtures of proteins can be simplified and then analyzed by mass spectrometry (*Figure 9.6*). An advantageous feature of this system is the ease with which it is integrated with downstream MS analysis, since each chip doubles as a modified MALDI plate (p. 56). Until recently, the *ProteinChips* needed to be coated with matrix prior to MALDI analysis, but the company recently released a new type of chip with the matrix compound incorporated into the surface chemistry. The chips can also be used to prepare conventional arrays (e.g. antibody arrays), allowing direct MS analysis of captured proteins (*Figure 9.6*).

9.2.5 Functional protein chips

Functional chips are arrayed with the proteins whose functions are under investigation. Unlike analytical chips, which are used for expression profiling, functional chips can be used to investigate many different properties of proteins, including binding activity, the formation of complexes and biochemical functions (*Figure 9.7*). As discussed above for antibody arrays, binding assays can involve direct labeling of proteins in the analyte, sandwich assays or label-free detection methods (Section 9.4). The two major problems limiting the development of functional chips are the difficulty in expressing large libraries of proteins and the difficulty in maintaining

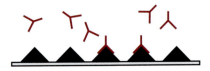

Figure 9.5

Some analytical arrays contain immobilized antigens, and are used to profile antibodies in serum and other analytes.

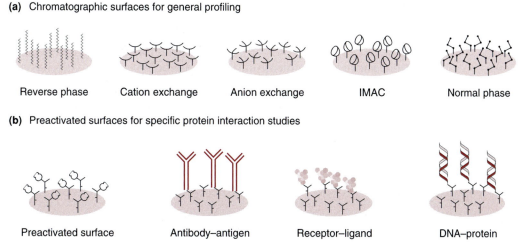

(a) Chromatographic surfaces for general profiling

Reverse phase   Cation exchange   Anion exchange   IMAC   Normal phase

(b) Preactivated surfaces for specific protein interaction studies

Preactivated surface   Antibody–antigen   Receptor–ligand   DNA–protein

Figure 9.6

Various ProteinChip Array Surfaces. Both (a) chromatographic surfaces and (b) preactivated surfaces are illustrated. Chromatographic surfaces are composed of reverse phase, ion exchange, immobilized metal affinity capture (IMAC) or normal-phase chemistries that function to extract proteins using quasi-specific means of affinity. Preactivated surfaces contain reactive chemical groups capable of forming covalent linkages with primary amines or alcohols. As such, they are used to immobilize specific bait molecules such as antibodies, receptors, or oligonucleotides often used for studying biomolecular interactions. Figure courtesy of Ciphergen Biosystems, Inc. (Fremont, CA). Courtesy of Scot Weinberger.

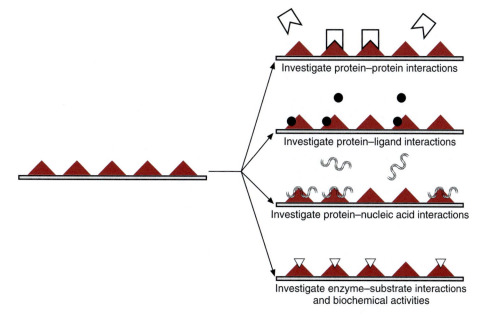

Investigate protein–protein interactions

Investigate protein–ligand interactions

Investigate protein–nucleic acid interactions

Investigate enzyme–substrate interactions
and biochemical activities

Figure 9.7

Some different uses for functional protein chips.

those proteins in an active state under a standard set of conditions. Functional chips containing up to 100 proteins have thus been available for several years and chips with specific functional classes of proteins, e.g. G-protein coupled receptors, are used to screen for particular types of interaction. However, the quantum leap to a whole-proteome chip has been achieved only recently and only for the yeast proteome. The Yeast ProtoArray, which was released commercially by Protometrix Inc., Branford, Connecticut in 2003, contains about 5000 proteins from *S. cerevisiae*. Some notable case studies involving the use of functional chips are presented in *Box 9.3*.

BOX 9.3

Functional protein chips: Case studies

Since 2000, several studies have been published involving the use of small- to moderate-scale functional protein arrays. One of the first reports described a universal protein array (UPA) comprising of a 12 x 8 cm nitrocellulose sheet with 96 protein spots (Ge *et al.*, see Further Reading). These represented 48 well-characterized human proteins (each spotted in duplicate to provide an internal control) including transcription factors, RNA-processing proteins and enzymes involved in DNA replication. The proteins were all expressed either in bacteria or using baculovirus vectors and were transferred to the sheet from a microtiter dish using a 96-well dot-blot arrayer. The array could be used to test protein interactions with proteins, nucleic acids and small molecules. Among other observations, it was shown that the phosphorylated version of the transcriptional activator protein PC4 bound to DNA more strongly than the unmodified version.

Another notable study, published by MacBeath and Schreiber in the same year (see Further Reading), involved the printing of proteins onto derivatized glass slides with a high spatial density. The proteins were attached covalently to the slide surface but retained their biochemical activities and interaction potentials. Several properties were tested, including protein–protein interactions (e.g. IκBa with p50), protein–ligand interactions and enzyme–substrate interactions. A rather different approach was used by Zhu *et al.* (2000) (see Further Reading) to study kinase activities in yeast. They produced a nanowell protein chip comprising of 140 microwells in silicone elastomer sheets placed on top of microscope slides (Section 9.3). Sixteen chips were coated with different substrates and then each well was probed with a different protein kinase along with radiolabeled ATP (119 of the 122 known and predicted kinases were studied). The experimental format was thus distinct from the usual idea of arraying different targets on the chip because, in this case, the chip was arrayed with identical targets and different substrates were applied at each address. These experiments confirmed many known kinase–substrate interactions and identified some new ones. The most surprising and provocative result, however, was that nearly a quarter of all the yeast kinases were capable of tyrosine phosphorylation even though they lacked the typical features of the tyrosine kinase family.

The most ambitious functional chip-based analysis carried out to date involved a prototype Yeast ProtoArray (p. 200) which contained some 5800 separate protein features. As discussed in the main text, yeast genes were expressed as His$_6$-tagged fusion proteins and the proteins were immobilized on nickel-coated slides using the affinity tag (see Zhu *et al.*, 2001; Further Reading). The chip was then probed with a selection of ligands, including calmodulin and a selection of phospholipids. This experiment revealed six of the 12 known calmodulin-binding proteins and 30 additional ones, and over 150 proteins that interacted with labeled liposomes containing specific phosphatidylinositides. Fifty of these proteins bound to specific classes of PIs and could be involved in PI-controlled signaling pathways.

The development of proteome-scale functional chips has demanded parallel advances in large-scale expression-cloning strategies. In the case of the yeast chip, this was achieved by systematically cloning each gene in an expression vector that allowed the protein to be expressed as a His_6-tagged GST fusion. About 95% of the yeast genome was successfully cloned in this manner and about 80% of the constructs were expressed as full-length, high-quality proteins. These proteins were isolated from cell lysates by GST pull-down (p. 141) and attached to Ni-NTA-coated glass slides via the His_6 tags. It is likely that bacterial proteome chips will follow the yeast prototype fairly rapidly, but proteome chips from higher eukaryotes will take longer to develop. Limitations include the lack of complete gene and protein catalogs, difficulties with large-scale expression systems and complications brought about by post-translational modifications. Unlike yeast and bacteria, where alternative splicing is rare or absent and post-translational modification quite limited in its extent, a large number of human genes undergo alternative splicing and most proteins are modified in multiple ways (Chapter 8). Therefore, although we have the complete human genome sequence, the proteome, with all its myriad complexities, is still rather like a black box. Even were the entire proteome to be cataloged, it would be difficult to find an expression system which was both amenable to the highly parallel formats required in proteomic research and suitable for producing all the correct post-translational modifications needed to study human proteins accurately.

The problem of maintaining proteins in an active state is also difficult to address. DNA chips have been astoundingly successful, but this is thanks in no small way to the very favorable properties of nucleic acids. DNA chips work on the principle of multiplex hybridization, where all the DNA probes are chemically similar so that a universal set of hybridization conditions can be used. Nucleic acids can be labeled uniformly, and can be tethered to solid substrates without interfering with their binding capabilities. In contrast, proteins are chemically and physically diverse, so it is difficult to envisage a universal set of conditions under which all proteins would adopt their native conformations, interact with their normal physiological ligands and display their normal biological activities. Proteins are difficult to label in a uniform manner, and labeling interferes with their normal range of interactions. Also, the act of immobilizing proteins on a solid support can also interfere with their biological activities. Finally, PCR can be used to amplify rare mRNA sequences as cDNA, therefore permitting the detection of very rare transcripts. There is no analogous procedure in protein analysis, which means that the detection of rare proteins relies solely on the sensitivity of the assay method.

9.3 The manufacture of protein chips

Protein chips containing arrays of immobilized protein probes (i.e. functional chips, antibody arrays and antigen arrays) are generally manufactured by the robotized spotting of proteins onto glass slides or other substrates. The substrates must be treated in such a way as to encourage proteins to bind without disrupting the secondary or tertiary structure, or losing their biochemical activity.

Most protein chips are made from coated glass slides, which are inexpensive and compatible with standard microarrayer contact printing apparatus. The surface of the slide is coated with a substance that either absorbs the arrayed proteins in a passive manner, or allows proteins to be cross-linked to the reactive surface. Nitrocellulose, agarose and poly-L-lysine fall into the former category, and nitrocellulose sheets can also be used as supports in their own right (*Table 9.2*). Proteins bind to the surface of such supports through nonspecific interactions and are oriented in a random manner. Cross-linking surfaces have been developed that provide either aldehyde, amine or epoxy groups that react with the primary amines of deposited proteins. Bifunctional thio-alkylene has been used to cross-link proteins to gold-coated slides, which are required for detection by surface plasmon resonance spectroscopy (see below). As for passive absorption, the protein molecules are arranged in a random manner and it is likely that a relatively large proportion of the immobilized proteins in both cases are either inaccessible or inactive due to linkages affecting important epitopes or functional residues. This problem can be avoided by using affinity tags to attach proteins to the chip surface. For example, in order to produce an antibody array with the antigen-binding domains of the antibodies exposed to the analyte, a recombinant staphylococcal protein A with five IgG-binding domains was covalently attached to the surface of a gold-coated slide. Antibodies bind to protein A via the Fc region, therefore at least one antigen-binding domain should be accessible to the solvent (*Figure 9.8a,b*). A similar principle applies to the use of His$_6$-tagged proteins, which can be immobilized in an oriented fashion to a chip surface coated with nickel-NTA resin (*Figure 9.8c,d*).

One disadvantage of coated glass slides is the tendency for the protein solutions to evaporate during chip manufacture, a problem that must be addressed by printing the chips in humidity-controlled chambers and/or using high concentrations of glycerol in the sample buffer. The protein *in situ* array (PISA) provides a potential solution to this problem because proteins are synthesized *in vitro* from isolated DNA sequences and immobilized onto the chip surface directly. Furthermore, various alternative chip formats have been developed to reduce evaporation (*Figure 9.9*). Several companies are investigating the production of chips with etched channels or wells, allowing proteins to be deposited within them to prevent them drying out. A similar strategy is the nanowell chip, in which the proteins are deposited into depressions in a polydimethylsiloxane surface fixed on the glass slide. This format also reduces cross-contamination and is very useful for biochemical assays in which several different reagents need to be added one after the other (*Box 9.3*). Weise and colleagues (see Further Reading) have developed nanowell chips wherein each well contains an 8×8 array of antibodies, which is particularly useful for the parallel application of many samples. Another format that reduces evaporation involves the use of polyacrylamide gel pads printed on the surface of the slide. The gel pads provide a porous, three-dimensional matrix into which the protein or capture agent can diffuse. The protein-binding capacity of such matrices is much higher than for other types of chip and the protein is maintained in an aqueous environment. However, these chips are more expensive to manufacture than the other types, and it is difficult to recover bound molecules from the gels for downstream analysis. Neither of the above chip formats is compatible with contact printing arrayers, and ink-jet technology is used instead.

Table 9.2 Properties of different surface chemistries used for protein chips. (PVDF, polyvinyldifluoride; NTA, nitrilotriacetate; PMDS, polydimethylsiloxane). Reprinted from Current Opinion in Chemical Biology, Vol. 7, Zhu and Snyder, 'Protein chip technology', pp 55–63, ©2003, with permission from Elsevier.

Surface	Attachment	Advantage	Disadvantage
PVDF	Adsorption and absorption	No protein modification requirement, high protein binding capacity	Nonspecific protein attachment in random orientation
Nitrocellulose	Adsorption and absorption	No protein modification requirement, high protein binding capacity	Nonspecific binding, high background. Low density arrays
Poly-lysine coated	Adsorption	No protein modification requirement	Nonspecific adsorption
Aldehyde-activated	Covalent cross-linking	High-density and strong protein attachment. High-resolution detection methods available	Random orientation of surface-attached proteins
Epoxy-activated	Covalent cross-linking	High-density and strong protein attachment. High-resolution detection methods available	Random orientation of surface-attached proteins
Avidin coated	Affinity binding	Strong, specific and high-density protein attachment, low background	Proteins have to be biotinylated
Ni-NTA-coated	Affinity binding	Strong, specific and high-density protein attachment, low background, uniform orientation of surface-attached proteins	Proteins have to be His$_6$ tagged
Gold-coated silicon	Covalent cross-linking	Strong and high-density protein attachment, low background. Can be easily coupled with SPR and mass spectrometry	Random orientation of surface attached proteins, tough to fabricate, not commercially available
PDMS nanowell	Covalent cross-linking	Strong and high-density protein attachment, well suited for sophisticated biochemical analyses	Random orientation of surface attached proteins
3D gel pad and agarose thin film	Diffusion	High protein binding capacity, no protein modification requirement	Tough to fabricate, not commercially available
DNA/RNA coated	Hybridization	Strong, specific and high-density protein attachment, low background, uniform orientation of surface attached proteins	Sophisticated in vitro production of labeled proteins

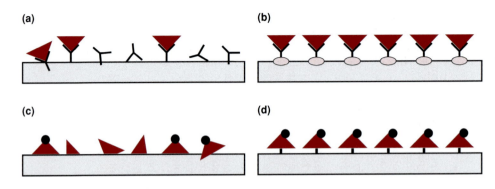

Figure 9.8

The importance of surface chemistry. (a) Antibodies will bind haphazardly to many surfaces via nonspecific bonds. Therefore, many of the antigen-binding domains are likely to be inactivated or obscured. (b) Coating the chip initially with staphylococcal protein A allows the antibodies to attach uniformly via the Fc regions, exposing the antigen binding domain to the analyte. (c) Similarly, proteins on functional chips are often inactivated due to random binding. The use of His_6-tagged proteins allows them to bind uniformly to a nickel-coated chip.

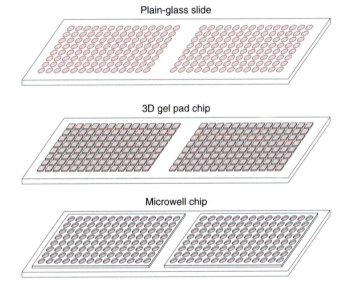

Figure 9.9

Different designs of protein chip – plain glass slides that are spotted using conventional contact-printing devices, gel pad chips that offer increased protein-binding capacity, and microwell chips, which allow multi-step reactions to be carried out. Reprinted from Current Opinion in Chemical Biology, Vol 5, Zhu and Snyder 'Protein arrays and microarrays', pp 40–45, ©2001, with permission from Elsevier.

9.4 Detecting and quantifying proteins bound to protein chips

Although functional protein chips can be used directly for the analysis of biochemical activities, both functional and analytical chips are used primarily to detect and characterize binding events. These may involve protein–protein, protein–nucleic acid or protein–small molecule interactions, and in each case a signal must be generated, detected and quantified.

There are three broad classes of detection methods (*Table 9.3*). In the first method, the analyte is labeled universally, either with a radioisotope, or an enzymatic or fluorescent conjugate, and the signal is detected directly from the bound analyte molecules on the chip. In the second method, the analyte is not labeled, but a sandwich reaction is used to detect molecules bound to the array and the signal is produced by the labeled detection reagent. Finally, there are several label-free detection methods that can be used to detect and/or identify proteins bound to capture reagents on the chip surface.

9.4.1 Methods that require labels

Although radiolabels and colorimetric assays can be used with low-density protein chips, fluorescent labels are safer, more convenient and provide a better spatial resolution. The label can be incorporated directly into the analyte or into a secondary detection reagent that is applied to the chip after it has been washed to remove unbound proteins. There are advantages and disadvantages to both methods. The advantage of direct labeling is that protein detection and quantification can be carried out in a one-step reaction, and multiplex analysis is possible (*Box 9.1*). A disadvantage of direct labeling is that not all proteins are labeled with the same efficiency, and the label itself can alter the structure of some proteins and interfere with their binding capabilities. These problems do not arise when a sandwich assay is used, so this approach may be preferable where accurate quantitation is needed. However, the main disadvantage of sandwich assays is the requirement for two antibodies recognizing different epitopes for each antigen captured on the chip, a problem that will increase in magnitude as the number of probes gets larger.

A variation of the sandwich assay is the immuno-RCA technique, which involves a tertiary level of detection by rolling circle amplification. The principle is that a protein, captured by an immobilized antibody, is recognized by a second antibody in a sandwich assay as above, but the second antibody has an oligonucleotide covalently attached to it (*Plate 10*). In the

Table 9.3 Summary of current detection methods used in protein microarray experiments. Reprinted from Current Opinion in Chemical Biology, Vol. 7, Zhu and Snyder, 'Protein chip technology', pp 55–63, ©2003, with permission from Elsevier.

Detection	Probe labeling	Data acquisition	Real time	Resolution
ELISA	Enzyme-linked antibodies	CCD imaging	No	Low
Isotropic labeling	Radio isotope-labeled analyte	X-ray film or phosphorimager	No	High
Sandwich immunoassay	Fluorescently labeled antibodies	Laser scanning	No	High
SPR	Not necessary	Refractive index change	Yes	Low
Non-contact AFM	Not necessary	Surface topological change	No	High
Planar waveguide	Fluorescently labeled antibodies	CCD imaging	Yes	High
SELDI	Not necessary	Mass spectrometry	No	Low
Electro-chemical	Metal-coupled analyte	Conductivity measurement	Yes	Medium

ELISA, enzyme-linked immunosorbent assay; CCD, charge-coupled device; SPR, surface plasmon resonance; SELDI, surface-enhanced laser desorption/ionization.

presence of a circular DNA template, a strand-displacing DNA polymerase and the four dNTPs, rolling circle amplification of the template occurs resulting in a long concatemer comprising hundreds of copies of the circle, which can be detected using a fluorescent oligonucleotide probe.

9.4.2 Label-free methods

Label-free methods use the intrinsic properties of proteins to report binding events on protein chips. Ciphergen *ProteinChips* can be used as MALDI plates and scanned directly by MALDI-TOF mass spectrometry to reveal bound proteins and, if possible, identify them by peptide mass fingerprinting (p. 60). The ionization of proteins bound to *ProteinChips* is enhanced by the properties of the chip surface, leading to more uniform mass spectra than possible with standard MALDI-MS analysis, a phenomenon described as surface-enhanced laser desorption/ionization (SELDI) (*Figure 9.10*). The quality of mass spectra is improved even further by incorporating the matrix compound into the chip surface, hence surface-enhanced neat desorption (SEND).

BIA-Core Inc. produces a range of protein chips on which protein interactions can be detected by changes in surface plasmon resonance (SPR). This is an optical effect that occurs when monochromatic polarized light is reflected from thin metal films. Some of the incident light energy interacts with the plasmon (the delocalized electrons in the metal) which results in a slight reduction in reflected light intensity. The angle of incidence at which this shadowing effect, the surface plasmon resonance, occurs is determined by the material adsorbed onto the metal film, which in this case is one or more proteins (*Figure 9.11*). There is a direct relationship between the mass of the immobilized molecules and the change in resonance energy at the metal surface, which can be used to study interactions in real time. Put more simply, when light is shone on a gold-coated glass chip from underneath, the angle of incidence that induces SPR will change when molecules bind to the chip surface, and the change will reflect the size of the interacting molecule. Direct coupling of SPR spectroscopy and mass spectrometry allows interacting proteins to be characterized.

Finally, atomic force microscopy (AFM) can detect protein interactions, albeit indirectly, if a binding event on the surface of a protein chip causes a change in surface topology. For example, this method has been used to detect the binding of an antibody immobilized on a thin gold film to a complementary anti-IgG by virtue of the change in height.

9.5 Emerging protein chip technologies

9.5.1 Bead and particle arrays in solution

The protein arrays discussed thus far in this chapter are two-dimensional devices that are manufactured with a fixed number of probes in specific positions. Each individual probe is identified by its spatial address on the array. A disadvantage of this format is the lack of flexibility – the only way to incorporate new probes is to fabricate a new array. One way around this problem is to release the array from its two-dimensional format and instead use beads in solution as the probes. Bead arrays (or solution arrays)

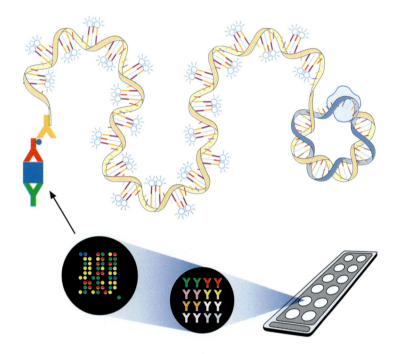

Plate 10

Sensitive protein detection using the RCA antibody chip. The chip is divided into sixteen teflon wells, each containing an array of 256 antibodies as probes. When a protein, represented by the blue square, is captured by one of the probes, it can be recognized using a second, biotinylated antibody (red), which is subsequently detected by a tertiary universal antibody connected to a circular oligonucleotide. A strand-displacing DNA polymerase can use this circular template, generating a long concatemer. Reprinted from Current Opinion in Biotechnology, Vol. 14, Kingsmore and Patel, 'Multiplexed protein profiling on antibody-based microarrays by rolling circle amplification, pp 74–81, ©2003, with permission from Elsevier.

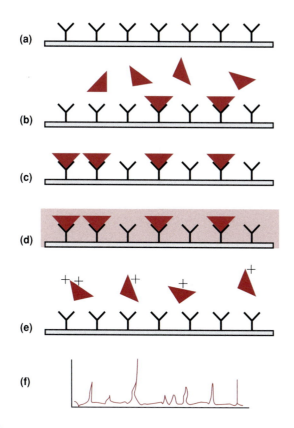

Figure 9.10

Principle of SELDI and SEND analysis. (a) In SELDI analysis, the protein chip (in this case preactivated and arrayed with antibodies) is exposed to the analyte (b) and captures antigens from the solution (c). The chip is then washed to remove unbound proteins and is coated with the matrix compound (d) before being inserted into the MALDI source of a mass spectromer. A pulsed laser beam causes the captured proteins to ionize (e), producing a mass spectrum (f). The uniform binding of the proteins to the chip produces mass spectra that are more uniform and reproducible than possible with conventional MALDI, allowing relative protein quantitation. In SEND analysis, the procedure is the same except that the matrix compound is included in the chip's surface chemistry. Therefore there is no need to add further matrix and matrix ions do not appear in the mass spectrum.

have all the advantages of solid phase arrays in terms of throughput and sensitivity, but have improved solution kinetics and are much more flexible in terms of the number of probes that can be used. The question is how to identify specific probes when they are free in the solution. Several answers have been put forward, including the use of fluorescence-encoded beads and barcoded metal particles.

Fluorescence encoding makes use of multiple fluorescent dyes at different concentrations to provide a unique spectral fingerprint for each bead. For example, the use of ten different fluorescent dyes would provide ten unique labels, but ten different dyes at ten different concentrations would provide 100 unique labels. Over 100 different fluorescent dyes are

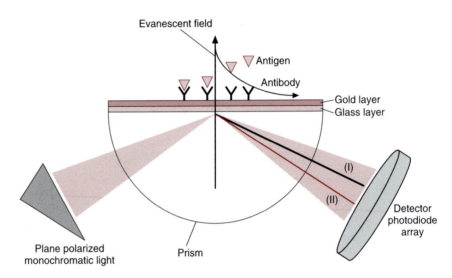

Figure 9.11

The principle of surface plasmon resonance spectroscopy. Plane polarized light is incident on a gold-coated glass chip containing immobilized antibodies (or other capture agents). A change in mass at the surface, caused by antigen binding, causes a change in the refractive index and thus the resonance state. This is reported by a change in the angle of the reflected light (I to II), which can be detected using a photodiode array. Reprinted from Enzyme and Microbial Technology, Vol. 32, Leonard *et al.* 'Advances in biosensors for detection of pathogens in food and water', pp 3–13, ©2003, with permission from Elsevier.

currently available and, by using a range of different concentrations, the system becomes rapidly scalable. Barcoding is a similar strategy in which metal particles, functionalized to accept antibodies or other proteins, are produced with a unique set of gold, silver and platinum stripes. The stripes are generated by carrying out electrochemical reductions with different metals and stripe width can be varied by controlling the current. This system also has potentially unlimited scale, the decoding step can be automated, and the particles can be combined with downstream analysis by fluorescence imaging or mass spectrometry.

9.5.2 Cell and tissue arrays

A lot of useful functional information is lost when proteins are extracted into solution for further analysis, including their spatial distribution and subcellular location. As discussed in Chapter 7, large-scale studies of protein localization have been carried out using a procedure in which adherent mammalian cells are grown on microarrays of cDNA expression constructs that have been treated with a lipid transfection reagent to promote DNA uptake. On such cell microarrays, cells growing immediately above each DNA 'spot' are able to express the cDNA and produce the protein, whose behavior in terms of subcellular distribution, oscillation in the context of the cell cycle and response to external stimuli can be observed by immunocytochemical staining and fluorescence microscopy (*Figure 9.12*).

Glass slide printed with cDNA in aqueous gelatin solution

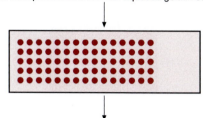

Each printed slide is incubated with mammalian cells and transfected

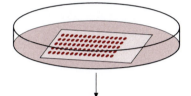

Detection assay performed on transfected cell microarray – only
positive cell clusters will show phenotype of interest

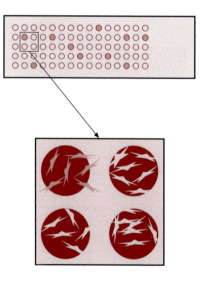

Figure 9.12

Preparation and use of cell arrays. Reprinted from Drug Discovery Today, Vol. 8,
Howbrook *et al.* 'Developments in microarray technologies', pp 642–651,
©2003, with permission from Elsevier.

Information about a protein's spatial distribution can also be obtained
by conventional histological examination but it takes a long time and
cannot be applied in a high-throughput manner. Tissue microarrays
resolve this problem by placing large numbers of tissue samples on microscope slides and allowing highly parallel *in situ* detection methods to
be applied under a constant set of conditions. Tissue microarrays are
constructed by taking needle biopsies of different specimens and embed-
ding these long, cylindrical tissue samples into blocks of paraffin in an
array structure. The block of paraffin is then cut into sections (up to 300
per block) producing many copies of the same array (*Figure 9.13*).

Donor paraffin block containing tissue specimen from which core
biopsies are taken

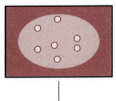

Recipient paraffin block into which an array of core biopsies are positioned

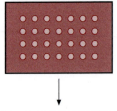

Recipient block containing core tissue biopsies is microtome sectioned

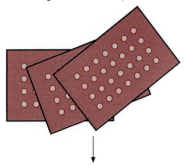

The sections are transferred to a glass slide for staining and analysis

Figure 9.13

Preparation and use of tissue arrays. Reprinted from Drug Discovery Today, Vol.
8, Howbrook *et al.* 'Developments in microarray technologies', pp 642–651,
©2003, with permission from Elsevier.

Advantages of this approach include the use of very small analyte volumes
and the fact that minimal damage is caused to the original specimen,
which can be subjected to conventional analysis if required.

Further reading

Braun, P. and LaBaer, J. (2003) High throughput protein production for
functional proteomics. *Trends Biotechnol* **21**: 383–388.

Campbell, D.A. and Szardenings, A.K. (2003) Functional profiling with
affinity labels. *Curr Opin Chem Biol* **7**: 296–303.

Cutler, P. (2003) Protein arrays: The current state-of-the-art. *Proteomics* **3**: 3–18.

de Wildt, R.M.T. (2000) Antibody arrays for high throughput screening of antibody antigen interactions. *Nature Biotechnol* **18**: 989–994.

Fang, Y., Lahiri, J. and Picard, L. (2003) G protein-coupled receptor microarrays for drug discovery. *Drug Discovery Today* **8**: 755–761.

Ge, H. (2000) UPA, a universal protein array system for quantitative detection of protein–protein, protein–DNA, protein–RNA and protein–ligand interactions. *Nucleic Acids Res* **28**: e3i–e3vii.

Gershon, D. (2003) Proteomics technologies: probing the proteome. *Nature* **424**: 581–587.

Haab, B.B., Dunham, M.J. and Brown, P.O. (2001) Protein microarrays for highly parallel detection and quantification of specific proteins and antibodies in complex solutions. *Genome Biol* **2**: 0004.1–0004.13.

Howbrook, D.N., van der Valk, A.M., O'Shaughnessy, M.C., et al. (2003) Developments in microarray technologies. *Drug Discovery Today* **8**: 642–651.

Jona, G. and Snyder, M. (2003) Recent developments in analytical and functional protein microarrays. *Curr Opin Mol Ther* **5**: 271–277.

Kingsmore, S.F. and Patel, D.D. (2003) Multiplexed protein profiling on antibody-based microarrays by rolling circle amplification. *Curr Opin Biotechnol* **14**: 74–81.

Lal, S.P., Christopherson, R.I. and dos Remedios, C.G. (2002) Antibody arrays: an embryonic but rapidly growing technology. *Drug Discovery Today* **7**: S143–149.

Liu, B., Huang, L., Sihlbom, C. et al. (2002) Towards proteome-wide production of monclonal antibody by phage display. *J Mol Biol* **315**: 1063–1073.

Lopez, M.F. and Pluskal, M.G. (2003) Protein micro- and macroarrays: digitising the proteome. *J Chromatogr B Analyt Technol Biomed Life Sci* **787**: 19–27.

MacBeath, G. (2002) Protein microarrays and proteomics. *Nature Genet* **32** (Suppl): 526–532.

MacBeath, G. and Schreiber, S.L. (2000) Printing proteins as microarrays for high-throughput function determination. *Science* **289**: 1760–1763.

Martzen, M.R., McCraith, S.M., Spinelli, S.L. et al. (1999) A biochemical genomics approach for identifying genes by the activity of their products. *Science* **286**: 1153–1155.

Nedelkov, D. and Nelson, R.W. (2003) Surface plasmon resonance mass spectrometry: recent progress and outlooks. *Trends Biotechnol* **21**: 301–305.

Phizicky, E., Bastiaens, P.I., Zhu, H., Snyder, M. and Fields, S. (2003) Protein analysis on a proteomic scale. *Nature* **422**: 208–215.

Schasfoort, R.B.M. (2004) Proteomics-on-a-chip: the challenge to couple lab-on-a-chip unit operations. *Expert Rev. Proteomics* **1**: 123–132.

Schweitzer, B. and Kingsmore, S.F. (2002) Measuring proteins on microarrays. *Curr Opin Biotechnol* **13**: 14–19.

Sreekumar, A., Nyati, M.K., Varambally, S. et al. (2001) Profiling of cancer cells using protein microarrays: discovery of novel, radiation-regulated proteins. *Cancer Res* **61**: 7585–7593.

Templin, M.F., Stoll, D., Schrenk, M., Traub, P.C., Vohringer, C.F. and Joos, T.O. (2002) Protein microarray technology. *Trends Biotechnol* **20**: 160–166.

Wiese, R., Belosludtsev, Y., Powdrill, T. et al. (2001) Simultaneous multianalyte ELISA performed on a microarray platform. *Clin Chem* **47**: 1451–1457.

Zhou, H., Roy, S., Schulman, H. and Natan, M.J. (2001) Solution and chip arrays in protein profiling. *Trends Biotechnol* **19**: S34–S39.

Zhu, H. and Snyder, M. (2003) Protein chip technology. *Curr Opin Chem Biol* **7**: 55–63.

Zhu, H., Klemic, J.F., Chang, S. et al. (2000) Analysis of yeast protein kinases using protein chips. *Nature Genet* **26**: 283–289.

Zhu, H., Bilgin, M., Bangham, R., et al. (2001) Global analysis of protein activities using proteome chips. *Science* **293**: 2101–2105.

Zhu, H., Bilgin, M. and Snyder, M. (2003) Proteomics. *Annu Rev Biochem* **72**: 783–812.

Applications of proteomics

10

10.1   Introduction

In the preceding chapters, we have discussed a range of different technologies that allow proteins to be studied on a large scale. These technologies can be applied in two major ways. The first type of application involves the systematic identification and quantitation of all the proteins found in a particular cell, tissue or organism. This approach lies at the core of systems biology and the ultimate aim is to provide a complete quantitative breakdown of the proteome including all post-translational variants. A more focused version of this approach is to find differences between related samples, i.e. differences in protein profiles that accompany changes in physiological states. The second type of application involves the investigation of protein functions and interactions, and includes a diverse range of experimental methods such as the analysis of protein sequences, structures, interactions and biochemical activities. When these global, discovery-driven methods are combined, they inevitably better our understanding of many biological processes. Already we are seeing how this new knowledge can be applied in medicine, agriculture and industry.

In this chapter we briefly explore how proteomics can be applied to solve real problems, focusing on drug development and healthcare because it is here that high-throughput studies of protein abundance and activity are having the largest impact. Indeed, most of the current investment in proteomics technology and research is funded by pharmaceutical companies, which see proteomics as a shortcut to the development of novel drugs and diagnostics. Proteomics can play an important role throughout the pharmaceutical research and development value chain, and is particularly powerful when used in combination with other genomics data, such as genome sequences, transcriptional profiles, single nucleotide polymorphism (SNP) catalogs and mutant libraries.

As well as its medical applications, proteomics is useful in the biotechnology industry for the characterization of microbes and plants that produce valuable metabolites, the analysis of genetically modified organisms, the study of genetic diversity, and the identification of proteins that protect plants and domestic animals from pests, diseases and environmental stress. Finally, proteomics can be used to provide novel genetic markers for the rapid mapping of uncharacterized genomes. In this way, we come full circle from genomes to proteomes and back to genomes once again.

10.2   Medical proteomics – disease diagnosis

10.2.1   Biomarkers

A biomarker is a biological feature of a cell, tissue or organism that corresponds to a particular physiological state. In a medical context, the most important biomarkers are those that appear or disappear specifically in the disease state (disease biomarkers), or those that appear or disappear in response to drugs (toxicity biomarkers, see later). There are many different types of disease biomarker, including the presence of particular pathogenic entities, disease-specific cytological or histological characteristics, gene or chromosome mutations, the appearance of specific transcripts or proteins, new post-translational variants, or alterations in the level of mRNA or protein expression. Molecular biomarkers, such as mutations, transcripts and proteins, are the most useful because they tend to appear well before the pathological symptoms of the disease, allowing early detection and prompt treatment. Furthermore, different biomarkers can sometimes be used to monitor the progress of a disease or its treatment.

As discussed in Chapter 1, proteins are advantageous biomarkers because the direct analysis of proteins can reveal characteristics, such as post-translational modifications, that cannot be identified by DNA sequencing or mRNA profiling. Perhaps more importantly, protein biomarkers can be assayed in body fluids, such as serum, urine, cerebral spinal fluid, saliva, synovial fluid and the aqueous humor of the eye. The ideal biomarker should be highly specific for a particular disease condition, a feature that can be established only by extensive validation in a broad population. Unfortunately, such biomarkers are rare and most candidate biomarkers are found in many different types of disease, perhaps with different expression levels in each case. A combination of relatively nonspecific biomarkers can, in some cases, provide a more specific disease index, and proteomics is potentially very useful in this context since it allows the expression profiles of hundreds of proteins to be studied in parallel. Many licensed tests that use proteins for disease diagnosis are ELISA-based systems that exploit protein biomarkers found in easily accessible fluids, so that the assay is noninvasive. In most cases, however, these assays have been developed after the fortuitous discovery of individual proteins that are overexpressed or ectopically expressed in the disease state. What proteomics can offer is the opportunity to compare the protein profiles of samples from healthy people and those with a given disease to identify protein biomarkers in a systematic fashion.

10.2.2 Biomarker discovery using 2DGE and mass spectrometry

Biomarker discovery was probably the first application envisaged for proteomics. As early as 1982, it was suggested that 2D gels could be used to detect quantitative differences in the protein profiles of healthy and disease samples, although at the time there was no easy way to identify the differentially expressed proteins that were discovered. This all changed in the early 1990s with the advent of mass spectrometry techniques that allowed proteins to be identified by correlative database searching (Chapter 3). The combination of 2DGE and mass spectrometry soon became the standard way to find potential new protein biomarkers. An initial strategy was to compare silver-stained gels by eye or using visual analysis software. Spots that were present on one gel and absent on another, or spots that showed obvious quantitative differences between gels, were picked and analyzed by mass spectrometry. The proteins contained within the spots were thus identified, and their relative abundance in different samples was confirmed using other methods (*Figure 10.1*). This led to the discovery of numerous potential disease biomarkers, many of which offered the prospect of diagnosis for different forms of cancer. There were also novel markers for heart disease, neurological disease and other disorders such as arthritis and hepatitis. The use of specialized databases to catalog and describe potential disease biomarkers is discussed in *Box 10.1*.

The discovery of cancer biomarkers using 2DGE and mass spectrometry has a long history, and some representative examples are shown in *Table 10.1*. Cancer has been the primary target for proteomic analysis because it is possible to obtain matched samples of diseased and healthy tissue from the same patient in sufficient amounts to carry out 2DGE (*Figure 10.2*). Good examples of this approach include the pioneering studies of Sam Hanash and colleagues, which identified various biomarkers that could be used to diagnose and classify different forms of leukemia (see

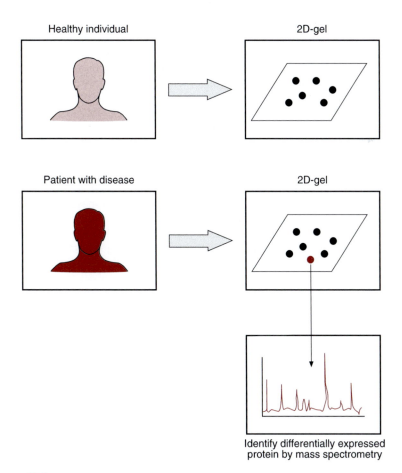

Figure 10.1

Identification of disease-specific biomarkers by 2DGE and mass spectrometry. After separation, proteins that are unique to the disease sample or significantly more abundant in the disease sample are selected for further characterization.

BOX 10.1

The role of databases in medical proteomics

Cancer

Hundreds of potential biomarkers and drug targets have been discovered by comparing tumors and healthy tissue, or through the comparison of body fluids from cancer patients and healthy individuals. Many pharmaceutical companies are now investing heavily in proteomic technology to accelerate the discovery of novel cancer markers and drug targets in their product pipelines. At a recent proteomics conference, held in Switzerland in July 2003, representatives of several academic institutions and pharmaceutical companies described their strategies and achievements in biomarker/target identification. Hoffmann–La Roche's adoption of laser capture microdissection in combination with 2DGE and mass spectrometry can be seen as a typical approach. In this case, the strategy has thus far produced over 100 proteins that represent potential biomarkers. Proprietary databases are a central component of such strategies. They are used to monitor the expression of potential biomarkers in patients, in order to study disease progression and the results of therapy. This type of analysis is essential to establish marker specificity and sensitivity, and thus to convert candidate markers into validated markers that are suitable diagnostics.

Several research groups have also established databases of 2DGE experiments, and more recently, profile patterns on protein chips, to provide data for marker validation and verification. One of the first examples was provided by Celis and co-workers, who established a 2DGE database in the pursuit of markers for bladder cancer. These investigators charted their systematic analysis of tumors, random biopsies, urine samples and cystectomies and deposited all the data, including annotated 2D-gels, in a central resource that can be accessed over the Internet (http://proteomics.cancer.dk/). Similar, although less extensive, databases have been established to archive protein expression profiles in lung cancer and prostrate cancer. Many other cancer-related 2D gels are available linked from the world 2D-PAGE index of 2DGE databases (http://us.expasy.org/ch2d/2d-index.html).

Heart disease

Several databases have been established to catalog 2D-gels of heart proteins, in order to accelerate the discovery of heart disease markers and drug targets. These databases catalog both human heart proteins and those from other mammals, allowing the proteomic analysis of animal disease models as well as the actual human diseases. Surrogate biomarkers have been discovered, for example, in a bovine model of dilated cardiomyopathy and in a rabbit model of myocardial ischemia, and these can be compared to human protein profiles to identify bona fide biomarkers for diagnostic or potential therapeutic development. The comparative analysis of human heart proteomes in health and various forms of heart disease has identified useful markers such as creatine kinase, dinucleotide dehydrogenase and ubiquinol-cytochrome c reductase. Such data can be accessed over the Internet, for example on the Heart 2D-PAGE database (German Heart Institute, Berlin) which identifies heart chamber-specific proteins and proteins expressed only in dilated cardiomyopathy (http://userpage.chemie.fu-berlin.de/~pleiss/dhzb.html), and in the Heart Science Centre 2D-PAGE database maintained by Harefield Hospital, UK (http://www.harefield.nthames.nhs.uk/nhli/protein/). Other heart-specific 2D-gel data can be accessed from the World 2D-PAGE index (http://us.expasy.org/ch2d/2d-index.html).

Other diseases

While cancer and heart disease have been at the forefront of disease proteomics, biomarkers have also been sought for many other types of diseases. Databases have been established for other human organs including the eyes, ears and teeth. Relevant databases include the LENS 2D-PAGE database maintained by Oregon Health & Science University (http://www.ohsu.edu/2d/2d.html), the Washington University Inner Ear Protein Database (http://oto.wustl.edu/thc/innerear2d.htm) and TOOTHPRINT, the proteomic database of dental tissues maintained by the University of Otago, New Zealand (http://biocadmin.otago.ac.nz/tooth/home.htm).

Table 10.1 A selection of protein biomarkers characteristic of different forms of cancer

Markers	Disease
Established	
CA125	Ovarian
Carcinoembryonic antigen	Breast, colon, lung and pancreatic cancer
α-Fetoprotein	Hepatoma and testicular cancer
Prostate-specific antigen	Prostate cancer
Novel, discovered using proteomics technology	
RHOGDI, glyoxalase-1, FK506BP	Invasive ovarian cancer
Annexin-1	Early prostate and esophageal cancer
HSP27, HSP60, HSP90, PCNA, transglein, RS/DJ-1	Breast cancer
PGP9.5, cytokeratins	Lung cancer
Hcc-1, lamin B1, sarcosine dehydrogenase	Hepatocellular carcinoma
Op18, nm23-H1	Leukemia
HSP70, S100-A9, S100-A11	Colorectal cancer
Keratins, psoriasin	Bladder cancer

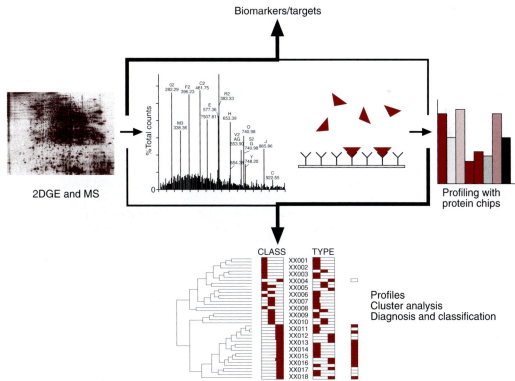

Figure 10.2

Overview of cancer proteomics. The comparison of tumor and nontumor tissue, or different types of tumors, can reveal biomarkers, therapeutic targets or diagnostic protein patterns. 2DGE is used predominantly to identify novel biomarkers, which are then developed into diagnostic immunoassays. Protein chips can be used to identify biomarkers, but are often used to generate pattern profiles which can be used in diagnosis and tumor classification.

Further Reading). One such study identified the protein stathmin (otherwise known as oncoprotein 18), which functions as an intracellular signal relay in the transduction of growth factor signals, as a reliable biomarker for childhood leukemia. The interesting feature of this particular protein is that only the phosphorylated form is implicated in the disease. Pioneering work was also carried out by Julio Celis and colleagues, who initially used 2DGE to study the changes in protein expression that occurred as cultured cells underwent growth transformation. The knowledge gained from this series of investigations was later applied to the analysis of bladder cancer (see Further Reading). Celis' group has discovered a number of markers, including different forms of keratin, which can be used to follow the progression of the disease from normal epithelium through the early transitional epithelium stage to the late squamous cell carcinoma. Another protein, called psoriasin, is shed into the urine of squamous cell carcinoma patients and thus has the potential to be developed as a validated biomarker for disease diagnosis. Breast cancer has also received much attention, particularly since proteins can be isolated from nipple aspiration fluid allowing noninvasive diagnosis. Several potential biomarkers have been identified through the comparative 2DGE analysis of bilateral matched samples of fluid taken from women with unilateral breast cancer (*Figure 10.3*).

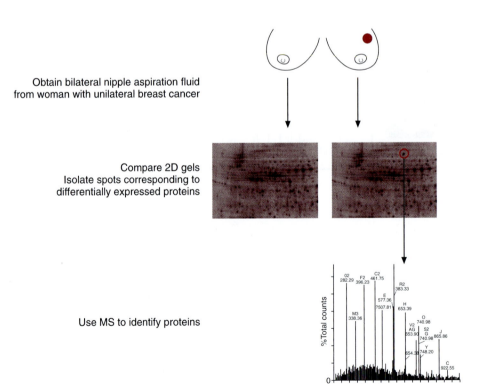

Figure 10.3

Novel biomarkers for breast cancer can be identified by the comparative analysis of nipple aspiration fluid from affected and nonaffected breasts in women with unilateral tumors.

Despite the many successes that have been reported, 2DGE has a number of disadvantages for biomarker discovery, including its low sensitivity and the requirement for relatively large samples. As discussed in Chapters 2 and 4, the information content of 2DGE can be improved through multiplex analysis, and the sensitivity can be increased through the use of novel protein stains, or by prefractionation of the sample prior to separation. As an example of multiplex analysis in biomarker discovery, Zhou *et al.* (see Further Reading) used difference gel electrophoresis (DIGE; p. 76) to compare esophageal squamous cell carcinoma and normal esophageal epithelium. Various strategies for prefractionation have also been tested in biomarker discovery projects, including approaches that select a particular component of the proteome for analysis or eliminate a certain fraction of the proteome during analysis. The selection of cell surface proteins on cancer cells by labeling the extracellular portion of such proteins on intact cells with a hydrophilic biotin reagent is an example of the first approach (Shin *et al.*, see Further Reading). In this study, labeled proteins were captured from whole cell lysates using streptavidin beads (*Figure 10.4*). An example of the second approach is the use of narrow pH range gels or simple chromatographic procedures that select proteins with particular physicochemical properties. In these cases, however, it is beneficial to use even larger amounts of the starting material to provide enough of the protein sample to facilitate the identification of low-abundance proteins. Unfortunately, most clinical samples are small and heterogeneous, and are surrounded by contaminating normal tissue, which makes the detection of useful biomarkers much more difficult. One way to address the problem of contamination is to use laser capture microdissection (LCM), a technique in which particular cell populations can be isolated under direct microscopic visualization (*Figure 10.5*). Although this combination of methods

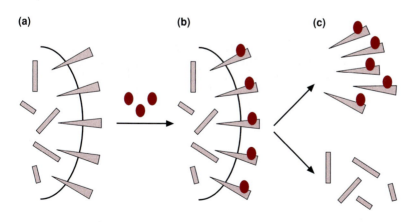

(a)   **(b)**   **(c)**

Figure 10.4

The cell surface sub-proteome can be isolated using affinity reagents that cannot penetrate the plasma membrane. (a) The cellular proteome comprises both cell surface and internal proteins. (b) A hydrophilic affinity reagent derived from biotin is added to intact cells, resulting in the universal labeling of cell surface proteins. (c) After disruption of the cells, the surface proteins can be captured using affinity chromatography with streptavidin beads, while the internal proteins are recovered in the eluate.

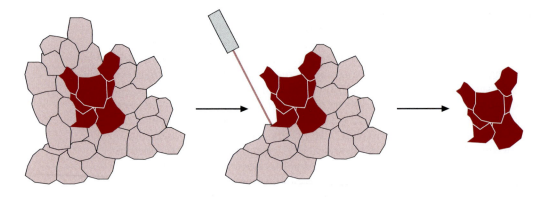

Figure 10.5

Laser capture microdissection uses a finely focused laser beam to select individual cells in a hetero-geneous tissue sample. In this example, dark tumor cells are being captured from a heterogeneous biopsy, which also includes normal cells.

has led to the discovery of several novel cancer biomarkers (e.g. glyoxalase-1 and FK506BP which are markers of invasive ovarian cancer cells), it remains difficult to produce sufficient amounts of starting material.

10.2.3 Biomarker discovery and pattern profiling using protein chips

In order to improve sensitivity, alternatives to 2DGE have been integrated into biomarker discovery programs. These include LC-MS methods, direct mass spectrometry of tissue sections (imaging mass spectrometry), the screening of expression libraries with autoantibodies specific for tumors or other diseases, and the use of analytical protein chips. While the first three techniques have been useful for the discovery of several individual biomarkers, protein chips could emerge as one of the most valuable technologies for high-throughput disease diagnosis. This is because hundreds of proteins can be analyzed simultaneously using very small sample volumes, facilitating the identification both of individual biomarkers and diagnostic protein patterns.

Protein chips have been used with success for the identification of individual biomarkers and are also useful as diagnostic tools once such markers have been identified. In Chapter 9, we discussed how antibody microarrays have been used to identify markers for colon cancer using dual fluorescence labeling (p. 200). Antibody arrays have also been used in combination with LCM to identify markers for oral squamous cell carcinoma and other forms of cancer. Broad-specificity capture chips can be used to profile healthy and disease samples by SELDI mass spectroscopy (p. 211), which occasionally leads to the direct identification of differentially expressed proteins. For example, several defensins have recently been identified as markers for the antiviral response of CD8 cells.

More often, however, differentially expressed proteins detected by SELDI cannot be identified directly, due to polymorphisms or variations in post-translational modifications. Under these circumstances, the overall pattern of protein expression can be a useful diagnostic tool, a method known as pattern profiling (*Figure 10.6*). Disease diagnosis is achieved by looking at the SELDI spectra produced by different samples, and the peaks on the spectra are diagnostic in themselves without necessarily identifying the proteins to which they correspond. In theory, this could provide higher sensitivity than the analysis of single biomarkers, which are often expressed in multiple diseases making a precise diagnosis difficult. This is especially true in closely related diseases, such as different forms of cancer or dementia. Sam Hanash and colleagues proposed the use of pattern diagnostics on 2D gels to classify different forms of leukemia in the 1980s, but protein chips offer the prospect of higher-throughput analysis with direct computer analysis of protein profiles using pattern-matching algorithms.

A useful example of SELDI pattern profiling is the early diagnosis of ovarian cancer, a disease that is usually detected at the late stage when cancer cells have already spread and the prognosis is poor. In the original study (Petricoin *et al.*, 2002; see Further Reading), mass spectra derived from the serum samples of women with ovarian cancer and from unaffected controls were used as a training set for a pattern-matching algorithm. A discriminatory pattern was identified, which was applied to another set of samples. This resulted in the correct diagnosis of all ovarian cancers (including 18 stage I cancers, where the prognosis is good because the neoplastic cells are still contained within the ovary) and a false-positive rate of only 5%. Similar algorithms have been used to diagnose breast and prostrate cancers. In each case, the sensitivity of the pattern-profiling method has been significantly higher than tests relying on the presence of single biomarkers, and in at least one study the sensitivity of the method has been high enough to achieve 100% correct diagnosis. This new approach to disease detection could revolutionize the clinical laboratory, providing the means to process more samples than before and detect diseases earlier and more accurately than is currently possible using ELISA methods. While similar methods have been developed using DNA microarrays to profile transcript levels (see Chapter 1), these can be applied only to tumor biopsies, since mRNA is not found in body fluids.

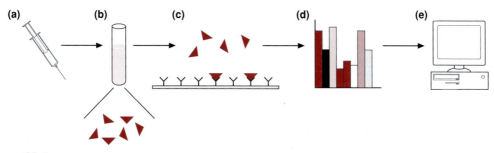

Figure 10.6

Protein patterns in disease diagnosis. A blood sample (a) contains many proteins (b), which can be captured and quantified on an analytical protein chip (c). The relative abundances of the proteins provide a unique signature, or fingerprint (d), which can be detected by specialized algorithms (e) and used to diagnose disease and classify different forms of tumor.

10.3 Pharmaceutical proteomics – drug development

10.3.1 The role of proteomics in target identification

The release of a new drug marks the end of a complex, lengthy and expensive process (*Figure 10.7*). It has been estimated that every drug candidate entering the clinic costs $70 million to develop and requires 250 employee years during the development process. Since many drugs fail at the clinical stages, the real cost of bringing a new drug to market is probably in the region of $700 million. Very few drugs recapture in sales the amount of money spent on their development. The drug companies have therefore been quick to embrace any new technology which increases the pace of drug discovery and reduces the attrition rate (the number of products abandoned during development), since attrition contributes most of the development costs. Such technologies include combinatorial chemistry, high-throughput screening, *in silico* screening, genomics and now proteomics.

Disease biomarkers represent proteins that are expressed specifically or preferentially in either the disease state or the healthy state. In many cases, such proteins appear or disappear merely as a consequence of the disease, but it is also possible that their presence or absence could contribute to the disease symptoms, i.e. they may also cause the disease. Where comparative proteomic analysis identifies proteins that are expressed only in the disease state, such proteins might represent not only useful biomarkers but also likely therapeutic targets. Biomarker discovery therefore provides fuel for the target identification stage of drug development (*Figure 10.8a*). Furthermore, where specific proteins are depleted in the disease state, these proteins could themselves be developed as potential drugs. Comparative proteomic analysis can therefore provide leads towards novel therapeutic proteins (*Figure 10.8b*).

As well as the direct comparison of healthy and disease tissues, another useful strategy in target identification is the analysis of protein profiles when particular cells, tissues or perhaps animal models have been treated with a regulatory molecule, such as a growth factor or cytokine. Since these molecules stimulate different forms of cell behavior, including proliferation, differentiation and adhesion, they can be useful in modeling the outcome of diseases. Examples of the above include the discovery of cytokine-regulated proteins in intestinal epithelial cells, the discovery of targets regulated by phorbol esters in erythroleukemia cells and the identification of phosphoproteins induced by epidermal growth factor treatment in HeLa cells. The last example is interesting because antibodies were used to isolate phosphotyrosine-containing proteins and comparative analysis was therefore facilitated by the selective purification of the

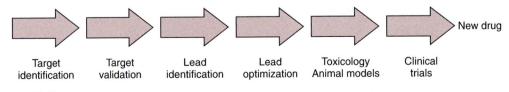

| Target identification | Target validation | Lead identification | Lead optimization | Toxicology Animal models | Clinical trials | New drug |

Figure 10.7

The major stages in drug development.

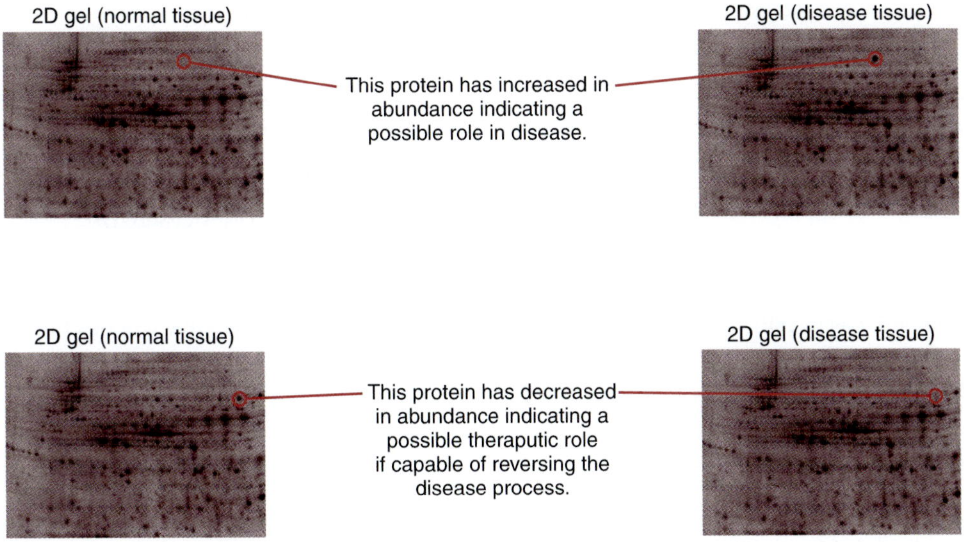

2D gel (normal tissue)

2D gel (disease tissue)

This protein has increased in abundance indicating a possible role in disease.

2D gel (normal tissue)

2D gel (disease tissue)

This protein has decreased in abundance indicating a possible theraputic role if capable of reversing the disease process.

Figure 10.8

The value of proteomics in target identification and the identification of potential protein thereapeutics.

phosphoproteome (Chapter 8). Potential drug targets in lymphocytes treated with interferon-α and interleukin-2 have also been identified in this manner.

Proteomics provides methods not only for the identification of new therapeutic targets expressed by the human genome in the disease state, but also offers many strategies for the identification of targets in the pathogen proteome, therefore providing leads in drug and vaccine development for infectious diseases (*Table 10.2*). The characterization of cell surface proteins or secreted proteins that are involved in infection or pathogenesis provides a rapid route to the identification of novel drug or vaccine targets. One approach is to separate the pathogen proteome by 2DGE and use hyperimmune sera from different patients to identify the immunodominant proteins. This subset of the proteome, the 'immunome', is likely to be a good source of drug targets as well as vaccine targets (since sites on these proteins are proven to be exposed to the host immune system). This strategy can also be used to identify proteins that are expressed in particular stages of the pathogen life cycle, as has been demonstrated in the case of the malaria parasite *Plasmodium falciparum*. Other advantageous strategies include the comparative proteomic analysis of pathogenic and nonpathogenic isolates of the same organism to identify pathogenesis-related proteins, or the comparative analysis of host and/or pathogen tissues before and after infection, to identify proteins specifically involved in host–pathogen interactions. The causative agent of tuberculosis, *Mycobacterium tuberculosis*, has been compared to its nonpathogenic relative *M. bovis* BCG, in order to identify proteins that

Table 10.2 A selection of 2DGE databases for microbes and plants

Database	Contents	URL
Department of Medical Microbiology, University of Aberdeen	*Haemophilus influenzae, Streptococcus pneumoniae* and *Neisseria meningitidis*	http://www.abdn.ac.uk/~mmb023/2dhome.htm
Cyano2Dbase	*Synechocystis* sp. PCC6803	http://www.kazusa.or.jp/cyano/Synechocystis/cyano2D/
Siena-2DPAGE	*Chlamydia trachomatis* L2	http://www.bio-mol.unisi.it/
European Bacteria Proteome Project (EBP)	*Chlamydia pneumoniae, Helicobacter pylori,* and *Mycobacterium tuberculosis*	http://www.mpiib-berlin.mpg.de/2D-PAGE/EBP-PAGE/index.html
Sub2D	*Bacillus subtilis*	http://microbio2.biologie.uni-greifswald.de:8880/
SWICZ	*Caulobacter crescentus* and *Streptomyces coelicolor*	http://proteom.biomed.cas.cz/
Various	*Borrelia garinii Francisella tularensis* LVS and *Mycoplasma pneumoniae* M129	http://www.mpiib-berlin.mpg.de/2D-PAGE/microorganisms/index.html
COMPLUYEAST-2DPAGE	*Candida albicans* and *Saccharomyces cerevisiae*	http://babbage.csc.ucm.es/2d/
Yeast Proteome Map	*Saccharomyces cerevisiae*	http://www.ibgc.u-bordeaux2.fr/YPM/
ANU-2DPAGE	Rice anther proteome, various tissues of the nodal legume species *Medicago trunculata* and *Sinorhizobium meliloti*	http://semele.anu.edu.au/2d/2d.html
CNRS / INRA / Bayer CropScience	*Arabidopsis* seed proteome	http://seed.proteome.free.fr/
The *Arabidopsis* mitochondrial proteome project	*Arabidopsis* mitochondrion	http://www.gartenbau.uni-hannover.de/genetik/AMPP
Samuel Roberts Nobel Foundation	*Medicago truncatula*	http://www.noble.org/2dpage/index.asp

are specific to the virulent strain. Comparative 2DGE analysis revealed 56 proteins specific to *M. tuberculosis* out of 96 spot differences, and 32 of these proteins were identified by mass spectrometry and are currently being investigated as novel vaccine targets. *In vitro* models of infection can be useful as long as they are physiologically relevant. For example, several models of tuberculosis infection have been established, including the Wayne model (where the bacterium persists in a nonreplicative state under conditions of reduced oxygen) and a disease model involving *in vitro* macrophage infection. In the latter case, 16 proteins were shown to be induced by infection and 28 were shown to be repressed.

10.3.2 Proteomics and target validation

Proteomics and other large-scale technologies have generated a boom in target discovery, but this has resulted in a bottleneck at the target validation stage. This is where supporting evidence is generated to show that interfering with the activity of the target protein will alter the course of the disease in a beneficial way. Compared to target identification, target validation is a low-throughput enterprise, since it can take 1–2 years to validate each novel target protein.

A wide variety of genomic and proteomic methods can be employed at the validation stage, including structural analysis, the investigation of protein interactions, expression studies to see if the protein generates an informative phenotype when overexpressed or suppressed, and the analysis of genetic variation in the target population. Targets with high levels of polymorphism within the population are usually unsuitable because the different variants are likely to show different responses to candidate drugs. In such cases, genetic and biochemical interaction studies may reveal potential interacting proteins, involved in the same metabolic or signaling pathway, which show less polymorphism and would represent more suitable targets. Another way that proteomics can be applied in target validation is the use of affinity-based probes to select proteins on the basis of their ability to bind particular small molecules (Chapter 9). Target proteins identified in this type of chemical screen are, in effect, preselected as susceptible to inhibition by small molecules, and are therefore more likely to respond favorably to candidate drugs. Affinity-based probes can be incorporated into cell-based and animal-testing programs and, as discussed below, can also be used as a starting point in the development of novel chemical entities.

10.3.3   Proteomics in the development of lead compounds

During the chemistry stages of drug development, certain proteomic technologies can provide a high-throughput approach for the identification and optimization of suitable lead compounds. For example, methods that identify protein–protein interactions can be used to screen lead compounds for interfering activity that would suggest useful physiological effects in the body. Functional protein chips can be used to assay protein–protein interactions *in vitro* in the presence and absence of potential lead compounds, allowing the rapid identification of molecules that prevent normal binding events. These molecules would have a significantly higher chance of interfering with protein interactions in living cells. When suitable leads have been identified, the same strategy can be used for lead optimization. In this case, protein interactions could be tested in the presence of selected chemical derivatives of the lead compound, to identify those with the most potent effects. Similar experiments could be carried out *in vivo*, using the yeast two-hybrid system and its derivatives to test for the disruption of protein interactions.

Structural proteomics also plays an important role in lead optimization, because the structural analysis of a potential drug target allows putative protein–small molecule interactions to be modeled *in silico* prior to experimental screening. Armed with structural information, researchers can use powerful computer programs to search through databases containing the structures of many different chemical compounds. The computer can select those compounds that are most likely to interact with the target, and these can be tested in the laboratory (Chapter 7). Other similar approaches include the preselection of target protein with affinity probes, allowing lead compounds to be designed on the basis of interacting molecular group, and the design of lead compounds on the basis of known ligands of the target protein. Such approaches eliminate the need for high-throughput screens of complex chemical libraries, and in principle allow lead compounds to be perfected using computers before any chemical screening is necessary. This is known as rational drug design, and has been successful in the development of a number of current drugs. The first drug produced by rational design was Relenza, which is used to treat influenza. Relenza was developed by choosing molecules that were most likely to interact with neuraminidase, a virus-produced enzyme that is required to release newly formed viruses from infected cells. Many of the recent drugs developed to treat HIV infections (e.g. Ritonivir, Indinavir) were designed to interact with the viral protease, the enzyme that splits up the viral proteins and allows them to assemble properly.

10.3.4   Proteomics and clinical development

Proteomics can be applied in studies that investigate mechanisms of drug activity and toxicity, both of which provide valuable data during the clinical stages of drug development. Adverse drug responses are the largest source of litigation in the US, and cost the pharmaceutical industry millions of dollars every year. Such effects often occur because the drug accumulates to toxic levels or is broken down into a toxic derivative, and in each case the clinical symptoms reflect unanticipated interactions between the drug or its metabolic byproducts and nontarget proteins in the cell. The result of drug toxicity is often a change in gene expression or protein abundance, which can be detected as a toxicity biomarker.

The study of protein profiles altered in response to drugs, using either traditional 2DGE or protein chips, has provided a great deal of data about the biochemical basis of drug activity and the pathways and networks upon which drugs act. Many different systems have been studied including acute promyelocytic leukemia cells before and after treatment with retinoic acid and Burkitt's lymphoma cells before and after treatment with 5′ azacytidine. This approach can be used not only to study human proteins or those in animal models of disease, but also the proteomes of pathogens to see how they respond to antibiotics. While expression proteomics shows which proteins are induced or repressed by particular antibiotics, interaction maps are useful in pinpointing hubs and redundant pathways. This can help to predict which combinations of drugs, acting on separate targets, will interfere most destructively with the pathogen life cycle.

Toxicity biomarkers have been discovered predominantly using 2DGE and mass spectrometry. A good example is calbindin, a calcium-binding protein that is depleted in the kidneys of patients treated with the immunosuppressant drug cyclosporin A. This drug is widely used to prevent organ rejection in children, but has devastating side effects including kidney toxicity, which occurs in up to 40% of patients. The toxicity is associated with the loss of calcium in the urine and the resulting calcification of the kidney tubules. A comparison of 2D gels from treated/untreated samples of rat and human kidneys showed a striking difference in the abundance of calbindin, and the loss of this protein following drug treatment provides a mechanistic explanation for the toxicity effect. Unlike humans, monkeys do not suffer cyclosporin A toxicity effects and proteomic analysis of monkey kidneys shows that there is no calbindin depletion following drug treatment. Studying the way in which monkeys metabolize the drug may therefore provide insight into novel ways to prevent side effects in humans.

10.4 Proteomics and plant biotechnology

10.4.1 Proteomics in plant breeding and genetics

Although biomedical applications dominate proteomics and are likely to do so for the foreseeable future, proteomics also has a long history in agriculture. Since the early 1980s, 2D gels have been used to study the extent of genetic variability in natural plant populations, and more recently the same techniques are beginning to be applied in the analysis of genetically modified crops. Proteomics has also been used to study plant development, physiology and interactions with other organisms, helping to identify proteins involved in defense and stress responses, and those expressed in improved agricultural varieties.

Among the earliest proteomic studies in plants were those performed by Zivy and colleagues to distinguish between different wheat varieties. Such experiments have been carried out in several important crops in addition to wheat, including rice, barley, sugarcane and pepper, as well as a number of tree species. Proteomics has also been used to study interspecific variety among cultivated wheats and other cereals. In the initial studies, several wheat species were analyzed by 2DGE, and the similarities and differences in the distribution and intensity of protein spots were used to calculate similarity indices. This allowed a phylogenetic tree to be constructed, which was found to be in excellent agreement with trees based on DNA sequences and classical taxonomy. As is the case for medical proteomics, a number of databases have been set up to catalog the proteomes of various plant species, including many of agricultural importance (*Table 10.2*).

A large number of proteomic studies have been carried out to investigate physiological processes in plants, often with the aim of identifying proteins corresponding to useful agronomic traits. In some cases, such studies have been used to compare mutant and wild-type varieties to characterize downstream effects of the mutation at the whole proteome level. For example, 2DGE has been used to study global differences between near isogenic pea lines differing only at the classical Mendelian locus *R*, which determines seed morphology. A comparison of *RR* seeds (round) and *rr* seeds (wrinkled) revealed extensive differences, affecting the abundance of about 10% of the proteome, agreeing well with the numerous biochemical and physiological differences that have been observed between these seeds in previous studies.

Proteomics has also been exploited to identify polymorphisms that can be used as genetic markers. Polymorphism occurs at three levels, described as position shifts (PS), presence/absence polymorphisms (P/A) and quantitative polymorphisms (sometimes called protein quantity loci, or PQLs). The first two types of polymorphism are useful genetic markers if they represent variant forms of the same polypeptide chain differing in mass or charge, but they may also represent different post-translational variants which are less suitable because this does not represent an underlying genetic variation at the same locus. Such markers have been used in wheat, maize and pine, for example, to generate comprehensive genetic maps also containing DNA markers. Quantitative polymorphisms are useful for identifying quantitative trait loci (QTLs) that cannot be pinned down by traditional map-based cloning or candidate gene approaches. The basis of the method is that protein quantitative polymorphisms that map coincidentally with QTLs can be used to validate candidate genes. An example is provided by the study of de Vienne *et al.* (see Further Reading). These investigators identified a candidate gene on chromosome 10 of maize for a QTL affecting drought response. The candidate gene was *ASR1*, known to be induced by water stress and ripening. Verification of the association was made possible because a protein quantitative polymorphism found during the comparison of 2D-gels from control and drought-stressed maize plants mapped to the same region; the quantitative polymorphism reflected different levels of the ASR1 protein under different drought stress conditions.

Most proteomic studies in plant biology have involved the comparison of healthy plants with those infected with pathogens, or stable plants with those exposed to particular forms of stress. Rice (*Oryza sativa*) and the model plant *Arabidopsis thaliana* have received most of the attention because the genomes of both species have been sequenced and extensive EST resources are available, facilitating the identification of proteins by peptide mass fingerprinting and fragment ion analysis (Chapter 3). Since rice is the most important food crop in the world, representing the staple diet for over 50% of the population, proteomics has been used to identify proteins that might affect traits of agronomic value in this species. For example, rice leaves treated with jasmonic acid, a known fungal elicitor, were compared to untreated leaves and 12 jasmonate-induced proteins were observed. Nine of these were similar to known pathogenesis-related proteins. The abundance of 21 proteins was found to change when rice plants were infected with the bacterial blight pathogen (*Xanthomonas oryzae* pv. *oryzae*) while 17 proteins were induced by infection with the blast fungus *Magnaporthe grisea*. The comparison of wild-type rice seeds and the seeds of a semi-dwarf variety revealed the specific expression of different forms of the storage protein glutelin in each type of seed. All these studies revealed proteins that might have specific roles in defense or agricultural improvement.

The most extensive proteomic analysis of a plant reported thus far was the systematic proteomic analysis of rice leaf, root, and seed tissue using both 2DGE and MudPIT methods (Chapter 2), reported by Koller *et al.* (see Further Reading). Over 2500 proteins were detected and identified, some of which were common to all three tissues and some of which were differentially expressed. This provided insight into the metabolic specialization of the different tissues, and allowed the identification of allergens in the seed endosperm, demonstrating that proteomics could be used as a general method to profile foods for allergens.

Interaction analysis has also been useful to predict functions for plant proteins. For example, flowering in *A. thaliana* is controlled by a closely related group of transcription factors whose DNA-binding domain is known as a MADS box. Similar transcription factors have been identified in other plants, but it is often difficult to determine their precise roles without painstaking analysis of mutant phenotypes. One shortcut is to assign functions based on conserved protein interactions. For example, the DAL13 protein of the Norway pine is a MADS box protein that could conceivably be the functional equivalent of any of the *Arabidopsis* proteins. In interactions screens, however, DAL13 interacted specifically with the *Arabidopsis* protein PISTILLATA, suggesting that DAL13 and PISTILLATA are functionally homologous (orthologs). A similar interaction screen, shown in *Figure 10.9*, has identified *Arabidopsis* SEPELLATA3 (SEP3) as the functional ortholog of petunia FBP2 and FBP5, since a conserved set of interactions is observed.

10.4.2 Proteomics for the analysis of genetically modified plants

One of the major applications of plant biotechnology is the development of genetically modified (GM) crops. In some cases, the crops are used as bioreactors for the production of valuable proteins or metabolites, but other crops are modified to improve their agronomic traits and are intended to be used as food or feed. Concerns about the safety of genetically modified foods revolve around the concept of substantial equivalence, i.e. whether the process of genetic modification has introduced any unanticipated (and undesirable) changes in the host plant. Such changes, resulting from the random integration of DNA into the plant

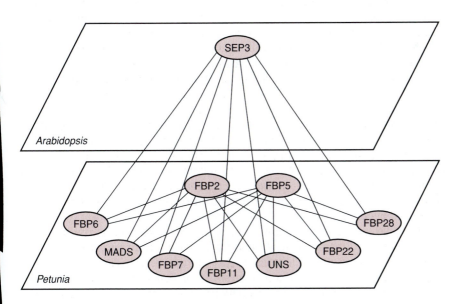

Figure 10.9

Heterologous interactions between SEPALLATA3 (SEP3) from *Arabidopsis* and petunia MADS-box proteins identified by the yeast two-hybrid system. The interaction partners of SEP3 are identical to those of the FBP2 and FBP5 proteins from petunia, indicating that SEP3 and FBP2 and FBP5 are orthologs. Abbreviations: FBP, FLORAL BINDING PROTEIN; pMADS, petunia MADS-box protein; SEP, SEPALLATA; UNS, UNSHAVEN.

genome and the influence this may have on endogenous genes, could include metabolic disruption and therefore changes in the concentrations of nutrients and potentially toxic compounds. Strategies for the comparative analysis of GM and non-GM crops often focus on specific compounds, such as particular nutrients, metabolites or toxins. However, in order to fully characterize any changes that may have occurred, it is necessary to use global and nontargeted approaches, including transcriptional profiling, proteomics and metabolomics (the global analysis of small molecules).

Proteomics potentially has an important role to play in food safety assessment because it allows changes in protein abundance and post-translational modifications to be identified, which cannot be detected using other global analysis methods. The use of 2DGE in food safety testing is being evaluated in several projects organized by GMOCARE, a working group established by the ENTRANSFOOD consortium (see Internet resources). Similarly, the UK Food Standards Agency is funding projects in which GM and non-GM crops will be compared using multidimensional column chromatography and ICAT-based quantitative mass spectrometry. An important component of these studies is the evaluation of natural proteomic variation within the model crops (potato and tomato) which will make GM-specific differences harder to detect.

10.4.3 Proteomics and the analysis of secondary metabolism

Plants produce a wide variety of chemical substances with very complex structures. These substances are known as secondary metabolites because they are not part of core metabolism, but they perform many useful functions, including defense against pathogens and attraction of pollinators. Secondary metabolites have been of interest to humans for centuries because they can be used as drugs, dyes, fragrances, nutritional supplements and flavors. Unfortunately, many of the most beneficial secondary metabolites are produced in such low quantities that their commercial extraction is unfeasible. Therefore, researchers have studied secondary metabolic pathways in an attempt to produce more of these desired compounds. A further hurdle is that secondary metabolic pathways are extremely complex, involving many enzymatic steps, extensive branching and cross-talk, and the compartmentalization of different steps in different cell types or organelles. Traditional methods to study secondary metabolism involve the step-by-step characterization of individual reactions using feeding experiments and labeled intermediates. Proteomics can accelerate discovery in plant secondary metabolism because it can identify not only enzymes, but also regulatory proteins and proteins involved in the shuttling of intermediates between compartments.

One of the best model systems for the production of useful secondary metabolites is the Madagascar periwinkle (*Catharanthus roseus*) which produces hundreds of alkaloids including the potent antineoplastic drugs vinblastine and vincristine (*Figure 10.10*). Proteomic analysis of *C. roseus* cell cultures under culture conditions known to affect alkaloid production has revealed five proteins whose abundance mirrors the level of alkaloid accumulation, suggesting either a catalytic or regulatory role. The common regulation of many of the genes involved in terpenoid indole alkaloid biosynthesis in *C. roseus* suggests that a useful strategy for

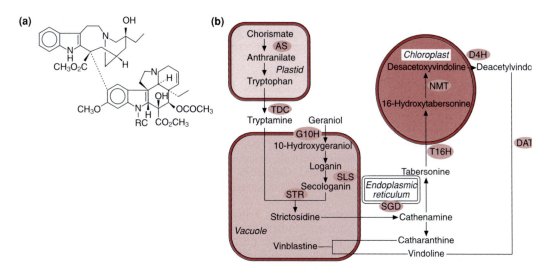

Figure 10.10

(a) The generic chemical structure of the alkaloid antineoplastic drugs vinblastine and vincristine (R = -CH$_3$ in vinblastine and -CHO in vincristine). (b) An abbreviated representation of the very complex and highly compartmentalized biosynthetic pathway for these compounds. Reprinted from Trends in Plant Science, Vol. 7, Immink and Angenent, 'Transcription factors do it together: the hows and whys of studying protein-protein interactions', pp 531–534, ©2002, with permission from Elsevier.

increasing the levels of alkaloids in this system would be to identify and manipulate transcription factors that control the expression of these genes. One such transcription factor, known as ORCA2, has been identified using the yeast one-hybrid system (p. 144) while another has been found in a screen involving insertional mutagenesis (p. 10). Proteomics has also been used to study the phytoalexin synthesis pathway in cell cultures of the common bean (*Phaseus vulgaris*), chickpea (*Cicer arietinum*) and tobacco (*Nicotiana tabacum*) following exposure to fungi or fungal elicitors such as cryptogein. Eleven spots on 2D gels were shown to increase in abundance after treatment of the chickpea cell cultures, and 23 proteins showed a change of abundance in tobacco cells. These included the two key enzymes phenylalanine ammonia lyase (PAL) and chalcone synthase (CHS).

Further reading

Alaiya, A.A., Roblick, U.J., Franzen, B., Brich. H.P. and Auer, G. (2003) Protein expression profiling in human lung, breast, bladder, renal, colorectal and ovarian cancers. *J Chromatog B* **787**: 207–222.

Barrett, J., Jefferies, J.R. and Brophy, P.M. (2000) Parasite proteomics. *Parasitology Today* **16**: 400–403.

Burbaum, J. and Tobal, G.M. (2002) Proteomics in drug discovery. *Curr Opin Chem Biol* **6**: 427–433.

Celis, J.E., Kruhoffer, M., Gromova, I. et al. (2000) Gene expression profiling: monitoring transcription and translation products using DNA microarrays and proteomics. *FEBS Lett* **480**: 2–16.

Hanash, S. (2003) Disease proteomics. *Nature* **422**: 226–232.

Hanash, S.M., Madoz-Gurpide, J. and Misek, D.E. (2002) Identification of novel targets for cancer therapy using expression proteomics. *Leukemia* **16**: 478–485.

He, Q.Y. and Chiu, J.F. (2003) Proteomics in biomarker discovery and drug development. *J Cell Biochem* **89**: 868–886

Jacobs, D.I., van der Heijden, R. and Verpoorte, R. (2000) Proteomics in plant biotechnology and secondary metabolism research. *Phytochem Anal* **11**: 277–287.

Jeffery, D.A. and Bogyo, M. (2003) Chemical proteomics and its application to drug discovery. *Curr Opin Biotechnol* **14**: 87–95.

Koh, H.L., Yau, W.P., Ong, P.S. and Hedge, A. (2003) Current trends in modern pharmaceutical analysis for drug discovery. *Drug Discovery Today* **8**: 889–897.

Koller, A., Washburn, M.P., Lange, B.M., *et al.* (2002) Proteomic survey of metabolic pathways in rice. *Proc Natl Acad Sic USA* **99**: 11969–11974.

Marko-Varga, G., Fehniger, T.E., (2004) Proteomics and disease - The challenges for technology and discovery. *J Proteomr Res* **3**: 167–178.

Ng, J.H. and Ilag, L.L. (2002) Biomedical applications of protein chips. *J Cell Mol Med* **6**: 329–340.

Petricoin, E.F. and Liotta, L.A. (2004) SELDI-TOF-based serum proteomic pattern diagnostics for early detection of cancer. *Curr Opin Biotechnol* **15**: 24–30.

Petricoin, E.F., Ardekani, A.M., Hitt, B.A., *et al.* (2002) Use of proteomic patterns in serum to identify ovarian cancer. *Lancet* **359**: 572–577.

Petricoin, E., Wulfkuhle, J., Espina, V., *et al.* (2004) Clinical proteomics: Revolutionizing disease detection and patient tailoring therapy. *J Proteomr Res* **3**: 209–217.

Petricoin, E.F., Zoon, K.C., Kohn, E.C., Barrett, J.C. and Liotta, L.A. (2002) Clinical proteomics: translating benchside promise into bedside reality. *Nature Rev Drug Discov* **1**: 683–695.

Shin, B.K., Wang, H., Yim, A.M., *et al*. (2002) Global profiling of the cell surface proteome of cancer cells uncovers an abundance of proteins with chaperone function. *J Biol Chem* **278**: 7607–7616.

Van Eyk, J.E. (2002) Proteomics: unraveling the complexity of heart disease and striving to change cardiology. *Curr Opin Mol Therapeut* **3**: 546–553.

Williams, M. (2003) Target validation. *Curr Opin Pharmacol* **3**: 571–577.

Wulfkuhle, J.D., Liotta, L.A. and Petricoin, E.F. (2003) Proteomic applications for the early detection of cancer. *Nature Rev Cancer* **3**: 267–275.

Zhou, G., Li, H.M., DeCamp, D., Chen, S., *et al.* (2001) 2D differential in-gel electrophoresis for the identification of esophageal scans cell cancer-specific protein markers. *Mol Cell Proteomics* **1**: 117–124.

Index